The Physician's Guide to Investing

Second Edition

The Physician's Guide to Investing

A Practical Approach to Building Wealth

Second Edition

By

Robert M. Doroghazi, MD, FACC

Columbia, MO

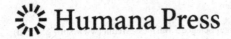 Humana Press

Robert M. Doroghazi, MD, FACC
115 Bingham Rd.
Columbia, MO 65203
USA
rdoroghazi@aol.com

ISBN 978-1-60327-543-9   e-ISBN 978-1-60761-134-9
DOI 10.1007/978-1-60761-134-9
Springer Dordrecht Heidelberg London New York

Library of Congress Control Number: 2009927126

Printed on acid-free paper

Springer is part of Springer Science + Business Media (www.springer.com)

Dedication

To my parents and grandparents
who taught me the value of a dollar
and to my sons John and Michael
two fine young men

Comments on the first edition of
The Physician's Guide to Investing:
A Practical Approach to Building Wealth

"You've really done a first-class job of telling your fellow doctors what to do in their financial life. In fact, your book should be required reading at med schools."

Warren E. Buffett, Chairman
Berkshire Hathaway

"This book should be a must read for every young physician finishing training and beginning a career".

George Meyer, M.D.
Practical Gastroenterology

"Dr. Doroghazi is a credentialed physician, a respected cardiologist, and a gifted writer addressing a crucial issue on the finances of physicians ... this book should be on the same shelf with *Gray's Anatomy*, Robbins and Cotran's *Pathological Basis of Disease*, and Goodman and Gilman's *The Pharmacological Basis of Therapeutics*."

Edward T. Creagan, M.D.
Mayo Clinic Proceedings

Foreword

As editor of *The American Journal of Cardiology* I am sent each year a number of books to review. In 2005, Bob Doroghazi's first book *The Physician's Guide to Investing: A Practical Approach to Building Wealth* appeared on my desk. I read the whole 228 pages the first night and was so intrigued that I purchased 5 other copies for friends. I learned that Bob Doroghazi had worked his way through both college and medical school graduating with high honors from each (Phi Beta Kappa and Alpha Omega Alpha). His internship and residency was at the Massachusetts General Hospital in Boston and his cardiology training was at Barnes Hospital in St. Louis. He was a practicing cardiologist in Columbia, Missouri, from 1982 until his retirement from medicine in 2005.

His first book was intended for physicians but it should not have been limited. This new book expands the first one. It tells us how to obtain our financial goals, how to avoid the pitfalls preventing this attainment, which specific assets are most worthy of our investments, and even comments on the importance of charity. Since 2006, Dr. Doroghazi has produced a monthly financial letter that I find extremely helpful. His new book incorporates some of the advice produced in these monthly letters. Although I found his first book highly useful, this new one is altogether a major step above the first one. I am glad that Dr. Doroghazi no longer practices cardiology and that he concentrates now fulltime on helping us all – not just physicians – achieve our financial goals.

William C. Roberts, MD
Editor in Chief, *The American Journal of Cardiology*
and
Executive Director, Baylor Heart and Vascular Institute,
Baylor University Medical Center
Dallas, Texas

Introduction

This book is unique. Although directed to physicians (and other high-income professionals such as dentists, veterinarians, athletes, artists and entertainers), it provides common sense and practical advice you will find nowhere else and that I believe will be profitable to all investors. I tell you how to avoid "The Doctor Discount" and being "The Mark", how to spot a con man, who you can and cannot trust, how to choose a piece of recreational property, why not to open a restaurant, and how to deal with real estate agents and bankers on your terms rather than theirs.

One review of the first edition suggested the subtitle "How to Avoid Making Dumb Mistakes" [1]. Quite true, and certainly very important, but this book is much more than that. I review general aspects of investing such as the power of thrift, the magnificence of compound interest, the malevolence of debt, the concept of risk, how to recognize real opportunities and when to buy and sell. I also review the topic of financial planning including the importance of paying off the mortgage early, how to fund your children's education and your retirement and determine your insurance needs.

This book will not tell you how to get "rich" because that should never be your goal. No one can define rich, and someone will always have more. But I do provide practical, common sense advice on how to attain your long-term goal of financial security, to be able to retire when you wish rather than continue to work because you must, and hopefully be able to afford a few of the finer things of life along the way.

Lack of financial instruction is the greatest deficiency of the medical establishment in our country, and I believe is indefensible. US medical school graduates, arguably the most competent, highly-trained professionals in the world, finish training in their 30s burdened with a six-figure debt and utterly defenseless in the real financial world. This can have a negative effect on their personal lives and adversely affect patient care.

This second edition is about a third longer than the first. My goal is to provide more details and insights, yet keep the book of a practical length to be easily read over a weekend or long plane flight. I suggest your spouse read this book. I have also added more anecdotes and personal observations in hopes of making this book more interesting than a run-of-the-mill financial tome.

I was a successful physician. I graduated with honors and trained at superior institutions. I am also a successful investor. Although I certainly made mistakes along the way, I did well enough in my personal money management to pay my own way through college and medical school, to own my home, vacation condominium, recreational property, various art work and collectibles and all of my personal belongings free and clear of debt, to fund my children's education, make significant charitable donations and accumulate sufficient assets that I was able to retire at age 54.

I am "second-generation American", all of my grandparents emigrated from Hungary between 1900 and 1921. Although I was born in 1951, I consider myself "first-generation Depression". The painful residual of that time was ever-present in our home. "Don't go into debt and save your money for a rainy day. We want you to have it better than we did (I do)". As this book goes to press early in 2009, it has clearly started to rain. The advice I provide in this book and in The Physician Investor Newsletter (see my website www.thephysicianinvestor.com; to sign up for a free 4 month subscription) should help keep you warm and dry.

Robert M. Doroghazi, MD, FACC
Columbia, MO

REFERENCE

1. Meyer G. Book Reviews: The Physician's Guide to Investing: A Practical Approach to Building Wealth. Practical Gastroenterology **29**: 63, 2006.

Acknowledgments

I would like to acknowledge Richard Lansing at Springer for recognizing the potential of this work and his help and support on both editions.

I would like to thank Scott Orr, Advisory Director of Jonesburg State Bank, Jonesburg, MO, for answering my questions and providing advice on banking-related issues.

I would also like to thank John John of ReMax-Boone Realty for answering my questions and providing advice on selected real estate issues.

Contents

I | On Track With Your Financial Goals

Chapter One
The Problem: Lack of Financial Instruction

It is customary to begin a discussion by defining goals. I reserve this for Chapter Two, with the remainder of the book devoted to how to achieve your financial goals.

I have chosen instead to start by defining the problem [1]. Every responsible parent begins to teach their children the importance of money from the time they ask for their first piece of candy or bubble gum at the confectionary. Meanwhile, our physicians, arguably the most highly trained professionals in the world, receive no instruction on how to manage or invest the hard-earned fruits of their labor.

United States medical schools graduate the best physicians in the world. The rich and powerful travel from the ends of the earth to our country for medical care. But when it comes to money, many of our wonderful, dedicated physicians are utterly incompetent.

The lack of financial instruction is further complicated by an utter disdain, bordering on overt revulsion, to any discussion of money, as if the person is just a pathetic money-grubber, unworthy of the fraternity of American medicine. It is almost as if the academic medical establishment wishes to keep physicians financially barefoot and in the kitchen. This is not only the greatest deficiency of our medical establishment, I believe it is indefensible.

The average medical student graduates with $140,000 in student loans. Since this is the average, many young physicians are

R.M. Doroghazi, *The Physician's Guide to Investing*,
DOI 10.1007/978-1-60761-134-9_1,
© Humana Press, a part of Springer Science+Business Media, LLC 2005, 2009

even further in hock (a non-intellectual but appropriately descriptive term). Add other sources of debt, such as marrying another indebted student (double your debt in one day!!), a car loan and mortgage or credit card debt, and as they begin their professional careers, already in their mid-to-late thirties, many physicians find themselves a quarter million dollars or more in the hole. This onerous amount of debt can have negative effects on all stages of a physician's career. I believe it can also compromise their ability to provide quality patient care.

I have previously suggested medical students and physicians-in-training receive their instruction on investing and personal financial management before completing training. I now recommend they receive this instruction as soon as they enter medical school. I can think of no reason to wait. The average college student graduates with almost $20,000 of student loans, and the beginning medical student is well aware that in less than four years this debt will be 5 times, or maybe even an order of magnitude, greater. Such an oppressive scenario can destroy any desire to be thrifty and, in plain and simple terms, respect for a dollar. Why make any effort to save $10, or for that matter, deny yourself any perk or luxury, when you are already $100K in the hole? I believe that part of a student's final debt total is due to exactly this mindset, bordering almost on a sense of entitlement. I do not think a medical student or physician-in-training with a six-figure debt should be buying a new car.

Delaying instruction on investing results in a further loss because of compound interest (*see* Chapter Three). Every dollar not saved and every extra dollar of debt is magnified by 50% after the four years of a medical education.

Six-figure debt, compounded by financial ineptness, can affect a physician's personal life, career choices and style of practice. Let me provide two real-life examples. The sister of a friend just finished her training at age 36 in a pediatric sub-specialty with almost $270K of student loans. A young professional with $90K of student loans married a house officer with more than $200K of debt. Add to this the mortgage on a very modest starter home. When telling me of her circumstances, she said "Bob, I don't know when we can afford to have children".

The stark reality is that these physicians will be lucky if they can just break even by age 50. They will then also realize they have only another 10 or 15 years to pay off the mortgage and any other debt, fund their children's education, and accumulate sufficient assets to retire. This very well may cause them, in a sense of near-desperation, to chase potentially higher return (and even much higher risk) investments to make up for lost time. In such a precarious situation, any problem, such as a drop in income, personal or family illness, or any major financial mishap, such as a secular bear market in stocks, could result in never achieving financial security, or, God forbid, declaring bankruptcy.

A physician may be forced to pursue a higher paying sub-specialty rather than a discipline that is more intellectually stimulating, and probably better for society, yet less financially rewarding, such as pediatrics or general practice. A survey by the non-profit Association of American Medical Colleges found that one-third of medical students say debt influences their choice of specialization (*Wall Street Journal*, 5/15/08). A physician may also choose to practice in an already over-served, more affluent area rather than a poorer area much more in need of their medical expertise.

I am also concerned that having to service large amounts of debt can affect a physician's style of practice. In a borderline (or maybe even not so borderline) case, it can become surprisingly easy to justify performing a highly remunerative cardiac catheterization rather than a less profitable exercise stress test. Performing un-needed procedures to service your personal debt is not in the best interest of the patient.

Businessmen who pull down a physician-range six-figure salary do so because they are good businessmen. Their business and money management skills and income increase pari passu (means to proceed at the same rate). In contrast, the time a physician enters practice is a very vulnerable period in their financial lives. Income can triple or quadruple in an instant, yet there is no reason to believe their money management skills are any greater than the day before. A salary that was previously just enough to get by and generate modest savings now becomes a monetary tsunami. Things that were previously just pie-in-the-sky now become an absolute necessity. Unfortunately, our society often places inappropriate social pressure on the young physician and their spouse to project a façade of wealth, and often take on more debt to do it. I prefer to impress people with my accomplishments and my character and charitable donations rather than the country club I belong to or the home I live in.

It is a fact; nature has dictated that physical, mental and emotional skills decline with age. Performing surgery and taking call at age 75 is just not the same as when you were 35. Be assured I am not criticizing elderly physicians. There are physicians in their 70s, 80s and even 90s who are better than I ever hoped to be. Likewise, they are not the same physician as when they were 40. If a physician is competent and wishes to practice into their 70s or beyond because of their love of medicine, I say more power to them. But if they are practicing after their skills have waned merely to make ends meet because of financial mismanagement is not a desirable situation for them or their patients.

I know of a general surgeon who practiced until he died in his mid-80s. For at least a decade before this, it was painfully obvious to everyone but him and his patients that he should not be performing surgery, or even practicing medicine. Eventually the hospital Chief of Staff had a talk with him relating everyone's concerns. Several weeks later the Chief of Staff said "Bob, what did you think about that talk we had two weeks ago"? Bob replied most sincerely "what talk". The story is as pathetic as it sounds. Lack of basic financial skills have put far too many of our colleagues in just such circumstances, which *is* harmful to their patients *and* degrading to them.

This overt resistance to any discussion of sound money management and investing occurs in a setting where the medical school establishment profits greatly from our capitalistic system. Medical schools generate significant profits from continuing medical education (CME) courses, and all sorts of arrangements with the private industry [2].

Administrators and faculty personally profit from speaking honoraria and consulting fees. Many serve on the boards of directors of for-profit corporations, such as pharmaceutical or biotech companies, medical instrument makers, and banks. Such positions are extremely lucrative. As a comparison, the compensation for just one year's service on the board of a publicly-traded company would usually more than cover the average medical graduate's student loans.

I believe the position of the academic medical establishment to deny medical students financial instruction is naïve, hypocritical, and indefensible. They should acknowledge that money is important. It is never as important as your patient. It is never as important as your family, your health, your freedom or your integrity. But it is important. Honest, hard work to make a good living is what America is all about. I know because I am proud to say that my family has lived the American dream. Financial security is important, it has its advantages. Financial instability can destroy your family and your health and harm your patients.

SUMMARY OF CHAPTER ONE

- *Everyone* should receive instruction on investing and sound money management.
- Lack of financial instruction is naïve, hypocritical and indefensible, and is the greatest deficiency of medical education in the United States.
- Instruction should begin as soon as students enter medical school.
- The average medical student graduates $140,000 in debt.
- Debt can influence a physician's choice of specialty, practice style and location.
- Financial mismanagement can cause physicians to practice longer than they should.
- A physician's personal financial situation can have an adverse effect on patient care.

REFERENCES

1. Doroghazi R M. Lack of instruction on personal financial management and investing in medical education. The American Journal of Cardiology **98**: 707–8, 2006.
2. Bok D. Universities in the Marketplace: The Commercialization of Higher Education. Princeton, NJ: Princeton University Press, 2003.

Chapter Two
Goals for Your Financial Return

It is very difficult to achieve what you want without having a well-defined goal. Expectations are important. Certainly with something as important as personal finances, one should define their goals and outline precisely how they plan to achieve them. I will start by defining reasonable investment goals. The rest of the book will detail how to achieve these goals.

This chapter has three sections. The first outlines an average return that can be anticipated from investments. The second section details returns that are attainable, but only with hard work and common sense. The last section describes returns that are unrealistic, and when promised, should immediately cause concern and alarm. The latter is especially important because it will allow you to quickly recognize the army of promoters and sometimes just plain crooks whose only desire is to separate you from your hard-earned money.

YOUR MINIMUM INVESTMENT GOAL

Over the long term, investors should anticipate a ten percent annual return on stock market investments. Some years this will be greater, some years less, and some years there will even be losses. But over the course of your investing lifetime, actually, your investing lifetime is your entire lifetime, your goal should be a ten percent annual return on non-cash investments.

R.M. Doroghazi, *The Physician's Guide to Investing,*
DOI 10.1007/978-1-60761-134-9_2,
© Humana Press, a part of Springer Science+Business Media, LLC 2005, 2009

Note I emphasize non-cash. There must always be sufficient cash to cover unexpected needs, debt service, and to take advantage of opportunities. It is the person with cash who can scoop up assets when they are cheap. But the price (the risk) of cash is that its long-term return is inferior to other investments, such as stocks or real estate. But in general, it is preferable to have a little more rather than not quite enough cash.

Ten percent is a round number but was not chosen at random. Over the course of the twentieth century, stocks in the United States returned an average of just under ten percent annually. Slightly more than half of the return, almost five percent, was due to capital appreciation, a number essentially equal to the growth of corporate profits over this time period.

Slightly less than half of this return, approximately four and one-half percent, was from the payout of dividends. But when inflation is factored out, decreasing the contribution of capital appreciation, the average annual return from stocks was approximately seven percent. Thus dividends represented almost two-thirds (62% to be exact) of the wealth created by corporations in the United States in the last century. I do not know how any other statistic can better emphasize the importance of dividends.

During the stock market bubble of the late 90s, it was thought that capital appreciation was all-important and dividends were of no consequence, sought only by old fogies who remembered the Great Depression. There was a new game in town, we were operating under new rules, a "new paradigm", old rules no longer applied. In the end, old rules always apply, that is why they are old rules. The old rule is that dividends are very important and they count a great deal. More information on dividend-oriented stocks can be found at the websites www.dividendinvestor.com and www.dividenddetective.com.

Why are dividends so important? Only by re-investing dividends can you realize "The Magnificence of Compound Interest" (see the next Chapter). Dividends are also cash in your pocket, to do with as you see fit. Cash from dividends can pay utility bills, the mortgage, your children's education bills and all the other expenses of daily living. Dividends are also important because investors believe that the payment of cash dividends is a reflection of a company's financial health. Investors treat a cut in the dividend as negative news about a company's future prospects, such that management will commit to increase dividends only when they are truly confident about their ability to maintain those dividends in the future. Financial analysts call this the "signaling theory of dividends." Simply stated, dividends are a signal about the future prospects for the company. Stable, and especially increasing dividends, are a general indicator of the financial health of a company.

Eventually a company must pay a dividend. If the price of a company's stock increases, but they do not pay a dividend, the only way to recognize this increase in value is to sell the stock. If the company continues not to pay a dividend, the only way the buyer can have cash to pay their daily bills is to sell the stock to someone else, and so on. Early in a company's history, their rapid growth phase, they may retain earnings for expansion, but at some time a dividend must be paid.

Stock prices may fluctuate markedly because of a change in the price to earnings (P/E) ratio. Investors are willing to pay more, or less, for what they anticipate will be a stock's earnings in the future. In the short term variations in P/E ratio are mostly expectations-driven and show a relatively poor correlation with an increase or decrease in corporate earnings. But over the long term, this variation in price to earnings ratio essentially disappears. In the end, what is left is the true value of the company – as represented by improved earnings – and the dividends that have been paid.

The minimum goal on your stock market investments is to capture the wealth created by corporate America (and increasingly, foreign economies), which in the twentieth century was an average compounded return of 10%. Considering the average physician's income, all that is required to live comfortably and retire when you wish is a little fiscal discipline and the avoidance of stupid mistakes, which is one of the principle points of this book. Financial security is important.

A REASONABLE INVESTMENT GOAL

With some work (actually with some hard work), common sense, and knowledge of where mistakes can arise, a fifteen percent compounded annual return on investments may be realized.

I choose fifteen percent for two reasons. The first is that it is attainable, you can do it. The second reason is that money will double in five years, due to the assistance of your greatest investment friend – compound interest.

Note this:

Year One $100 × 15% = $115
Year Two $115 × 15% = $132
Year Three $132 × 15% = $152
Year Four $152 × 15% = $174
Year Five $174 × 15% = $201

A little work, compound interest and patience can result in financial security.

A simple way to determine how quickly money doubles is the rule of 72. Divide the rate of return into 72. Money growing at 10% per year doubles in 7.2 years. In the example above, money growing at 15% per year doubles in just under 5 years.

Before concluding this section, I must emphasize that investing is a three-step process.

1. Earn money
2. Do not spend all of the money (for some people this is problematic)
3. Invest the money

For example, one physician saves $10,000 and hits an investment grand slam, realizing a 25% return, resulting in $12,500 at the end of the year. You are more thrifty, save $15,000, and realize the standard 10% return. At the end of the year this is $16,500. It is virtually impossible for great investing to overcome poor saving habits. The easiest way to accumulate wealth and attain financial security is save money on a regular basis and invest it wisely. Savings equals investment. **The best investors are the best savers**.

AN UNREASONABLE INVESTMENT GOAL

There are some truly gifted investments geniuses, such as Warren Buffett, George Soros and a handful of others, who have been able to generate returns of greater than 20% for prolonged periods of time, but they are literally one in a million. Of importance as it relates to this discussion is that such people will have bona-fide, verifiable results with reputations and references to match. If you should be lucky enough to find one of these truly gifted legitimate investment wizards, just hitch your star to theirs and hang on for the ride.

The point of this section is to think of a 20% return as an almost magical number in the investment world. If anyone comes to you saying they will make, almost guarantee, a twenty five percent, thirty percent or more annual return on an investment, but they do not have a track record to prove it, just tell them to forget it. It is as pure and simple as that. They could conceivably be the next Buffett or Soros (possible, but literally one in a million), but more likely they are bogus and just wish to relieve you of your money.

Here is the essence of what I feel is one of the difficulties that physicians experience with investing, and which I will detail in the remainder of this book. Physicians do not wish to be left out. They feel their great intellectual gifts, qualities that can result in being the greatest neurosurgeon, cardiologist or oncologist in the world, automatically apply to areas outside of medicine. The ability to save a life does not necessarily imply the same ability to evaluate a real estate investment or read a financial statement or determine the potential of a natural gas property in Wyoming. It just does not.

No one was blessed with greater intellectual gifts than Sir Isaac Newton. In 1687, he published *Principia* (*Mathematical Principles of Natural Philosophy*) which outlined the basic laws of gravity. Newton developed the calculus (credit also goes to Gottfried Wilhelm von Leibniz for his simultaneous and independent work on the calculus) to provide the mathematical quantification of his theories. Although in later years Newton was Master of the Royal Mint, and helped implement John

Locke's revolutionary idea to fix the value of coinage [1], he lost a great deal of money on the South Sea Company, one of history's most classic investment manias. Newton said "I can calculate the motions of heavenly bodies, but not the madness of people."

Do not worry about being left out. Chances are a million to one that anyone, especially someone you do not know, or have never heard of, who has no previous verifiable results, who tells you, who assures you, who guarantees you, a twenty percent or more return on your investment, will not. Just forget them. Instruct them to leave and not to come back.

SUMMARY OF CHAPTER TWO

- Reasonable anticipated long-term return on investment   10%
- Return attainable with work and common sense   15%
- Promised, but unattainable, return that should cause alarm   30%
- Dividends are very important.
- Beware of the "new paradigm". Old rules are important.
- Investing is a three-step process. You must make money and not spend it. Only then do you have money to invest.
- The best investors are the best savers.
- Being a physician does not make you smart at everything.

REFERENCE

1. Lewis N. Gold: The Once and Future Money. Hoboken, NJ: John Wiley & Sons, 2007.

Chapter Three
The Magnificence of Compound Interest

Einstein referred to compound interest as the Eighth Wonder of the World (see Table 1 for the Seven Wonders of the Ancient World). How did this scientist, from all of my reading, a somewhat absent-minded individual with no particular investment prowess, come to make this comment, which merits the third chapter in this book and a detailed discussion?

Just examine Einstein's most famous field equation: $E = mc^2$. A tiny amount of mass, compounded, compounded, and compounded, again and again and again, results in an unbelievable amount of energy.

A person was once challenged to come up with a saying that applied to everything. The result was "this too shall pass." Why does this comment apply to all situations? Because it describes an absolutely inevitable event – the passage of time.

The economy changes, tax rates increase or decrease, the party in control of the White House or Congress changes, the

Table 1
The Seven Wonders of the Ancient World

The Pyramids of Giza
The Pharos (Lighthouse) of Alexandria
The Temple of Artemis in Ephesus
The Mausoleum at Halicarnassus
The Colossus of Rhodes
The Hanging Gardens of Babylon
The Statue of Zeus at Olympia

R.M. Doroghazi, *The Physician's Guide to Investing*,
DOI 10.1007/978-1-60761-134-9_3,
© Humana Press, a part of Springer Science+Business Media, LLC 2005, 2009

stock market goes up or down, natural or man-made catastrophes occur, but the passage of time and compound interest
are absolutely inevitable. Compound interest is all investor's
greatest, most powerful tool, their best friend. Compound interest has the same power to generate wealth as Einstein's equation does to generate energy. The only requirements are money
to invest and patience. Consider this equation:

$$\$ \times C.I. \ (compound \ interest) = \$\$\$\$\$\$\$\$\$\$\$\$\$\$\$$$

Unfortunately, if you are in debt, compound interest pos-
sesses the same power to confiscate your wealth. A home mortgage is compound interest in reverse, and a homebuyer with a
30-year mortgage pays several times the price for the home over
the life of the mortgage (*see* Chapter Sixteen).

Examine Table 2 from the work of Richard Russell of the *Dow
Theory Letters* (more on Russell later). Each investor puts aside
$2,000 per year, compound at the average anticipated rate of
return of 10%. All interest and dividends are re-invested, and
thus re-compounded. As mentioned in the last chapter, without
dividends, and without reinvesting the dividends, there can be
no compounding. Investor B puts aside $2K a year for seven
years, from age 19 through 25, and then stops. He never invests
another penny (this is just an example, you should never stop
investing). Investor A starts at age 26 and invests $2K per year
for the next 40 years. Look who wins. Absolutely amazing.
Einstein and Richard Russell are right.

I will give another example of the power of compound interest. Queen Isabella spent $30K to finance Columbus. His voy-
age opened up another world, an amazing investment for
humanity (at least from the European point of view). But Warren Buffett suggested that it was a poor investment for Her
Majesty. In a letter Buffett wrote at age 32 on "The Joys of
Compounding," he suggested that if Queen Isabella had taken
the $30K, invested at four percent compounded annual interest
(this is the intrinsic value of money, lent out in a zero inflation
environment to a customer who will repay the loan, the rate
paid on the British Consol(idated) bonds during the 18th and
19th centuries), by the 1960's the Queen's investment would

Table 2
The Power of Compound Interest

Age	Investor A Contribution	Year-end Value	Investor B Contribution	Year-end Value
1–18	$0	$0	$0	$0
19	$0	$0	$2,000	$2,200
20	$0	$0	$2,000	$4,620
21	$0	$0	$2,000	$7,282
22	$0	$0	$2,000	$10,210
23	$0	$0	$2,000	$13,431
24	$0	$0	$2,000	$16,974
25	$0	$0	$2,000	$20,872
26	$2,000	$2,200	$0	$22,959
27	$2,000	$4,620	$0	$25,255
28	$2,000	$7,282	$0	$27,780
29	$2,000	$10,210	$0	$30,558
30	$2,000	$13,431	$0	$33,614
31	$2,000	$16,974	$0	$36,976
32	$2,000	$20,872	$0	$40,673
33	$2,000	$25,159	$0	$44,741
34	$2,000	$29,875	$0	$49,215
35	$2,000	$35,062	$0	$54,136
36	$2,000	$40,769	$0	$59,550
37	$2,000	$47,045	$0	$65,505
38	$2,000	$53,950	$0	$72,055
39	$2,000	$61,545	$0	$79,261
40	$2,000	$69,899	$0	$87,187
41	$2,000	$79,089	$0	$95,905
42	$2,000	$89,198	$0	$105,496
43	$2,000	$100,318	$0	$116,045
44	$2,000	$112,550	$0	$127,650
45	$2,000	$126,005	$0	$140,415
46	$2,000	$140,805	$0	$154,456
47	$2,000	$157,086	$0	$169,902
48	$2,000	$174,995	$0	$186,892
49	$2,000	$194,694	$0	$207,561
50	$2,000	$216,364	$0	$226,140
51	$2,000	$240,200	$0	$248,754
52	$2,000	$266,420	$0	$273,629
53	$2,000	$295,262	$0	$300,992

(continued)

Table 2 *(Continued)*

Age	Investor A Contribution	Year-end Value	Investor B Contribution	Year-end Value
54	$2,000	$326,988	$0	$331,091
55	$2,000	$361,887	$0	$364,200
56	$2,000	$400,276	$0	$400,620
57	$2,000	$442,503	$0	$440,682
58	$2,000	$488,953	$0	$484,750
59	$2,000	$540,049	$0	$533,225
60	$2,000	$596,254	$0	$586,548
61	$2,000	$658,079	$0	$645,203
62	$2,000	$726,087	$0	$709,723
63	$2,000.	$800,896	$0	$780,695
64	$2,000	$883,185	$0	$858,765
65	$2,000	$973,704	$0	$944,641
Less Total Invested		($80,000)		($14,000)
Equals Net Earnings		$893,704		$930,641
Money Grew		11-fold		66-fold

Reprinted with permission: Dow Theory Letters, Inc., Richard L. Russell

have grown to two trillion dollars. By today, this would have grown to just about fund our national debt. Buffett's point is that even (apparently) small amounts of money should be invested with great care because of the amazing potential afforded by compound interest. Compound interest is the reason "time is money".

The more frequent the compounding of your money, the greater the return. For example, on a Certificate of Deposit, the rate of interest may be 4.0%, but because of the quarterly (every 3 months) compounding, the Annual Percentage Rate (APR) is 4.06%. This is the real rate of return. When you are in debt, more frequent compounding has the opposite effect, to your obvious detriment.

I once heard a physician make the statement – "you can make investment mistakes when you are young because you can make it up later." That is not correct! In fact, there are several significant problems with this statement.

- It suggests arrogance.
- It presumes that a physician will continue to make a signifi-cant amount of money in the future, a possibly faulty assumption.
- It suggests a lack of respect for money, another problem that afflicts some physicians.
- Finally, and most importantly, it ignores the benefits of com-pounding. It is more financially punishing to make mistakes early as compared to later in life. Profits made and com-pounded on early successes will more than make up for a bad late-career investment while missed opportunities and bad investment decisions made early in life will **NEVER** be recovered.

The money will not be made up later. It will never be recouped, never. The thought that you will ever "catch up" is an intrinsically flawed concept. Just examine Table 2. You must be more careful, not more careless, with money when you are younger. You have less investing experience, and can and will make more mistakes. But as it pertains to this subject, the younger the investor, the more valuable your money because of the power of compound interest. You must make more than $60 at age 65 for every one dollar lost at age 23. It is almost depressing to consider all the money spent unwisely when you were young and what it would have grown to now. Considered from another prospective, the money generated from an hour's work at a minimum wage job at age 23 is more valuable than that generated by a physician working for more than an hour at age 65.

I opened a Roth IRA for my younger son Michael on his high school graduation from the Culver Academy (Culver, IN). I then made Michael and older son John (graduated Choate Rosemary Hall, Wallingford, CT) the following offer: I will match whatever you put into a Roth IRA. At a young age they are introduced to compound interest, I am encouraging them to save, they are not just being given money, and when they are 50 years old they will have some serious money in the bank. I encourage you to make the same offer to your children and grandchildren.

Getting rich quickly sounds neat and glamorous and does occur occasionally. If it happens, consider yourself fortunate. But the desire to get rich quickly is much more likely to result in grief than in the big pay off. The easiest way to accumulate real wealth, your best chance of attaining financial security, is to work hard, save your money, and with the help of compound interest, do it the easy way. Get rich slowly.

SUMMARY OF CHAPTER THREE

- Compound interest is your most valuable investment tool. It is inevitable.
- Even seemingly small amounts of money have amazing potential.
- The more frequent compounding of your money, the greater the return.
- The younger you are, the more valuable your money.
- Lost money will *never* be recouped.
- Offer to match your children's and grandchildren's contribution to a Roth IRA
- Get rich the easy way. Get rich slowly.
- Compound interest is why "time is money".

II Avoid Being Diverted from Your Financial Goals

Chapter Four
Arrogance, Ego, Greed and Envy

It is it is impossible to be a successful investor, in fact, to be successful at much of anything in life, without controlling greed. Everyone, whether they are willing to admit it or not, has had quite thorough first hand experience with greed. Should these comments seem misplaced, try to impartially analyze the greatest failures of your life. There is a good chance that greed was one of the principal culprits.

I make no pretensions that I can adequately discuss greed, nor unfortunately, as it relates to this discussion, that I have any solutions that would otherwise seem obvious. One conclusion, though, is clear. Inability to control greed will result in financial ruin.

I am sure you feel these comments about greed apply to everyone but you. You are hard- working, honest and diligent. You treat your patients with respect. You are a good and loving parent and spouse, an upright member of the community. You have everything that anyone would want, including a great income and the respect of your patients and colleagues. You have rightfully earned all of the success that you now enjoy. Well, Martha Stewart probably felt the same way. She was convicted of multiple felonies and spent time in jail trying not to lose an amount of money infinitesimally small in comparison to her fortune. Peter Lynch, to get tickets for something he could have watched on TV, now has a black mark on his name (*see* Chapter Thirty-Eight). Let's be honest. It was due to greed.

R.M. Doroghazi, *The Physician's Guide to Investing*,
DOI 10.1007/978-1-60761-134-9_4,
© Humana Press, a part of Springer Science+Business Media, LLC 2005, 2009

Unfortunately, greed can be as subtle as it is powerful. You do not need to commit a crime to experience the financially devastating destructive capacity of greed.

The vast majority of the movie-going public probably feels that George C. Scott's greatest role was "Patton." But as it relates to this discussion, I feel he gave an outstanding performance in "The Flim-Flam Man." At the beginning of the movie, Scott, the flim-flam man, tells Michael Sarazin, "Greed's my line. Greed, and 14-karat ignorance. They never let you down ... you can't jip an honest man." The flim-flam man is able to succeed because he plays upon the greed of the sucker. In the end, the greedier the person, the greater the flim-flam man's chance of success.

I will spend more time discussing arrogance, ego and envy. I admit at the outset that to discuss things such as this, in the manner I do, may appear overly blunt. Discussing the basic failings of humans is always difficult. But I truly believe the poor investing judgment and wasteful spending displayed by some physicians relates to their inability to appreciate the malevolent power of arrogance, ego, greed and envy.

I suggest you read *Profiles in Folly: History's Worst Decisions and Why They Went Wrong* [1]. One of the unifying themes of failure is arrogance: The Titanic is unsinkable, the Germans will never breach the Maginot line (they didn't, they just went around it), the Iraqis will greet us as liberators, Custer didn't need to wait for reinforcements. A little humility will save you a great deal of money.

This book discusses many points of value to all investors. This chapter, and several others, are directed more to the physician investor, and other professionals such as dentists, veterinarians, artists, athletes, entertainers and airline pilots, who make their living by having a skill or talent that results in a high level of remuneration but that does not necessarily require a high degree of business skill.

Physicians are extremely bright, in fact, often brilliant. They usually graduate at the head of the class. Things just seem to come so easily. They train for many years and eventually acquire a talent to save lives. They can cure cancer, treat heart attacks and save dying infants. They can diagnose an illness they have never seen before and may have read about only once twenty years ago. Doctors can be miracle workers. This ability both requires and creates self-confidence.

This can also be the problem. Physicians think they are invincible. They think they are faster than a speeding bullet, more powerful than a locomotive and that they can leap tall buildings in a single bound. You may recognize this as the introduction to the Superman TV series of the 1950s starring George Reeves and Phyllis Coates and later Noel Neill. Physicians often have the (mistaken) assumption that their amazing ability to impact life and death automatically results in the same capacities and abilities outside medicine. It does not!!

There is a fine line between self-confidence and arrogance. Physicians all too often think that just because they are a physician, possibly even the best physician in the world, that this tremendous talent, mental capacity and ability automatically applies to everything else in their life, including investing. Physicians sometimes have no idea of their limitations. This type of arrogance and ego can result in investing disaster.

Let me give an example. An intelligent, prominent physician must have investments, a net worth, and material goods commensurate with their position and image. In simple terms, a "big shot" doctor should be rich and look rich. Ego can and often does trump financial sanity.

A physician will never be the richest person in town. This goal in and of itself suggests arrogance, ego and greed. In a practical sense, a physician can make only so much money because there are only so many hours in the day. A physician can bill only for services directly performed. I once read that the secret to becoming truly wealthy is to be able to make money while asleep (investments can do this but a physician cannot) and to be able to make money from the labor of others. A businessman with employees can make money from the labors of others, but a physician cannot.

A physician must immediately give up the idea of being the wealthiest person in town, or rich. How much money is enough? No matter how much you have, someone will always have much, much more. How do you even define rich? Being rich should never be your goal. Rather, physicians make enough money that they just need to be wise – and control arrogance, ego, greed and envy – to be able to live a life of financial security. This should be your goal – financial security.

I suggest you read *Green With Envy: Why Keeping Up With the Joneses is Keeping Us In Debt* [2]. Boss does a nice job in recounting real-life stories to show how honest, good, hard-working people can be seduced by envy that is financed by debt. My advice: Don't be jealous of what other people have, just be content with what you have. People would be far happier if they realized there are some things they just cannot afford.

I believe more money is lost in the hospital doctor's lounge, or other similar settings where physicians tend to congregate and talk, such as at a party or the country club, than anywhere else. It is in such situations that the emotions of arrogance, ego, greed and envy overwhelm sanity.

Let me digress for a moment. Note that I will routinely throughout this book say "he." As I have spoken with more female physicians regarding their investments, it is clear they are much more levelheaded than their male counterparts. My impression is the female physicians who are not good with finances recognize and accept it, appropriately making them risk averse. More significantly, I do not believe I have ever heard a story of a female physician who has done the stupid things that some male physicians have done to lose millions of dollars or declare personal bankruptcy.

There would be no better place for male physicians to begin than by listening to their wives. I would at the same time encourage, actually challenge, wives to become more involved in investing decisions since by co-signing they are equally liable. In essence, a spouse has veto power. Do not be afraid to use it!! A wife must not be intimidated by her brilliant, forceful, ego-driven, but financially inept physician husband. I would go even further to say there are situations where the man should stick to the practice of medicine and allow his wife to control the purse strings and manage the investments. I know many excellent male physicians who do exactly this, and it works out fine. To my knowledge, no one has ever shown that the gene for financial success resides on the Y chromosome.

To return to the previous thought. A physician who is the epitome of the trained professional believes he must have investments and material goods that match his medical prowess. A prominent, brilliant physician must have equally grand investments. How can you brag about a passbook savings account, a money market fund or a Certificate of Deposit? Good Lord what an embarrassment that would be! Or income-averaging, sending a check every month, into a Standard & Poors (S&P) 500 Index mutual fund. Where is the glory in that? Such investments are clearly not adequate for an important, prominent physician.

Only an investment that sounds really cool, exciting, or chic, available only to a few, which returns 25 or 30% a year, or even more, and of course is in some way tax-advantaged or even tax-free, is an investment worthy of a prominent physician. To some people a glamorous investment that does not make money is more desirable than a dull, mundane investment that is profitable. To remind you, the goal of investing is not to impress others, it is to make money. In the end, people will be more impressed by an investment that makes money than a glamorous loser.

The above statements may seem ill-advised and intemperate. But they are absolutely true, and perfectly capture the mindset of those who most needs to read this book, but almost certainly will not. This chapter is not about logic. It is about the antithesis of logic, about the base emotions of arrogance, ego, greed and envy that seem to be at the root of so many of the problems that plague some physicians with their investments. Jack was always looking for those magic beans that would grow a stalk to the heavens. There are no magic beans.

It almost seems that some physicians are attracted to the chic, glamorous investments so they can gloat. A year or two later the doctors who were boasting do not tell you the investment was a complete bust. Alarmingly, yet distressingly predictable, they are describing yet another can't-miss investment that is certain

to make 30% or even 50% or more a year. Some people unfortunately never learn. And because of the previous loss, they must
"make it up" on the next investment. This tends to initiate a
cascade of more poor investments. Never "double-down" on a
loser.

This is in contrast to the successful physician investors who
are content with their unexciting, ho-hum, even boring, mundane investments that are earning ten to fifteen percent a year.
These physicians will be the ones who can retire when they
wish rather than continue to work because they must. In fact,
I would recommend that the young physician seek out the
opinion and advice of the older successful physician investors.
In my experience, such physicians are delighted to help their
junior colleagues any way they can. Just ask.

The people who promote such grandiose, can't-miss investments know very well how to play to the physician's soft emotional underbelly. One angle is exclusivity. Any steelworker or
secretary can purchase a CD at the local credit union or invest in
a mutual fund. But an investment available to only a select few
people is clearly superior. Exclusivity plays to ego. It is a basic
human emotion. One reason to belong to a Country Club,
whether you are willing to admit this to yourself or not, is
because of exclusivity. The more expensive, and thus exclusive,
the Country Club, the better. The same with investments.
Investments available only to a select few, such as those requiring a substantial minimum amount, say ten thousand dollars or
more, are worthy of a prominent physician.

The second chapter detailed a minimum anticipated return
on investment, a return that may be realized with hard work,
and most importantly, a return that when promised should
immediately cause alarm. This alone should help separate the
solid opportunities from the bogus schemes.

When it is assured, guaranteed (you should know well from
your training as a physician that no one can guarantee anything) that an investment can return thirty percent or more a
year – just say no thank you and leave. But this works again
and again. Remember – "fool me once, shame on you, fool me
twice, shame on me." Everyone makes mistakes, but you

should learn from your mistakes. It is terrible when physicians continue to be enticed into bogus schemes but it is invariably due to arrogance, ego and greed.

It is essential to cut your losses (*see* Chapter Thirty, When to Sell). This is difficult psychologically but must be done. Start by going to the nearest financial institution and purchase a FDIC/ FSLIC-insured Certificate of Deposit. You may not be able to brag to your colleagues about a CD, but you will have money in the bank.

Do not be concerned about being "left out". Another physician tells you of a deal he knows of that is so "sweet", so sure to make millions, that he will be able to retire in five years. And if you miss this opportunity you will still be slaving away, taking call on nights, weekends, and holidays, ten years later. In fact, it was hearing the following true story that stimulated me to write this book. I have done my good deed for the day (for the year) if I can prevent just one person from suffering a similar fate. (I must point out that none of those who invested live in Columbia, or to my knowledge, the State of Missouri).

A group of physicians (one absolute sign of a loser is when all of the potential investors are physicians, *see* Chapter Twenty-Five) were approached by a non-US citizen (you must be very wary of investing with foreigners, see also Chapter Twenty-Five) regarding a fantastic investment opportunity in South America. The physicians were to put up some cash and sign some notes. After barely an hour of discussion and questions (actually very few "soft" questions, the physicians did not wish to offend the man who was about to lead them to a life of financial and personal misery and despair) the majority of the physicians signed the contracts – contracts that were not even in English. I will repeat that in case you missed it. The contracts were not even in English. One of the physicians who did not invest in this "fantastic opportunity" is the one who related this story to me.

The deal went south (a terrible pun, but very true). Each physician lost between three and ten million dollars. Three and ten million dollars! A lifetime of hard work, an entire lifetime. These physicians will be working until they are seventy just to get out of debt. And it was their fault, and their wives! Think of the pain. They attended college for four years, medical school for four years, three to seven more years of training and then will work sixty or more hours a week for another twenty-five or thirty years. The nights, the weekends, the holidays, the time away from their spouse, their children and their grand-children. They have made millions of dollars in wages and are still in debt! Their lives, their family's lives, and possibly their mental and physical health are destroyed.

One physician was later asked why he participated. He said that if his partners had retired in five years in luxury he would kick himself. To lose ten million dollars just not feel left out. Pathetic.

But do not feel sorry for them. It is safe to say they would not have shared the profits had things gone well. Their motives were simple – arrogance, ego, and especially greed. The "Big G" as a local businessman friend of mine calls it. They wished to be rich, to retire early, to be big shots, to have more money than everyone else and to be able to boast about how well they had done. They were skinned, and it was because of arrogance, ego, and greed. This happens too often. Please, please, do not let it happen to you.

SUMMARY OF CHAPTER FOUR

- Greed is the most powerful and malevolent of your investment enemies.
- Greed can be as subtle as it is powerful.
- Just being a physician does not make you an expert at everything.
- Your goal is not to be rich, but to have financial security.
- A forceful spouse can help prevent investment mistakes.
- Forget glamour. The goal of an investment is to make money, not impress others.
- Jack found out that there are no magic beans.
- Do not be concerned about being left out.
- Do not be jealous of what others have. Be content with what you have.

- People would be happier if they realized there are some things they just cannot afford.
- The best investment you can make is not making a stupid investment that was motivated by arrogance, ego, greed or envy.

REFERENCES

1. Axelrod A. Profiles in Folly: History's Worst Decisions and Why They Went Wrong. New York: Sterling, 2008.
2. Boss S. Green with Envy: Why Keeping Up with the Joneses is Keeping Us in Debt. New York: Warner Business Books, 2006.

Chapter Five

The Mark and the Doctor Discount

My favorite "Far Side" cartoon shows two deer in the woods. The one on the right has a huge red symbol on his chest that looks terribly like a bull's eye and the other deer says "Bummer of a birthmark, Hal."

Many salesmen, business people, and in fact a good number of people in general feel that physicians have this big target on their chest that says, "I'm The Mark". Unfortunately, it is both true and often well deserved. In fact, the basic reason for writing this book is to help prevent you from being "The Mark."

How can you avoid being "The Mark?" The nuts and bolts of accomplishing this are related throughout the book, but I provide some basic practical tips:

- Accept the fact
- Seek help from a pro

ACCEPT THE FACT

The first step is to accept the fact. As you know, the first reaction of a patient when told they have a major illness is denial. Do not deny it! You may be a hard-working, superbly trained, absolutely brilliant physician, but many people consider you "The Mark."

I can give no better example of a physician being considered "The Mark" than a story I heard in the doctor's lounge. One

R.M. Doroghazi, *The Physician's Guide to Investing*,
DOI 10.1007/978-1-60761-134-9_5,
© Humana Press, a part of Springer Science+Business Media, LLC 2005, 2009

physician was teasing another (actually, one of his partners). Bob said to Bill, "Remember when you bought your first SUV. It had snowed the day before, you were in your scrubs and you walked into the dealer's showroom with your wife and small children. You said you needed to buy a four-wheel drive vehicle and you needed to buy it today. It was dreary and the salesman probably thought he was going to have a bad day. Then he saw you walk in, the sun suddenly began to shine and he thought this might not be such a bad day after all". Bill was clearly up to the task and replied, "I probably made his month."

These physicians are both my age and can joke about this sort of thing because their experience has allowed them to gain insight into this problem that so often afflicts physicians.

Do not proudly announce to people, especially salesmen, they are dealing with a physician. Do not introduce yourself as Dr. so and so. An MD degree may carry weight at a scientific meeting, but in many business situations the other person just sees $$ signs and that big target on your chest. If you wear your scrubs out when conducting business, you may as well hang a sign around your neck saying "I am a chump" because you are. Physicians are "The Mark."

If you feel you are being patronized or taken for a patsy because you are a physician, just leave. If dealing with this person cannot be avoided, make it clear to them you are offended. Now they are on the defensive.

One comment that should immediately put you on guard is being referred to as a "rich doctor." This person thinks they see that bull's eye on your chest and is zeroing in for the kill. To use this term is clearly a sign of disrespect, and is no different than making a derogatory generalization about a racial or ethnic group. Never lower your guard with people who use the term "rich doctor."

A local businessman acquaintance drove by as I was cutting the lawn. I stopped and walked to the street to say hi. As I approached the car, he rolled down the window and said, "I didn't know that rich doctors cut their own grass!" Without hesitation I replied, "That's why I am a rich doctor."

Similar comments include "this is not much for a doctor" or "you should be able to afford this." How in the heck does anyone know what I can afford? Comments such as this show about as much insight as a physician telling a patient "this won't hurt" just before inserting a chest tube without the benefit of any anesthetic.

I was in a group where I had to sit by someone. Shortly after meeting him, I was making conversation and mentioned I had a condo at the Lake of the Ozarks. He said "all rich doctors have a condo at the Lake". I said to myself "watch out, Bob".

About a month later, I mentioned that the credit card company called that day asking me to confirm a $17,000 charge that was posted from a foreign country. Of course, someone had stolen my card number. He said "That's not much for a doctor". I did not even attempt a response. I learned long ago never to argue with people dumber that you, because you can't win. He has further confirmed my initial impression with several other vulgar remarks.

Another comment I have found to be both patronizing and insincere is "we need to have you over sometime, or we need to go out to eat sometime". Sometime, of course, means never.

SEEK HELP FROM A PRO

Physicians are especially poor negotiators. There are many reasons for this. Physicians are often dealing in an area outside of their expertise, a problem well detailed in many other areas of this book. Physicians do not understand patience as businessmen do. A physician's time frame for decision-making is typically less than a day, and is often measured in hours, minutes or even seconds, such as ventricular fibrillation or biopsying a mass that is actually the aorta, resulting in blood hitting the ceiling or the wall. A businessman's time frame of decision-making is usually measured in weeks, months or even years. The patient businessman can out-wait the brilliant and decisive, but impatient, physician.

The easiest remedy is to hire someone to negotiate for you. Admit that negotiation is not within your area of expertise and seek appropriate assistance.

There is a man in town who has a full-time job completely unrelated to the automobile. But his passion is cars. He buys them, sells them, fixes them up, reads car magazines, and knows the blue book by heart. It is not an exaggeration to say that he knows as much about cars as a physician knows about medicine. A friend told me of him. Whenever I want to buy or sell a car, I call him, tell him exactly what I want, including color and options, and it's done. He goes to multiple dealers, shops around my trade-in and negotiates the deal. I just show up at the time of purchase to pay and sign papers. It is not an exaggeration to say that car dealers hate to see him walk in the door. I pay him a fee and he takes care of everything. Not only does he save me hours of time, but I am terribly impatient, and I am not a particularly good negotiator. He easily saves me hundreds or even thousands of dollars on each and every purchase.

I had this gentleman and his wife over recently for supper. He is an African-American who grew up in the still-segregated Mississippi of the 1940s. When he was 6 or 7, fishing at a pond owned by his father's employer, he thought he had a snag, but proceeded to reel in a 6 lbs bass, the largest ever caught there. The owner offered him $5 for the fish if he could claim he caught it. My friend said "sure".

When the gentleman looked in his wallet, he had only three ones and a ten. He said to my friend "here are three dollars".

My friend said "Sir, you said five dollars, not three dollars". He got the ten dollar bill!!

To quote Caeser "Fortune favors the bold".

My friend assures me he has seen situations where the price was increased when a salesman discovers they are dealing with a physician. I have heard the same from other people. The "Doctor Discount" works, my dear readers, because some physicians are so arrogant that the salesman knows they will score big-time.

My friend also expands this point further by saying that women routinely face a similar problem with negotiations in general and especially when buying automobiles. Even if a woman is knowledgeable, a good businesswoman, and a good negotiator, it is often difficult to command a salesperson's, especially an auto salesman's, respect. A female physician would appear to be at a double disadvantage. I would suggest that, in appropriate circumstances, a female physician be accompanied by a male, if for no more than "muscle or backup."

Another person who can help with negotiating is a family member, or very close friend, who is an astute businessperson. Otherwise my recommendation for negotiating any significant investment or contract is to consult a lawyer. Their fee will be dependent upon the time they spend, but in general it is worthwhile. If a six-figure purchase or investment is being considered, the savings could easily be thousand of dollars.

There are other reasons besides price where a lawyer's input is helpful, such as the terms. Once a deal is done, it is done. Everything must be negotiated up front and obtained in writing. It is possible to receive a reasonable price but terms that are terrible (*see* Chapter Twenty-Six). This could result in significant losses down the line. Details count and they count a great deal. Lawyers should also be able to identify anything that is not on the up-and-up. When they express concerns, heed their advice. To disregard such advice would be similar to a man obtaining annual blood tests for PSA then not following up when an abnormality is found.

A local businessman relates one circumstance where it can be to a physician's advantage to be considered "The Mark." Because physicians often have cash available for investment they may be presented with more opportunities. A local physician has been able to purchase several pieces of real estate at distressed prices because the sellers needed to move quickly and the physician had cash, or borrowing capacity. But this requires tremendous patience and good judgment to invest only in the few situations that do represent real genuine opportunities.

SUMMARY OF CHAPTER FIVE

- Physicians are considered "The Mark." Accept the fact.
- Do not hesitate to hire someone to negotiate for you. It is not a sign of weakness.

- Salesmen often do not have the same respect for a female as they do a male.
- To be referred to as a "rich doctor" is a sign of disrespect.
- The "Doctor Discount" is when people find out you are a physician and raise the price.

Chapter Six

It's Not Much, I Can Afford to Lose It: The Concept of Risk

In medicine we are continually admonished not to make guarantees, but I will make one here. If you take the attitude of the title of this chapter, you will lose more money than you originally thought possible, and possibly even everything.

How much should you be willing to risk? The answer is both practical and psychological. One dollar, one thousand dollars, one hundred thousand dollars, where do you draw the line? The only correct answer is zero. There is no reason to "risk" anything unless you believe the expected profit more than compensates the risk. To provide a medical analogy: How much can an alcoholic safely drink? The only correct answer is nothing.

John D. Rockefeller used to give away dimes, when they were still silver, real money. He would say "this is the interest you receive on a dollar in one year". His lesson was what seems like a tiny amount of money is actually the fruits of labor of a dollar for a whole year.

-Do not confuse risk with loss. Even the (apparently) safest investment with the best risk/reward ratio can result in a loss. This happens to even the greatest investors. I am referring to risking money, in essence, gambling with money. The vast majority of physicians would abhor the thought of being seen buying a lottery ticket or playing the quarter slots in a casino, yet they do the exact same thing when they "gamble" with

R.M. Doroghazi, *The Physician's Guide to Investing*,
DOI 10.1007/978-1-60761-134-9_6,
© Humana Press, a part of Springer Science+Business Media, LLC 2005, 2009

investments. Do not make any investment unless you are as sure as possible that the projected return more than compensates for the risk, that is, generates an acceptable profit.

Also be aware of the difference between uncertainty and risk. With uncertainty, you do not know what will happen in the future. With risk, you still do not know what will happen, but you do have some idea of the different possibilities, the likelihood that they might occur, and how they can be managed.

Say an investment in an oil well was structured as a limited partnership with a minimum investment of $10,000. Drilling began immediately after the investment was made and within two months you would know if it is a dry hole or a gusher. If it is a dry hole the $10K is gone. If they strike oil, the payoff could be 5 to one or greater. After dreams of turning $10K into $50K in two months, and being able to brag about an oil well in the doctor's lounge or at the country club, you decide to "risk" it. But the well was dry and the investment a complete loss.

If you have an investment portfolio of $100,000, you have just lost a full year's return. Remember sums that seem small or inconsequential have amazing potential because of the power of compound interest. If your child is one year old, what in 17 years will fund more than half of their college education has been squandered.

Now, consider this situation in a different light. Suppose you hire a geologist who believes the probability of striking oil on the property is 10%. This is still a risky investment, but you now have the information to make a rational decision. A 10% probability of achieving an investment worth $50K gives the investment an expected value of $5K (0.1 × $50,000 = $5,000). So the risk of a $10K investment is not worth the expected profits.

To make wise investment decisions under conditions of risk, you must have an idea of the possible future outcomes and the likelihood that each outcome might occur. If you do not know, consider retaining an advisor (The advisor's fee must also be considered). If you still do not know the probabilities of making or losing money on an investment, do not invest. Invest only when you anticipate an appropriate profit.

Take Texas Hold'em. A player is dealt two hole cards, followed by five community cards, the first three are dealt together and called the "flop", the next card is the "turn", and the last community card is the "river" (the colorful terms are part of the magnetism of the game). Players can bet after their hole cards, and after each dealing of the community cards. The player uses his two hole cards and the community cards to make the best 5 card hand.

Say you are dealt the ace and eight of clubs (two pairs, aces and eights, are the "Dead Man's Hand", so named because it was Wild Bill Hickok's hand when he was gunned down). The flop comes queen of hearts and king and four of clubs. One more club, and you will have a flush (five cards in the same suit, a powerful hand).

Your chance of hitting a flush on the turn are 9 (the number of clubs still in the deck) over 47 (the total number of cards still in the deck), or exactly 0.191. Should you not catch a club on the turn, your chance of catching one on the river is 9 over 46, or 0.195. Thus your cumulative chance of catching one club with two cards to go is 0.386 (0.191 plus 0.195), about $1\,^3/_4$ to 1 odds.

After the flop, the pot is $3,000. Your opponent bets $500. If you call, you are betting $500 to win $3,500, providing you with expressed (or pot) odds of 7 to 1. Because your chance of getting a flush with 2 cards to go is much better, you wisely call (but do not raise here with a drawing hand).

The turn is the nine of diamonds. No help to you (or probably to him either). There is one card to go. The pot is $4K, and your opponent again bets $500. For $500, you can win $4,500, or 9 to 1 odds, far in excess of your 4 to 1 (0.195) chance of catching a flush. Note that had your opponent made a larger bet, say $4,500, and denied you adequate odds, you would have been forced to fold.

The river – a 7 of clubs. Yes! (Be sure not to get excited). You not only hit a flush, but you have the ace, which means you have the highest possible flush. Since the other cards on the board preclude a hand stronger than a flush, you have the "nuts" (a non-anatomical Texas Hold'em term which means you have an unbeatable hand). Your goal now is to extract the maximum amount from your opponent without causing him to fold (For an elegant discussion of the risk/reward ratio, and a solid introduction to Texas Hold'em, I suggest Dan Harrington's books [1–3].

Several points. First, gambling is when you play hunches that have no basis in fact. In this example, by knowing the exact odds, the risk/reward ratio, you were able to make an intelligent, informed decision on how to play the hand. You "invested" in a situation where your chance of a successful outcome was in excess of your risk. Of course, no one wins all the time. But, if you only play when the odds are in your favor (and that *is* the *only* time you should play), over the long-term you should be able to generate a positive return.

You also must consider implied odds. This nebulous and unquantifiable concept says that, using the above example, although going into the last card you had only a one in five (0,195) chance of hitting a flush, if you were successful, considering you had the ace, you would win a large pot. If you do hit it, it would be a big win.

The lesson is that this is how you should evaluate all investments, on as risk/reward basis. Gambling is gambling. Participating in this hand was an objective assessment of the potential of generating a positive return on your investment.

Even with appropriate efforts to identify, handicap and manage risk, playing a "long shot" is rarely worthwhile. Consider the racetrack. A horse that should be at the glue factory goes off at 50–1. A $2 bet pays $100. After finishing your third beer you realize that putting down a C-note on the nag could pay $5,000. You know you are unlikely to win, but are seduced by the huge potential payout. After all, one win at 50–1 odds will make the night. In addition, winning against such odds and with such a large payout allows you to brag to your friends. Winning $2.10 on a $2 show bet on "Dr. Bob" is nothing compared to winning $200 on a $2 bet at 100–1 odds on "Tony the Bull!" (Because the standard bet is two dollars, in years past $2 bills circulated freely at the track).

The problem is that your chance of winning against such odds is less, usually much less, than even the quoted odds of 50–1. In reality, even the one huge payout is rarely sufficient to make up for all of the losses. In a practical sense, when betting on long shots, people usually run out of money before they hit the big score. And even if they do hit it big, they continue on until losing it all back. Avoid long shots at the racetrack and in investing, they rarely pay off.

When I was growing up, my family would often get together to play Hungarian poker (we still do occasionally). The big winner for the evening could be anyone, but my grandfather was the consistent winner. He would only bet when he knew he had a strong hand. My father and uncles would tease him and say, "Dénes, you only bet on the lead pipe cinches." He would just smile and say "igen" (yes in Hungarian) as he scooped up the pot.

I will conclude with a story and a several quotes from Warren Buffett. From time to time Buffett would get together for a weekend with friends and business associates to play golf and bridge and exchange ideas. At one session, Jack Byrne, Chairman of GEICO (a large holding of Berkshire Hathaway) proposed that for a "premium" of $11, he would pay $10,000, almost 1000–1 odds, for anyone who could make a hole-in-one over the weekend. Only one person did not take the bet –Buffett. The man, almost a billionaire at this time (the early 1980 s), would not risk $11 for a chance to win $10K. He realized that the odds of him making a hole-in-one were so remote that even a 1000–1 payoff was not worth the risk. Buffett noted that because of the power of compound interest to turn seemingly small sums into much larger ones, he treated an $11 wager exactly as he would an $11,000,000 investment.

Buffett notes that investing is not like diving, a greater return is not awarded for a more difficult investment. Take the easy ones, don't force it. He also said "Charlie (Munger, his principal associate at Berkshire Hathaway) and I detest taking even small risks unless we feel we are being adequately compensated for doing so." Buffett is worth billions and he detests even a small risk. I suggest that you take his advice seriously.

SUMMARY OF CHAPTER SIX

- There is no reason to "risk" any amount of money.
- Seemingly small amounts of money have amazing potential.

- EDC-Every Dollar Counts.
- A good investor must be able to identify, assess and manage risk.
- All investments should be evaluated on a risk/reward basis.
- Avoid long shots.

REFERENCES

1. Harrington D, Robertie B. Harrington on Hold'em: Volume I: Strategic Play. Henderson, NV: Two Plus Two Publishing, 2004.
2. Harrington D, Robertie B. Harrington on Hold'em: Volume II: The Endgame. Henderson, NV: Two Plus Two Publishing, 2005.
3. Harrington D, Robertie B. Harrington on Hold'em: Volume III: The Workbook. Henderson, NV: Two Plus Two Publishing, 2006.

III Principles for Achieving Your Financial Goals

Chapter Seven
Define Specific Goals

Few things that are really significant, that are truly important, that are a major part of your life, just happen. Financial security does not just happen. It requires years of detailed planning and discipline to put the plans into effect. Even if you receive a major financial windfall, such as an inheritance or winning the lottery, it will be gone in short order unless there is a plan on how to husband such a largesse.

As a note, I hope no physician plays the lottery. The French philosopher Voltaire (François Marie Arouet) called the lottery "a tax on stupidity."

There is one and only one time to start planning both your near-term and long-term financial goals, and that is right now. Today. It is never too late to start. Every day that goes by robs you of your most powerful investment tool, that magnificent friend of compound interest.

Spend time on the subject, as much time as you and your spouse can spare. I suggest one hour *per week* as an absolute minimum. People will spend hours planning a vacation or researching the purchase of a depreciating asset, an article of consumption, such as an automobile or a boat, and then not spend ten minutes researching a five or six-figure investment. Money that took months or years to accumulate is squandered because you rely on what someone else tells you rather than spend the appropriate amount of time and effort to research the investment for yourself.

R.M. Doroghazi, *The Physician's Guide to Investing*,
DOI 10.1007/978-1-60761-134-9_7,
© Humana Press, a part of Springer Science+Business Media, LLC 2005, 2009

Goals must be identified and should include, at a minimum, the topics in the next section, including paying your bills, buying and paying off your home, your children's education, insurance needs, and funding your retirement.

You may have other wishes and desires. You may love to fish, hunt, or just hike through the woods, so at some time you would like to purchase a suitable piece of recreational property (*see* Chapter Thirty-Two). Family members besides your children may require significant financial assistance. Your parents may have spent all of their time and resources helping you obtain your medical degree. If you should ask them, I am sure they will tell you that they were happy to do it, they would do it again any day, and they are proud of you for being a doctor. Your parents could be in their 50s or 60s with minimal savings and you feel it is your responsibility to help them financially. I think it is. Or you could have a sibling with special needs. Who is going to provide their financial support when your parents die? Considering that you are a well-educated, successful person who earns a great wage, you take it upon yourself to provide financial support for your special-needs brother or sister when your parents pass away. If you do this, you are to be congratulated.

Or you may have some personal desires. You have always dreamed of an around-the-world trip. Your passion is collecting coins or stamps or antique furniture. My personal library numbers more than 1,200 volumes (I have read almost all of them), and I buy 5 to ten books a month. I have run out of rooms to build more bookshelves. In two or three years I would like to build a library addition on my home. And considering that I live on Bingham Road, I would like to have a George Caleb Bingham portrait to hang in it.

Or you would like to leave a legacy, maybe a scholarship fund or even an endowed professorial chair. Something that, in either a small or possibly even large way, makes humanity a little better. My family has endowed the Doroghazi Clinical Teaching award at my medical school Alma Mater, the University of Chicago. Believe me, it is a good and satisfying feeling and something one can be proud of.

Realizing such goals and desires requires significant planning. Since life rarely goes according to plan, you must re-evaluate your situation, the progress of your general plan, and at regular intervals make whatever changes are necessary.

SUMMARY OF CHAPTER SEVEN

- Start to plan your financial future today.
- It is essential to identify your financial needs and goals, only then can you make appropriate plans to achieve them.
- Include charity in your long-term goals.

Chapter Eight
Thrift

I strongly encourage you to read *The Millionaire Next Door: The Surprising Secrets of America's Wealthy* [1]. It is not a book on investing, but rather one of the best, if not the best, books ever written on thrift. I am convinced it can save the average physician $10K or more a year. I also recommend that your spouse and children read it.

I mention several times that investing is a three-step process:

1. Earn money.
2. Do not spend it (i.e. – thrift).
3. Invest the money.

THRIFT IS THE MOST CRUCIAL PROCESS IN THE ACCUMULATION OF WEALTH.

The reason is that it is the variable over which you have the most control. For example, it may be difficult or even impossible to increase your income significantly. If you are just some regular Joe or Jane working in the vast majority of jobs in our society, the only way to increase your income is by changing jobs (difficult or impossible, especially with unemployment currently on the rise) or getting a second job.

For a physician, it may be just as difficult, or even impossible over the short term, to increase your income. If you work in an

R.M. Doroghazi, *The Physician's Guide to Investing*,
DOI 10.1007/978-1-60761-134-9_8,
© Humana Press, a part of Springer Science+Business Media, LLC 2005, 2009

academic setting, or large clinic or similar organization, you are on a salary. Even if you are in a fee-for-service private practice and are willing to see more patients, the ability to increase your income may be limited by the competition and is limited by the number of hours in the day. Even if you wish to see more patients, it may take months or years to ramp up your production significantly. You could take more call, but you would need to be pretty desperate to consider this. In essence, if you truly wish to increase your income, you must find a different job or accept a significantly different life style.

How about increasing the return on your investment? That is one of the principal objectives of this book, but is a very long-term process. Over the course of several years it is very possible to increase your return on investment, but over the short term it is impossible. In fact, trying to force such an issue is much more likely to result in a loss rather than a profit. You do not just wake up Monday morning and say, "I want my investments to return 15% instead of 5%." That is just not how it works.

But how much you spend can be changed both drastically and instantaneously. Some physicians spend all they make, and sometimes even more. You can spend less – 10%, 30%, 50% less – and you can do it today. Thrift is the most important variable in the accumulation of wealth because it is the one over which you have the most control.

Arrogance, ego, greed and envy are in constant conflict with thrift. A successful physician, making a quarter million dollars a year or more, does not wish to appear "cheap or stingy or tight or chintzy," or whatever other similar term may be applied. The people who apply these terms to one who is thrifty are often the spendthrifts, who are wasteful of their money. The preceding terms only apply to those who will not spend money when it should be spent. I suggest you read about Hetty Green, the "Witch of Wall Street", who accumulated more than 100 million dollars around the turn of the last century but caused her teenage son to have a leg amputated because she would not pay his medical bills. Or you make more than half a million dollars a year and have three sons who enjoy the Boy Scouts, but you will not donate one hundred dollars even when solicited by another physician. This is how I would define cheap or stingy.

I hope the reader is able to garner many points, both general and specific, from this book. In the end, if there is only one point that you can remember, I suggest the following. If you can say:

THIS IS TOO EXPENSIVE, I CANNOT AFFORD THIS

You may never be rich or wealthy, but you will *never* be poor. You should always have something to eat, clothes to wear, and a roof over your head. If you can say, "I cannot afford this" you have taken the first step to a lifetime of financial security.

To be careful with money, which is the term I prefer, is not to be cheap, but is wise. No matter what the level of your income and no matter how much money is in the bank, if you do not have respect for money you will not have it for long. It is those who do not have respect for money that are most likely to succumb to the army of charlatans that prey on physicians.

You must always be cognizant of thrift, but an especially vulnerable time in a physician's financial life for excessive or unnecessary spending is when they complete training and start practice. Income may triple or quadruple in an instant. All those years of hard work, sacrifice and delayed gratification have finally paid off. It is appropriate to spend more at this time because you have finally reached your goal. The problem is that you can loosen up too much. Unless you are careful spending can easily outstrip income. What was previously just a dream now becomes an absolute necessity. Your previous vehicle was a $12K three-year-old used car. Your next car should be a $25K new car but you say "what the heck, I can afford it" and buy a $45K set of wheels (and borrow $35K to do it). It is very easy at this time for your appetite to easily outstrip even the significant increase in your income.

I will give several examples of how I define being careful with your money. I take French lessons from an ex-patient. She gave me the following example of thrift. Her father had a stable job during the Depression, and although they were not by any means rich, all of their basic needs were covered. They were the only family on the block with a telephone and one of the few families on the block to receive a daily newspaper. They were instructed to read the paper carefully, fold it nicely with no wrinkles, as four or five other families would be reading it after they finished. This was especially so of the classified section, as there may be a help wanted advertisement for a job so sorely needed by one of their neighbors. The Great Depression was a terrible, painful time but it did teach those who lived through it a respect for the basic necessities of life that is often absent in our society today.

I loved to sleep at my grandmother's on Friday night. Saturday morning she would give me 25¢ for baseball cards. Each pack of five cards was 5¢. If I purchased all 5 – 5¢ packs at once – i.e. 25¢, there was a penny tax. My grandmother would not give me the extra penny for tax. (This is an example of both generosity and thrift. These virtues are not mutually exclusive). Instead, my instructions were "Bobby, buy three packs (i.e. 15¢ and no tax), open them, say something like "wow, these cards are great, I don't have any of these guys" and then buy the other two packs". After I did this on several occasions, the owner of the confectionary, who knew my grandmother very well, said "Bobby, your grandmother won't give you the extra penny for tax, will she?" I said "no Mrs. Lambert, she won't!" After that, I was able to just plunk down my quarter, buy all five packs of cards at once, and Mrs. Lambert would ring them up as separate purchases.

I use this story in all of my talks. After a presentation three years ago, a man in his late-20s came up and said "I am the youngest of nine children. My grandparents came over from Italy. When we were given money for candy, we received the exact same instructions to save that penny tax". I think many immigrants are so careful with their money because they remember how things were in the "old country".

Thrift is similar to being on a diet. It requires eternal vigilance. You can watch your snacks and serving sizes all week, exercise daily and then go out on Saturday night and chow down with a 5,000 calorie meal, negating the hard work of the previous week. You can do a nice job watching the pennies, nickels, and dimes and then make one purchase (often impulsive) and blow the budget for an entire month or more. Be careful.

Talking about food, do not go shopping when you are hungry. Besides the obvious grocery shopping, studies have shown that in general you spend more money when you are hungry than when you are satiated. So the next time the family plans to do some power shopping (the very thought should cause you to break out in a sweat), stop at McDonalds on the way to the mall and you might save 20%.

What amount of money is too little to be concerned with? I suggest EDC – every dollar counts. If you do not respect a dollar, then there will be no respect for one hundred dollars. If you do not respect one hundred dollars, then there will be no respect $1,000, and so on. When you are walking along the sidewalk and see a penny under the parking meter, do you pick it up? It is not the amount that is important, it is the act (I am told these pennies are very lucky).

Years ago a colleague made the following comment. It is simple but elegant and sums up the power of thrift.

I MARRIED A GOLD MINE. MY SPOUSE IS THRIFTY.

Although I admit I am not as conscientious as I used to be, I still use coupons whenever possible. At least a dozen physicians or their wives thought they were the only ones who spent the time and effort to clip coupons and were "relieved" after they read this book to discover they were not alone. You need not be concerned that you will waste a million dollars when you are willing to expend the effort to save $1 with a coupon. It just will not happen.

Earlier I noted investing is a three-step process. The first step is to make money. Physicians are very adept at this. Sometimes it seems that the money will flow forever, almost as easily as opening a faucet. The second step is to save it, i.e., not spend the money. Only then is there money to invest.

How much should you save? John D. Rockefeller suggested fifty percent of your income. When my boys were growing up, I paid them $30 to mow the lawn. As soon as they finished, they received $15 cash, their's to use as they saw fit. We set the other $15 aside. They never "expected" or "missed" it, because they never saw it, it went straight to the bank. It became their habit to save 50% of their lawn money. Make savings your habit.

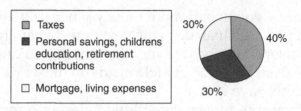

Fig. 1. Approximate distribution of total income.

Saving 50% of your after-tax income is also quite possible for a high-income wage earner such as a physician. Our average physician makes $250K a year (*see* Figure 1). Forty percent goes to taxes, leaving $150K. Half of the remainder after taxes, six thousand two hundred and fifty dollars per month, is invested ($75K a year). This amount includes saving for the children's education (*see* Chapter Seventeen), personal non-retirement savings and pension contributions. The remainder, the other half of income left after taxes, $6,250 a month, is for living expenses. After a mortgage payment of $2,902 a month (*see* Chapter Sixteen) there is still more than $3,300 a month of after-tax, after-mortgage money available for living expenses. Couples raise families of two to four children, with all children acquiring a college education, on a total pre-tax, pre-retirement, pre-mortgage, pre-savings, salary of $3,300 per month.

Note the amazing rewards in ten years (*see* Table 1) of getting into the habit of saving and investing.

Table 1
Rewards of Saving 50% of After-Tax Income

One year	$75,000 × 10% = $82,500
Two years	($82,500 + 75,000) × 10% = $173,250
Three years	($173,250 + 75,000) × 10% = $273,075
Four years	($273,075 + 75,000) × 10% = $382,882
Five years	($382,882 + 75,000) × 10% = $503,670
Six years	($503,670 + 75,000) × 10% = $636,537
Seven years	($636,577 + 75,000) × 10% = $782,691
Eight years	($782,691 + 75,000) × 10% = $943,360
Nine years	($943,460 + 75,000) × 10% = $1,120,306
Ten years	($1,120,306 + 75,000) × 10% = $1,314,837

Compounded at 10% per year.

If you enter practice at age 35, the above approach has generated more than one million dollars in savings by age 45 for you, your retirement and your children's education. A fortune, and your home is paid off. Financial security is attainable, but discipline is required.

If one desires the biggest, fastest car, the most expensive clothes, an airplane, the biggest vacation home and all other sorts of flashy things, this is their decision. This is not a criticism of those who choose this lifestyle. People who spend their money in this way are the ones who bring much of the color and excitement to the world. I admit that if everyone's personality were like me the world would probably not be quite as lively (but it would be safer). In the end, people get what they want. If your desire is financial security, considering a physician's income, it is a Darryl Dawkins (Chocolate Thunder) shatter-the-backboard slam-dunk. If you want to appear rich and important, with all of the luxuries, do not expect financial security. In *The Millionaire Next Door* Stanley and Danko refer to the big spenders with sublime comment of "big hat, no cattle." If you do wish to splurge a little, to loosen up, do it after there is a million dollars in the bank and after the mortgage has been retired.

This talk of thrift is not to completely discourage you from spending money to obtain the finer things of life. To the contrary, these are the things that add color, zest, enjoyment and satisfaction to one's existence. Everyone agrees on what the finer things are, it is usually just a matter of price. Purchase all of the finer things you wish, just make sure it is within your budget and after you have achieved financial security.

Being thrifty also does not mean you live a boring, miserly, rag-tag existence. To the contrary! I submit it is thrift, being careful with your money, that allows you to purchase the finer things. When my home was built in 1939, it was the most expensive home in Columbia ($25,000). It is elegant and decorated with nice art and collectibles. I have a four bedroom condo at the Lake of the Ozarks, and, with a friend, a 73 acre piece of recreational property with a 20 acre lake, both of which generate considerable enjoyment for me and my relatives and close friends. Everything is paid for free and clear. At least part of being able to afford these nice things is that I find the free coffee in the doctor's lounge just as tasty as the $32 per gallon brew at Starbucks.

This may or may not come as a surprise, but patients are acutely aware of how physicians spend their money. This is especially true if one lives in a smaller community. Patients realize how hard a physician works and most (but not all) expect them to have a higher standard of living. It is almost expected that a celebrity should flaunt their money, and it is almost expected that a physician should not. An occasional patient is drawn to the appearance of wealth (they often have the same personality), but generally patients do not like it. As the old saying goes "patients prefer that their doctors drive Buicks rather than Cadillacs."

The majority of patients make a mere fraction of a physician's income. Ten percent of $250K is $25K, an amount probably greater than your nursing tech makes. Even just 20% is $50,000, which is probably about what your nurse makes. And as you know, some patients must decide between food and utility bills or buying their medications. Your bill to a patient for $1,500 could represent two years of their savings, or even their entire life savings. They may even be forced to borrow to pay the bill. Or they may be walking into your office to make the twenty-dollar monthly payment on their bill as they see you park your new $100,000 car.

Sometimes when making a purchase, I consider how long it took me to earn the amount to be spent, not as a Cardiologist in private practice, but at my wage at previous jobs. When I was 6, I went with my father when he cut lawns. When I was 11 or 12, I started to cut them myself. The usual pay per lawn was $3, and that included raking, sweeping, and trimming, which was done with hand shears (I believe that the inventors of the weed whacker, power edger, and leaf blower have done such a service for humanity that they should be awarded a special Nobel Prize). When I turned 16 I began working at Graham's Book Store in Granite City, IL. My starting salary in 1967 was $ 1.59 ½ per hour. In the summers between years at college and between college and medical school I worked at Granite City Steel (now a division of United States Steel (X). The base wage in 1970 was $2.66 per hour. Labor was a "two point" job, each point was worth an additional 7 cents an hour. A "bonus" brought the total wage to approximately $3.00 an hour. Now, when considering a purchase, rather than thinking of how many patients I had to see, I consider how long I had to work for Mr. Graham or how long I had to shovel slag or chip fire brick off the walls of the soaking pits in the blooming mill at Granite City Steel to make the money. It does provide a little perspective.

Or compare your income to that of your parents or grandparents, especially if they were working class people. It is very possible you would be embarrassed to tell your parents you make more in two or three weeks (even adjusted for inflation) than your father made in his best years as a foreman at General Steel, or after the Commonwealth (as the plant was also called) closed, that he made as a janitor at the local high school, or that the return on your investments in a good month is more than your parents were able to save in their life.

TURN OUT THE LIGHTS

I am a second-generation American. All five of my grandparents (my mother's father died of the consumption when she was four years old, my grandmother then re-married) were immigrants from Hungary, coming to the United States between 1900 and 1921. I also considered myself "first-generation Depression." Although I was born in 1951, the residual of that painful time was ever present in our home. "Don't go into debt. Don't buy stocks. Keep your money in a pass-book account. Don't go into debt (it was repetitive). Don't go in or out too much (In-again-out-again-Finnegan as my mother would say) because it lets in the cold or warm air. Clean your plate, and turn off the lights when you leave a room".

When the boys were growing up, I always made them turn out the lights. If they came up from playing downstairs and the lights were still on, I sent whoever came up last back down to turn them off. Now when I visit my sons, *they* will send *me* back into a room if I have not turned everything off (*Forbes*, 9/04/06-an auto-off feature on your home lights could save $150 a year).

I mention this to make both a general and a specific point. The essence of thrift is not to waste any resource. Do not buy things you do not make adequate use of and use to the fullest things you purchase. Although this example involves only pennies, it will illustrate the point. You go to the store to purchase a six-pack of imported beer for $8.50. Thus each beer costs $1.42. However, you recently joined a warehouse club with an annual fee of $25. Because they purchase in quantity and can pass on the savings directly to you, a case of 24 beers is $25.00, or only $1.04 per beer. Cool, what a bargain, a savings of almost 27% on each beer. But you do not drink beer, you just keep it available for guests. One year later there are still eleven beers and they are stale and flat (although after the first one they seem to taste fine). Remember to include the annual fee when calculating how much was "saved" on the case of beer. Make sure a bargain really is a bargain. A purchase at any price is not a bargain if you do not make use of the product.

A straightforward example of using what you have to the fullest would be if you belong to a club or organization that requires a minimal expenditure over some period of time to maintain your membership in good standing. Many country clubs require so much be spent on food every month or every quarter. You will be billed the minimum whether you go to the club or not. If you do not use the minimum you may as well flush the money down the toilet because you are receiving absolutely nothing in return. If you consistently do not meet the minimums, then consider dropping the membership.

As a corollary, before you join a country club or buy a condo along a golf course where there are golf fees each month, run the numbers to see how much it will cost per hole. Unless you play a great deal (difficult if you are a busy physician), the cost per hole should make you reconsider. And if you move away and cannot sell the condo, you still owe the golf fees. It is analyzing the finances of situations such as this that separates those who can accumulate wealth from those who just spin their wheels.

A disclaimer: In the first edition the title of this section was "Clean Your Plate". Considering the obesity problem in our society, many thought I should change the headline, and I agree. Please do not get me wrong: I still get nervous at the thought of wasting food, I just make sure I do not put too much on my plate.

Now, would you like to save one-quarter to one-third on your restaurant bills? When was the last time you ate out and finished everything – the bread, the appetizer, the salad, the main dish, and the desert? I suspect you rarely finish everything you pay for. Try ordering less, often much less. You will save money and not over-eat. Split the appetizer, and/or the salad, and/or the entrée, and/or the desert. In many restaurants, the servings are too large anyway. In fact, before ordering remember to ask the waiter the portion size. If you take children out to eat, I am sure that food, and what you paid for it, is being wasted.

My sons John and Michael, daughter-in-law Diana and I were just in Chicago for four days to present the Doroghazi Clinical Teaching Award at The University of Chicago, Pritzker School of Medicine. On the first day there, I said "Look, I want us to have a good time, but we are going to some pretty expensive places, we really need to watch what we order". We did a great job. We also had a good time, and no one complained they were hungry.

You may say you always bring home a doggie bag. In general, this is not an option when traveling. I would also point out you are eating some pretty expensive leftovers that are never as good reheated as they were when originally served, especially fish.

My recommendation to save a significant amount of money on your restaurant bills and/or be able to eat out more often is to only order enough food so that you can "clean your plate."

I remind you that thrift is the ninth point of the Boy Scout Law.

SUMMARY OF CHAPTER EIGHT

- Thrift is the most important variable in the accumulation of wealth.
- You must not spend money in order to have money to invest.

- Remember these phrases:
- I CANNOT AFFORD THIS.
- I MARRIED A GOLD MINE, MY SPOUSE IS THRIFTY.
- Do not allow your spending to increase more rapidly than your income.
- A physician should be able to save 25–50% of their after-tax income.
- People get what they want. You should want financial security.
- Make saving your habit.
- Do not allow ego to turn you into a spendthrift.
- Turn out the lights when you leave a room.
- Thrift is the ninth point of the Boy Scout Law.

REFERENCE

1. Stanley T J, Danko W D. The Millionaire Next Door: The Surprising Secrets of America's Wealthy. Marietta, GA: Longstreet Press, 1996.

Chapter Nine

Invest in What You Know

How many of the following questions can you answer correctly? Guesses are not allowed, you either know the answer or you do not.

1. What is rhinotillexis?
2. You have been retained as an expert witness for the defense in a medical malpractice case. The plaintiff's attorney says "Doctor, how much are you being paid for your testimony"? How should you respond?
3. In what disease would you see "die rote blute welle"?
4. Who is credited with the description of hereditary elliptocytosis?
5. In what organ do you find the fissures of Santorini?
6. What specialist would be consulted in a patient with a phlyctenule?
7. What is the difference between congenital and acquired Horner's Syndrome?
8. What is the significance of p<.05?
9. Are most patients with trichotilomania male or female?
10. What percentage of women with pre-eclampsia suffer a mis-carriage?

You are a bright, successful, well-trained physician and I bet you did not know that rhinotillexis is using your finger to pick your nose. I chose topics from most major areas of medicine so

R.M. Doroghazi, *The Physician's Guide to Investing,*
DOI 10.1007/978-1-60761-134-9_9,
© Humana Press, a part of Springer Science+Business Media, LLC 2005, 2009

that hopefully everyone answered at least one question correctly. You may even have gotten two or three right, either because of reading extensively or perhaps a fact was remembered from medical school days. You just scored only 20 or 30 out of a possible 100 on a seemingly simple medical quiz.

(The best answer to #2 is "Sir or Madam, I am being paid for my time, not my testimony". I will let you look up the answers to the rest of the questions so you will learn more).

Presume you are a neurosurgeon and the computer-generated report of the EKG on your patient is abnormal. In fact, you are the premier neurosurgeon in the world in the treatment of saccular aneurysms. Rich and powerful people will travel any distance and pay any fee to seek your expert care. But what about the abnormal EKG? You recognize this is not within your area of expertise so you wisely obtain a Cardiology consultation. By seeking a consultation you admit that your knowledge and skill is not all-encompassing, in fact, that it does not even extend to other areas of medicine. One of the world's premier neurosurgeons has been stopped by a simple EKG with the interpretation of "possible left atrial enlargement and non-specific ST-T wave changes. No previous EKG for comparison."

A physician's amazing knowledge and expertise in one area of medicine does not make them an expert in everything. It certainly does not automatically imply they are an investment wizard. To think otherwise is arrogant, and will cost you money.

Answer the following questions:

1. In the futures market, what are contango and backwardation?
2. What is the current vacancy rate of commercial property in the West End of Boston as compared to Jamaica Plain or Natick?
3. When can you use accelerated as compared to straight-line depreciation?
4. What was the first Exchange Traded Fund (ETF)?
5. Which Hartland statue is most valuable: Stan Musial, Dick Groat, Ted Williams, Mickey Mantle or Henry Aaron?
6. What is a Collateralized Debt Obligation (CDO)?

7. Which George Caleb Bingham painting would be most desirable to own? (Bingham lived here in central Missouri and I live on Bingham Road) "Portrait of Mrs. Robert Beverly Price" (an ancestor of my next door neighbor), "Lighter Relieving a Steamboat Aground" (hangs in the White House) or "The Squatters" (in the Boston Museum of Fine Arts)?
8. What is the current exchange rate, to the third decimal point, of the euro/yen?
9. Is the Tobin Bridge in Boston named after the Tobin who developed the Q ratio?
10. What is used to calculate the per-acreage payment for land placed in the Conservation Reserve Program (CRP)?
11. For extra credit. Who invented the ticker tape?
12. For double extra credit. The streets on the Monopoly board have their origin in what eastern city?

It is quite possible you did not know the answer to any of these questions. But I assure you that someone does. When investing there is someone who knows as much about any particular area as a physician knows about their area of medicine. They are just as bright as a physician. They graduated at the head of their college or business or law school class. They work and study just as hard as a physician (Actually, considering the new rules, they often work harder than physicians). They read books and journals and go to seminars just as physicians do. They discuss investments with others just as physicians discuss cases with their colleagues. If you invest in their area of expertise, you will be competing directly against them. If you do not know as much as they do, you will lose!! Remember this equation: Knowledge = Money.

A physician's great intellect, their tremendous knowledge in an area of medicine, may make them the greatest physician in the world. But it does not make them expert at everything. This feeling of intellectual invincibility is one of the physician's worst investment enemies.

Invest in what you know. If you do not understand stocks, bonds, real estate, collectibles, art or whatever, then do not buy it. It really is that simple. If all you understand is a Certificate of Deposit, then invest in a Certificate of Deposit.

Many of the greatest companies in the world succeed because the principals of the business know what skills they possess, but more importantly, realize their weaknesses, what skills they lack. One person often has the business/financial/management skills and the other the technical/engineering skills. Examples include Sloan and Kettering at General Motors (I am sure every physician has heard of Memorial Sloan Kettering in New York), and Hewlett and Packard. These men succeeded just as much by realizing what they did not know, when to defer to the expertise of others, as by their own tremendous abilities and desire for success. Andrew Carnegie said the secret of his success was that he surrounded himself with people smarter than he was. It is just as important for a physician to realize the limits of their expertise and knowledge.

A friend and I own a piece of land. Because I like to do it, I conduct the basic business. Although I physically keep the check book, we both must sign all checks. We both also appreciate that his inter-personal skills far surpass mine and would make Dale Carnegie (pronounced differently and no relation to Andrew Carnegie) jealous. Two or three times a year we need to meet with someone to discuss issues that have come up. Aside from introductions and maybe a few questions, he does all of the talking, and things work out fine. Our skills compliment each other's nicely.

Beware of peer pressure. This is especially critical for a young physician just beginning practice. I am sure that at some time the following scenario will occur. An older physician will describe an investment that is so glamorous, so exclusive and so prestigious that only a few truly sophisticated and savvy investors (presumably such as him) can participate. Of course, it is essentially guaranteed to return twenty-five or thirty percent a year and requires no cash up front. A young and impressionable physician, who at this state of their investing career understands only a passbook savings account and US Savings Bonds, can easily be awed, or even intimidated, by a (seemingly) more knowledgeable senior physician discussing such an investment. And then this physician will say, "Bob, you should really consider this investment. Several other heavy-hitters in practice have already signed up (intimating he is a heavy-hitter and you will also be one should you participate)". It is at this moment that the young physician's judgment and self-confidence will be put to the test. Do not be pressured. You may feel stupid and embarrassed but just say no thank you. A year or two later what appeared initially to be a paltry return on your bank account will look like a gold mine in comparison to the complete loss of their glamorous investment.

Remember this equation: Knowledge = Money. An investor can and will make money if they know more about an investment than the person they are dealing with. They will lose money if the other person is more knowledgeable. Or consider the situation from this point of view: Whenever you buy or sell anything, the person on the other side of the deal is almost always a professional.

How can you determine where to invest? It is really quite simple. What do you like? It is essential not to "force" yourself to like something or pursue something just for the hope that it may be profitable. It will not work but more importantly it will not be profitable. Instead, just keep looking until you find an area that does captivate your interest and that is fun, something you like so much that you can't wait to get some free time so you can do more with it. Your passion will also be your greatest chance for profit.

Do you already possess detailed knowledge in an area? How do you gain expertise in any area? The same way you acquire expertise in medicine – study and hard work.

What do you like? Do you have any hobbies or interests? Did you collect anything growing up? I collected baseball cards and could name the National and American league batting champions and home run champions from 1920 through 1970. Growing up in the St. Louis area, I was a Cardinal fan. Stan Musial, Ken Boyer, Bob (Super) Gibson, Lou Brock and Curt Flood (see below) were my heroes. I could not believe one city was lucky enough to have both Harry Carey and Jack Buck as announcers. I can still name all 25 members of the 1964 (World Champions),

1967 (World Champions) and 1968 Cardinal teams (they should have been World Champions. I still think Gibson's performance in Game One is second only to Don Larsen's perfect game as the best World Series game ever pitched). So I collect baseball cards and sports memorabilia.

Your family has had a farm for four generations. Certainly you and your family know the value of farmland. Buy farmland as an investment.

You can look for investments in the area in which you are already an acknowledged expert, i.e., medicine. I was a Cardiologist. Who has the best pacemaker? Who makes the best stent? (Note that just because a company has the best product does not make their stock a good buy. Price is always important). If you are a surgeon, did you buy Intuitive Surgical (ISRG) after hearing of or using one of their robotic devices? A nephrologist friend recognized the potential of erythropoetin and made millions (yes, millions) of dollars investing in Amgen (AMGN).

What about medicine in general? Does the pharmaceutical representative describe a new product that could be a blockbuster or do they proudly announce their company has just released the fourteenth angiotensin-converting enzyme inhibitor (ACE Inhibitor) on the market? What about health maintenance organizations (HMOs), for- profit hospital chains, drug distributors, temporary staffing agencies, subspecialty management groups and so on? This is already your area of expertise. It is not an exaggeration to say that a practicing physician may know more about these issues than Wall Street analysts.

I use the above discussion only to illustrate the point. I have not owned any health care stocks for more than a decade. I believe that the next great wave of progress in medicine has not yet presented itself, as confirmed by the dismal performance of the stocks of the big pharmaceutical companies.

A great way to find ideas for investments is in your daily life. Peter Lynch repeatedly notes this as an important source of his investment ideas (*see* Chapter Thirty-Eight). You and your family walk into a restaurant chain that is packed. The food is quite good and reasonably priced and the service is good, or even great. Consider investing in their stock, but only after more research, of course. You pay $110 for a pair of shoes that fall apart in three months. Do not buy the stock of that shoe manufacturer. If you are a wine connoisseur and a vineyard that produces a superior wine at a reasonable price and is well-managed is coming public, consider purchasing their stock. In fact, you should visit the vineyard and speak with the owner. Even if you do not purchase the stock, I am sure you would have a good time.

In August 2003, I went to Las Vegas for a convention. I had not been there before and was impressed. While walking down the Strip, passing literally dozens of spectacular hotels, I remembered that the annual meetings of American Heart Association and American College of Cardiology had become so large that there were only four or five cities with enough hotel rooms and facilities to service such a large group. When I returned to the hotel, I picked up an issue of *Barron's*, which had an interview with the director of the Invesco Leisure Fund. Guess what city he said had become the #1 conventional destination in the United States? Yes, Las Vegas. He pointed out that there are more then 150,000 hotel rooms in a relatively small area, the weather is usually good and there is obviously plenty to do. He focused specifically on Mandalay Resort Group (MBG). They had just completed the largest single convention center in the country and I knew that they had initiated a 2.5% dividend earlier in the year. The dividend had been raised twice. I did more research on Mandalay Bay. They were a well-run, very profitable company and their focus on luring convention business fit nicely with my observation and impression. I purchased the stock that week. In late June 2004, MGM Grand announced an offer to buy Mandalay Bay. I sold the stock that day for a gain of 95% (plus the dividends paid in the interim). It is possible to get investment ideas, and make money, by events in your daily life.

Two years ago I noted that the financials of Gamestop (GME) looked extremely favorable. I consulted my video game experts, sons John and Michael. They shopped at Gamestop, said the stores had nice traffic, and liked the basic business model and service. I purchased a small position and made a few bucks.

Are you really knowledgeable about computers? Who makes the best computer? A physician friend who is very knowledgeable in this area purchased Dell (DELL) early in its growth phase and made a significant amount of money. Who is the best software manufacturer? What company sells junk?

To become a successful investor, do exactly what you did to become an expert in medicine. Find an area you truly like, that captivates your interest, that becomes your passion, and specialize. Become as knowledgeable in that area as possible, and then stick to it. I cannot emphasize this enough. You do not need to be knowledgeable in everything or even knowledgeable in many areas. Just be very knowledgeable in one area.

Curt Flood's first year in St. Louis was 1958, the year I began to follow the Cardinals. His last year was 1969, the year I graduated high school. I loved Flood. He hit for a high average and I believe was a better defensive centerfielder than Willie Mays, although Mays clearly had more power and a better arm. I met Flood in 1960 or '61 at a Temple in St. Louis, where he made an appearance with linebacker Bill Koman of the recently arrived from Chicago football Cardinals.

Flood was a man of great personal pride, who chose to challenge baseball's reserve clause after his trade to Philadelphia following the 1969 season. It ruined his career – he *would* have made the Hall of Fame had he continued to play – and gained nothing for him, but did open the door for free agency, which has profited all pro athletes since [1].

SUMMARY OF CHAPTER NINE

- A physician's great knowledge and intellect does not make them expert at everything.
- Knowledge = Money.
- Being a successful investor requires hard work. It does not just happen.

- Invest in what you know and like.
- Your passion will be your greatest chance for profit.
- Investing is like medicine, the greatest chance for success is to specialize.
- Watch for investments where you are already an expert – i.e., medicine.
- Beware of peer pressure.
- You can get great investment ideas from your daily life.

REFERENCE

1. Snyder B. A Well-Paid Slave: Curt Flood's Fight for Free Agency in Professional Sports. New York: Viking Press, 2006.

Chapter Ten
How to Identify Real Opportunities

Your goal should be to realize a ten to fifteen percent, or more of course, if possible, annual return on investments. To realize this goal it is mandatory to be able to recognize real opportunities. They do exist. The second chapter not-withstanding, there will be chances to make investments that can return fifteen or twenty percent, or sometimes even more per year. Only three or four such investments are needed for a lifetime of successful investing. How can you recognize these true, real opportunities when they do arise?

I will make two suggestions. The first is practical, a simple rule of thumb The second fits my personality and psyche, but does have a very considerable basis in fact and at a minimum will generate ideas that will allow you to formulate your own criteria. I cannot emphasize this later point enough. Do not do just what I say, do not do just what anyone says, or you will make mistakes. It is mandatory for you to make your own investment decisions (see the next Chapter).

HOW OFTEN DO REAL OPPORTUNITIES ARISE?

For some time I kept a daily journal. It was interesting and fun. I not only recorded the events of the day, but as it relates to this discussion, I also tried to analyze what had happened. This

R.M. Doroghazi, *The Physician's Guide to Investing*,
DOI 10.1007/978-1-60761-134-9_10,
© Humana Press, a part of Springer Science+Business Media, LLC 2005, 2009

allowed me to gain some insight into many things, such as who can and cannot be trusted (*see* Chapters Twenty and Twenty-Three).

I once looked back through my life to determine what opportunities ⁓ financial, personal, social, and professional – I had taken advantage of (some) and what I had missed (many). It was an epiphany. Here is the first point of this chapter – real opportunities occur infrequently. Sometimes twice a year, sometimes a real opportunity does not arise for several years. On the average, real investment opportunities occur approximately once a year.

This will tremendously simplify your investing life. Real opportunities do not occur every hour, every day, every week. That is just noise, non-statistically significant jiggle. Let them go by. Do not jump at everything, in fact, jump very rarely. Simple patience may not even be sufficient. Tremendous patience is mandatory. Real opportunities only occur once a year.

You read the *Wall Street Journal*, *Barron's* (my personal favorite), *Forbes* or whatever financial publications interest you. There are financial shows on the television and NPR on the radio. An infinite amount of financial information is available on the internet. Your stockbroker calls with a tip or suggestion (*see* Chapter Thirty-Eight for Swensen's opinion of full-service brokers), a salesman calls with an opportunity (hang up immediately), or you talk with friends who mention something. You are literally bombarded with hundreds of (apparent) opportunities. The more you read, see and talk to people, the more possibilities for investments arise. Pay attention to those that seem interesting, study for yourself, but remember that the absolute overwhelming majority of these apparent opportunities will prove disappointing. A rule of thumb: Only ten of one hundred opportunities are even worth spending time to investigate, and only one in ten is worthy of an investment. Remember that number, one in one hundred.

Some time ago I read a statement by Warren Buffett (*see* Chapter Thirty-Eight). He said that a person only needs to make twenty or thirty investment decisions in their lifetime. Of course he is right. The importance of patience seems to be a recurring theme for success in almost all aspects of life. As it relates to investing, I define patience as one real investment opportunity a year.

HOW TO RECOGNIZE REAL OPPORTUNITIES

I discovered that whenever I had to talk myself into anything it invariably failed. If I equivocated, I wasn't sure. I said yes, then no, then yes, if someone else had to talk me into something, it was always a loser. Always! I have come to the point that when I am thinking about an investment, if I have any doubts, large or small, definable or just a gut feeling, it is time to say no and move on.

When I look at something and say instantly, "this is the greatest thing since sliced bread" – these are the winners. There is no equivocating or wringing of hands. The decision is so easy. Every time I have this feeling the investment is not always a winner. No one has winners all the time. But every time I did have a successful investment I had this feeling from the outset.

This also means that I never second-guess myself. Life has enough problems without beating yourself up over such things.

Let me make several analogies to illustrate this feeling of when you are sure, when you are convinced from the outset. I will begin with sports. Even from the bleachers, where I prefer to sit, it is possible to see the batters eyes light up when the pitcher hangs a curve ball belt high, right down the middle of the plate. Here comes a pitch, twenty miles an hour or more slower than a fast ball, but it does not curve or move at all. It just sits there like a lollipop, seemingly begging to be rocketed into the bleachers (hopefully where I am sitting). It is thrown so poorly that the batter can count the stitches (there are 108 (double) stitches on a major league baseball, the first and last are hidden, so a batter with a good eye can count only 106) and read the name of the league president on the ball. This is the major league equivalent of Little League T-ball.

Ted Williams was a great hitter and a great student of hitting. Williams divided the strike zone into little squares (they would now be called pixels) and estimated what he could hit with a pitch in each area of the strike zone. Belt high, inside corner, a pitch he could pull, better than .400. Low outside area of the strike zone, about .200. Williams also had a tremendous number of walks. He let the balls out of the strike zone and the pitches of low yield but in the strike zone go by. He was patient and waited for the ones he could hit for a .400 clip. However, in baseball, three strikes and you are out. Williams eventually was forced to swing even at the pitches of low yield if there were two strikes and the ball was in the strike zone.

This is the beauty of investing. You can take ten, twenty or even a thousand pitches and they do not count against you. Just keep your money in a money market, a passbook, or a Certificate of Deposit. The money earns some interest, but more importantly, nothing is lost. Just wait for the belt high hanging curve ball on the inside corner of the plate and then swing as hard as you can.

Because I am a *very* impatient person, and I realize this, I have thought a good deal about patience. Impatience is good when you need to get things done quickly, such as with a very ill patient. Impatience is not good when investing. I would suggest that an appropriate synonym for patience could be pain. It can be difficult to wait, sometimes it actually hurts. Years can pass in an instant whereas seconds, minutes and hours may seem like an eternity.

You have saved enough for an investment. You are fairly knowledgeable about real estate and begin to look at some properties. You read the real estate section of the local paper each Sunday and have spent four afternoons or evenings in the last two months looking at property with a real estate agent or just driving by on you own. There were several that were OK and one that looked pretty good but you just could not quite talk yourself into making the purchase. Another month passes and you continue to look. Now the money is starting to burn a hole in your pocket. You want to get this investment out of the way so that you can move on to something else. Cool your jets, you must be patient.

A stock was purchased a year ago at 37. It now trades at 32. You are convinced it is a good company in a good sector, and you know from past experience that you often identify trends before others. But you find it increasingly difficult even to look up the daily closing price because it is down almost fifteen percent one year after the purchase. Or you sold some stocks for a profit because you felt the market was over-priced. However, the market remains over-priced and your money is just sitting in (unexciting) cash earning only 1 or 2% interest. More new money is coming in all the time. Patience is painful. But to be a good investor you must often just wait and wait and wait. And wait.

Even after several large investments, Warren Buffett is still sitting on billions of dollars in cash at Berkshire Hathaway (BRK). He realizes it is being under-utilized, but says "It's a painful condition to be in, but not as painful as doing something stupid."

Let me provide an example from history of how painful, yet necessary, patience can be. In the third century BCE, the city of Carthage, on the northern cost of Africa, battled Rome for dominance of the Western Mediterranean. In the first Punic War, the Carthaginians forces were commanded by Hamilcar Barca. In the Second, and more famous Punic War, the leader of the Carthaginian Army was Hamilcar's son Hannibal.

Theodore Ayrault Dodge considered Hannibal to be the greatest General of antiquity, superior even to Alexander or Caesar [1]. Hannibal repeatedly mauled the Romans, and at Cannae in June 216 BCE, put the entire Roman army, except the Consul Varro who fled, a total of almost 70,000 brave stouthearted Roman warriors, to the sword.

It was the Roman dictator Quintus Fabius Maximus who eventually devised the strategy to defeat Hannibal. The strategy was simple – not to fight him. Offense and aggression were in the Roman's blood. To decline battle, to display continuous caution, to remain forever on the defensive, was equated with weakness. The Romans began to doubt Fabius and lose faith in his strategy. He was even tagged with the sobriquet "Cunctator", the Delayer. It was only after years, and more stinging defeats at the hands of Hannibal, that the Romans realized the wisdom of the patience of Fabuis Maximus (The Fabian Society, which favors gradual, incremental change as compared to revolution, is so named to honor his methods).

Before moving on, let me make a general point. As you will see throughout this book, I make many references to the classics, history and other non-financial material. The classics are the classics because their wisdom and beauty is eternal, and since there are only rarely any new ideas, the study of history is essential. Many of the great investors note that they are more likely to generate profitable ideas from their non-financial, general reading than from a stock report from a brokerage firm.

Now I will provide a medical analogy of patience. You are a cardiac surgeon. It is of no consequence how often you operate, a successful result is all that matters. You evaluate an 88-year-old man with left main and three-vessel coronary artery disease, unstable angina pectoris, and a left ventricular ejection fraction of twenty five percent. You pass. You evaluate a 65-year-old female who suffered an inferolateral myocardial infarction six days before that is now complicated by a ruptured papillary muscle resulting in wide-open mitral regurgitation. An intra-aortic balloon pump is inserted to stabilize her hemodynamics and she is intubated. You pass. You evaluate a 62-year-old who looks 92 because they continue to smoke. Their blood gases and pulmonary function tests are terrible. They have closed all of their grafts, including both internal mammary grafts, from their two previous surgeries and are now in need of their third bypass operation. They have no conduit remaining. You pass. You evaluate an otherwise healthy 11-year-old girl with a secundum atrial septal defect (ASD). The chance of a successful outcome is 999 out of 1000. After making sure she is not a candidate for a catheter-based device, you operate. Recognizing real opportunities can be that easy, but patience is clearly mandatory.

Warren Buffett says real opportunities are so obvious that they will "grab you by the throat."

I was once invited to speak to a group of physicians in a community more than an hour from Columbia. When the physician called to extend the invitation, I said, "Jack, you can give this talk as well as I can." He said, "Bob, you live more than 50 miles away, that makes you an expert."

Real opportunities do not just arise elsewhere. They can occur locally, literally in your back yard. Real opportunities can occur in Bay City, Michigan, Weston, Ohio, Collinsville, Illinois or Columbia, Missouri, just as they can occur in New York, Boston, Chicago or San Francisco. In fact, because they are local you can have a significant advantage by discovering them before everyone else does.

For example, there are several artists in Columbia of note. I fell in love with Paul Jackson's work as soon as I saw it (www.pauljackson.com). Paul is the youngest person ever elected to signature membership in the American Watercolor Society, beating out by several months the great Winslow Homer. I think Paul is a genius and I have six of his works. The cover of this book is not a photo, it is one of Paul's watercolors.

Larry Young won the bronze medal in the 50 K walk in both the 1968 and 1972 Olympics. I find the elegant simplicity of his sculptures enchanting (*see* www.youngsculpture.com) and recently purchased one. Real opportunities can occur anywhere, including right down your street.

Kirk Kirkorian has made billions through investing, mostly in real estate and hotels in Las Vegas. Every few years he will make a purchase or a sale. The article I read about him made an analogy to an alligator lying on the bank with its mouth wide open. The alligator just sits there, motionless, still and relaxed, soaking up the sunshine, not wasting any energy chasing potential prey. It just waits and waits and waits. And if it has to, it just waits some more. Finally something walks right into its mouth and it just clamps down those powerful jaws and swallows.

A successful investor must be patient. And I have just supplied, in both time frame and psychology, a practical definition of patience.

SUMMARY OF CHAPTER TEN

- Real investment opportunities occur only occasionally, approximately once a year.
- Only one in one hundred opportunities are worthy of an investment.

- Likewise, real opportunities may occur anywhere and any time. Keep your eyes open.
- The study of non-financial material, from the classics, history and science to your daily newspaper, can generate profitable investment ideas.
- Real opportunities should be so obvious that you never have to "talk yourself" into them.
- Patience is difficult because it is painful.

REFERENCE

1. Dodge T A. Hannibal, A History of the Art of War among the Carthaginian and Romans down to the Battle of Pydna, 168 BC, with a Detailed Account of the Second Punic War. Boston: Houghton–Mifflin, 1891, Boston: Da Capo Press, 1995.

Chapter Eleven
Make Your Own Investment Decisions

Allowing someone else to make your investment decisions has the potential for complete financial devastation and ruin. I believe this ranks with arrogance, ego, greed and envy and the seductiveness of debt in its capacity to cause catastrophic harm.

Rasputin, which translates roughly as "debauched one" or "licentious", was a Russian monk (born Grigory Yefimovich Novykh) who held a pathological influence over Czarina Alexandra, and thus indirectly on her husband Czar Nicholas II [1]. The Romanovs, the last Russian royal family, were ultimately deposed and shot by the communists. Beware of the "investment advisor" who wants to control everything, who wants to make all of the investment decisions. Physicians have lost their entire life savings with such people because they stopped making their own decisions and blindly did whatever these "Rasputins" suggested.

This chapter will help differentiate the Rasputin-like promoters, often mere flim-flam men, from legitimate investment advisors and money managers. Allowing a professional to manage a portion of your portfolio can be extremely profitable. Using their knowledge and expertise, they make the specific investment decision. However, you have made the strategic decision to allow them to manage your money, but only after very considerable evaluation of them and their firm. It is

R.M. Doroghazi, *The Physician's Guide to Investing,*
DOI 10.1007/978-1-60761-134-9_11,
© Humana Press, a part of Springer Science+Business Media, LLC 2005, 2009

mandatory that they have good references and that their results are verifiable. There should be *no record whatsoever* of improprieties. If a person has had any problem with a regulatory agency, such as the Securities and Exchange Commission (SEC), or, in my opinion, anything besides a traffic violation, they should be avoided. There are so many solid, straight-as-an-arrow people out there that there is no reason to work with tainted material.

I believe many physician investors would be well served by working with wealth management advisors at a brokerage, bank, trust, investment bank or large, private firm. The usual fee is around 1% of the assets under management. Not only will you be working with legitimate people, but you will have the best chance to realize at least market-mimicking returns. You should also be provided with broad advice, from your insurance needs to apparently mundane but important things, such as reminding you to videotape the assets of your home for insurance purposes. An important plus of such advisors is that they should also help you avoid doing stupid things, such as participating in a blatantly worthless limited partnership or opening a restaurant.

The easiest way to separate legitimate investment managers from the Rasputin-like characters is to use the same decision making process that you use when evaluating a patient. Take a history, examine the patient, order tests, and if required, obtain a consultation. Sometimes additional reading is required on the subject and sometimes one or several colleagues are asked their opinion. You gather facts and make a decision.

The business term for this process is due diligence, which basically means you look at everything. The legitimate investment advisors expect this from sophisticated investors and are not offended. To the contrary, they are glad to comply, to show you they are worthy of your business. If someone gives you any heat at all when you ask for such information, it is time to move on. It is when this process is abrogated that catastrophes can occur.

Presuming such professional investment managers are legitimate does not guarantee success. Because losses can and do occur, especially over a short period of time, it is essential not to place too great a percentage of your net worth with any one manager.

Before moving on, let me make one important point concerning investment managers. They may boast that they beat the averages, such as the DJIA or the S&P 500, by some percentage each year, or that they out-performed ninety percent of their peers over some period of time. This is quite desirable when the market is up, but it is of little use when the market is down. From 1929 to 1932, the DJIA lost almost 90% of its value. Benjamin Graham, the father of value investing, beat the averages by almost 20% over this period but still lost 70% of his capital [2]. This is not successful investing. The goal of investing is to make money.

Now let me describe the Rasputin-like characters who must be avoided at all costs. They want to manage everything, they want all of your money. Rather than suggesting a CD or cost-averaging into the S&P 500 index fund or paying down debt, they suggest placing all of your money into a limited partnership. Can you guess the name of the general partner? Of course, Rasputin! The partnership will be structured with a $50 K initial payment and the investor will sign two $50 K notes, one due in one year and the other in two years.

The deal will not involve stocks, bonds or a traditional real estate investment such as a duplex down the street. Rather it will be a highly leveraged real estate development, an oil well, or a start-up company where he is the board of directors, or a deal in a foreign country such as an ostrich farm in China or a tax shelter in Bermuda. The pay off will be sometime in the future, or more likely, never. And as soon as you have more money to invest another deal will be available.

Allowing someone to make all of the investment decisions essentially gives them control of your money. Giving someone control of your money allows them to rob you. And they will.

The reason such people can assume a position of control is because they know how to manipulate arrogance, ego, and especially greed. These Rasputins promise big returns, 25 or 30% a year or more, that are (somehow) tax-free to boot. Such investments make spectacular conversation for the doctor's lounge and cocktail parties and only a very few select people can invest with this man. Do not underestimate the persuasive power of these Rasputins. Their ability to gain peoples' complete confidence and trust can be astounding, absolutely mind-boggling. If someone tells you they have an investment advisor who is more spectacular than Superman, you should run in the other direction. There is no Superman.

Jó Isten (Good God in Hungarian). Please do not allow this to happen to you. Accountants, and especially lawyers, are good at recognizing these kinds of scams. Ask their advice, and if they say no, it is mandatory not to proceed.

I have so far refrained from using, and I promise I will never again mention, the adage "beware of things that sound too good to be true." Everyone has heard this many times yet few seem to pay attention. Rather than continually repeating this clearly ineffectual phrase, I spend a good portion of this book specifically defining with numbers, examples and circumstances, what is "too good to be true."

Never invest in anything just because someone else does. Remember when you were small. One of the principle arguments you voiced to your parents to obtain permission to do something was "but Johnnie's parents let him do it so why can't I." Of course, even before you had finished, the traditional reply was "if Johnnie's parents let him jump off a roof, would you jump too?"

Even if Warren Buffett has purchased a stock, you must evaluate the investment for yourself. As a practical matter, it is also very unlikely you will be able to obtain the same price that Buffett paid (as seen with Buffett's recent investments in Goldman Sachs (GS) and General Electric (GE). Even if someone you know personally and whose opinion you respect has invested, you must still evaluate the investment for yourself. This person could be wrong or the investment just may not be suited for you.

Most importantly, do not allow just plain name-dropping to induce you into any investment. You are told by the promoter that both Jay Leno and David Letterman have put large sums into this investment (I use these two names only because they are well-know personalities. I have no idea of their investing capabilities). Such name-dropping must immediately raise a red flag. In fact, I would almost go so far to say that when this type of "hype" is used you should probably just walk away. Is this all that the salesman/general partner can say about the investment? What counts are the fundamentals of the business, the competition, the amount of debt, etc. I am not impressed one bit by who else has chosen to invest. You must make your own decisions.

Likewise, do not allow your name to be used to induce others to invest. In fact, no one else should ever know that you are even interested in any investment. At a minimum, this is very indiscreet. What I invest in is my business and absolutely no one else's. If I choose to tell someone else, that is my decision. If someone name drops your name, you must be forceful and make it clear that this cannot be tolerated and is unacceptable. In my opinion, financial information is as private at medical information.

One time I allowed my name to be used when an investment was being sold to others, essentially an endorsement. In the end, I was terribly embarrassed. And it was my fault. I will not make that mistake again.

In the end it is just like anything else in life – you must make your own decisions. You can and should seek other people's council (It is a strength, not a weakness, to ask for advice. Other people are flattered when you seek their opinion), placing more or less weight on their advice depending upon their credibility, but in the end you must make your own decisions.

Obviously, you must gain confidence in your ability to evaluate investments. The only way to do this is by making an investment. You can watch or monitor something forever, you can even practice using fictional accounts. But until a commitment is made, until you invest with real money, you will never really learn. There are few better ways to learn about investing than to lose a *few* (notice I emphasize few) of your hard-earned bucks. To borrow a phrase from Notre Dame football coach Knute Rockne "One loss is good for the soul. Too many losses is not good for the coach".

It is obviously mandatory to start small. The importance of starting with small investments not only makes common sense, but also has a basis in statistical probability know as The Theory of Gambler's Ruin. Even the world's greatest gamblers have losing streaks, and these streaks could conceivably be long enough and severe enough to wipe them out, thus Gamblers Ruin. The equation to determine the potential for ruin includes variables for hourly win rate, standard deviation and size of bankroll [3]. Thus, for an inexperienced investor (lower win rate due to greater probability of a losing investment) greater standard deviation (larger amount placed on each investment) and smaller bankroll (smaller net worth) there is a finite probability of ruin that is actually much greater than you might imagine. For repeatedly poor investments that represent too great a percentage of your total net worth, gamblers ruin is inevitable!

But as you gain experience and become more confident in your ability to objectively evaluate an investment, the amount of each investment can and should be increased. Note I did not say "risk" more on each investment. You should never "risk" anything (see Chapter Six). And when your increasing knowledge and experience indicate that a real opportunity has been identified, go for it!

There is another very practical reason to make your own investment decisions. With only rare exceptions, every investment will sooner or later be sold. If you did not know the reasons that the investment was made initially, it is impossible to judge if these factors have changed sufficiently such that a sale of the asset is indicated. There is no mechanism for risk control.

The last reason to make your own decision would seem purely psychological, but it is also quite practical. If an investment results in a loss, it is essential to analyze the situation to determine the cause(s) of failure. If someone else made the investment decision, you will never learn from your failure. But hopefully you will learn to be the one to make the decisions in the future.

SUMMARY OF CHAPTER ELEVEN

- You may seek the advice of others, but in the end, you must make your own decisions.
- Avoid any money manager with a tainted history.
- Giving someone control of your money allows them to steal from you.
- Use due diligence to choose your investment advisor.
- The goal of investing is to make money. Beating an average is immaterial.
- Do not place too much money with one investment manager.
- Do not invest just because someone else has.
- It is mandatory to start somewhere, but you must start small.
- As you gain confidence you can increase the size of your investments.
- The risk of Gamblers Ruin is much greater than you appreciate.
- Risk control mandates intimate knowledge of an investment.

REFERENCES

1. Axelrod A. Profiles in Folly: History's Worst Decisions and Why They Went Bad. New York: Sterling, 2008.
2. Graham B. Benjamin Graham: The Memoirs of the Dean of Wall Street. Ed by Chatman S. New York: McGraw-Hill, 1996.
3. Carlson B. Blackjack for Blood: The Card-Counter's Bible, and Complete Winning Guide. Las Vegas, NV: Pi Yee Press, 2001.

Chapter Twelve

Documents Required for Financial Security

This is the most boring, BUT, probably one of the most important chapters of this book. It is just not easy to make humorous, glib or clever comments about why you need a safe-deposit box or how long to keep your tax records. Using the tortoise and hare analogy, this is clearly tortoise material, the mundane things you need to make it to the finish line. To borrow terms from classical music, this chapter would be played somewhere between andante (moderately slow) and adagio (moderately slow but moving).

BUDGET

This is not a personal legal document but is a prerequisite for any successful financial plan. Businesses and corporations keep detailed and exact records of receipts and expenses. They also make projected budgets to anticipate income and expenses in the future.

You must know how your money is being spent. To keep a daily expense record to the penny is impractical, ponderous and not required, unless you are having problems paying your daily bills. However, to keep a detailed record of expenses over a short period of time, such as one month, can be quite illuminating. I have not kept a detailed budget in

R.M. Doroghazi, *The Physician's Guide to Investing*,
DOI 10.1007/978-1-60761-134-9_12,
© Humana Press, a part of Springer Science+Business Media, LLC 2005, 2009

years, but I would encourage you to do so if you wish. You can be sure I watch the checkbook and bills closely.

When you look at your exact expenditures it is much easier to identify areas where money can be saved. You subscribe to four magazines (or medical journals) but really read only one, the other three just sit on the coffee table and are thrown away unread. Cancel those three subscriptions. Once or twice a month you use an ATM that is out of your bank's network. Charge = $1.25. If this is done 20 times a year, the charge is $25.00. You receive one or several premium cable channels. Is it really worth the extra fifteen or twenty (or more) dollars a month on top of the already very expensive basic cable charge? This is $180–$240 dollars of after-tax money a year.

Or the expenses may be much larger. You have something for enjoyment and relaxation, such as a horse or a boat or a motorcycle. Are you using them enough to justify the expense? You have season tickets to a sporting event but because of call, working late and the children's activities, attend only one-third of the games. It will be difficult, especially if you have had the tickets for many years and have taken every opportunity to improve the seat location, but consider letting them go. It is often possible to use friend's tickets for one or two games a year, especially if they are physicians, since they have the same time constraints as you. As a practical matter, a physician is typically delighted to do such a favor for a potential referral source. If you want to go to a game, purchase tickets for the games that you can attend, otherwise, just watch them on TV.

Budgets are also required so that you will have cash available to pay bills when they come due, the concept of cash flow. You may have $1M in CDs at the bank, but if a bill for $5K is due on the 29th of the month and you do not get paid until the 5th business day of the next month, and there is only $1K in the checkbook, you do not have the cash to pay your bills on time. I will discuss more on the nuances of cash flow in Chapter Fifteen, Paying Your Daily Bills.

RECORD KEEPING

I examined more than a dozen books on the general topic of financial planning to prepare for this book. The one I found most useful was the 2008 edition of *The Road to Wealth: A Comprehensive Guide to Your Money* by Suzy Orman [1]. The book is quite detailed, and makes many points that are disarmingly simple and amazingly practical. I strongly suggest you purchase this book as the core reference source in your financial library. A variety of points made throughout this book, especially on topics with many rules and regulations, such as Funding Your Children's Education (Chapter Seventeen), Insurance (Chapter Eighteen), and Funding Retirement (Chapter Nineteen), rely on Ms. Orman's book as the main source.

There may be other books that are better, but you cannot read everything. In fact, this brings me to a point I have found very useful in my daily life; when you find what you are looking for, stop looking. I could have read every book ever written on financial planning, but I found the one that answered my questions and I stopped there (*see* Chapter Thirty-Nine on my observations about a physician as an executive).

It is mandatory to keep adequate records. The first category is legal documents that concern major events in your life. These should be kept in a safe deposit box (the fee for the safe deposit box should be deductible as an investment expense, consult your accountant) and includes things such as birth certificates, passports, deeds, power of attorney, etc.

Tax returns should be kept for at least six years. Records of your investments should be kept at least six years. Major financial documents should be kept for as long as applicable.

Good record keeping protects you. If you are audited by the IRS and your records are sloppy or non-existent you are in "for a world of hurt." There will be interest and there could be fines and penalties.

Honest disagreements can and do arise on things as simple as a monthly newspaper bill or credit card statement or things as major as a significant business dealing or investment. If you have everything in writing you have the best chance of protecting your interests. Keeping good records also enhances your credibility so that when there are gray or ambiguous situations you are more likely to receive the benefit of the doubt.

In the end, what records should be saved? I suggest everything.

WILL

I am not a legal, tax, or accounting expert so I have taken significant pains throughout this book to avoid giving anything but the most superficial of advice in these areas.

All adults should have a will. Your goal is to keep your estate out of probate, out of the courts. Consult your lawyer.

PERSONAL FINANCIAL STATEMENT

There are two general reasons to have a personal financial statement. The first is to accurately tabulate your assets and liabilities. There can be surprises. Sometimes people are worth more than they think, sometimes less. I recommend that the statement be updated every year. This way you can accurately monitor your financial progress, or possibly, lack of progress.

The second reason is banks require this when applying for a loan. A bank will not loan money without a detailing of your income, assets, and liabilities (In the now busted credit market, sub-prime mess, people secured "liars loans". As the name implies, applicants lied about income and assets and the banks made no effort to confirm the data. Lenders are now moving back towards more traditional lending practices. If history is a guide, they may well overshoot, causing a credit crunch). By having a prepared financial statement, you will save the time and drudgery of having to fill out a different statement for each bank. It will make your financial life easier.

Below is an outline of my personal financial statement. I have found this statement not only meets my needs but it includes almost all of the information that banks, or other lenders, routinely request (*see* Figure 1).

Name

Address

Phone Number

Fax Number

E-mail Address

Occupation   You   Spouse

                    Medical Doctor

                    Work Address

                    Work Phone

                    Work Fax #

                    Work E-mail

Duration of Employment

Social Security #

Marital Status

Children   #1   #2   etc.

Birthday

Social Security #

ANNUAL INCOME AND TAXES

See tax returns from specific years

RETIREMENT ACCOUNTS

IRA   _____

KEOUGH   _____

PENSION/PROFIT SHARING   _____

401 K   _____

TOTAL – RETIREMENT ACCOUNTS   _____

Fig. 1. Personal financial statement.

NON-RETIREMENT, CASH OR EQUIVALENTS

Checking Accounts   _____

Passbook Savings   _____

Stocks/Mutual Funds   _____

Bonds/Bond Funds   _____

U.S. Savings Bonds   _____

Certificates of Deposit   _____

Other   _____

TOTAL, NON-RETIREMENT CASH   _____

COLLECTIBLES

Art, Antiques   _____

Anything with   _____

Significant Value   _____

TOTAL COLLECTIBLES   _____

PERSONAL PROPERTY

Automobiles   _____

Boat   _____

(Value of Personal Property not included in calculation

 of Net Worth)

NON-RETIREMENT, NON-CASH

Partnerships

        A)   Limited   _____

        B)   LLC   _____

        C)   Other   _____

Closely-Held Companies   _____

Your Practice   _____

Practice-Associated Real Estate   _____

TOTAL, NON-RETIREMENT, NON-CASH   _____

Fig. 1. (*continued*)

REAL ESTATE

Home   _____

Vacation/Second Home   _____

Any Other Real Estate   _____

    A)   Farm   _____

    B)   Rental Property   _____

TOTAL, REAL ESTATE   _____

INSURANCE

Life   _____

Disability   _____

INDEBTEDNESS

	Monthly Payment	Loan Balance	(if Rental Property Income)
Property			
Lender			
Student Loan(s)			
Car Loan			
Investment Loan			
Any other Secured or			
Unsecured Note			

TOTAL INDEBTEDNESS   _____

*(Note – all credit card and similar accounts are routinely paid in full each month)

* – If you can say this.

TOTAL NET WORTH

RETIREMENT ACCOUNTS   _____

NON-RETIREMENT, CASH OR EQUIVALANTS   _____

NON-RETIREMENT, NON-CASH   _____

COLLECTIBLES   _____

REAL ESTATE   _____

    SUBTOTAL   _____

    DEBT   Subtract   (_____)

FINAL TOTAL

Fig. 1. (*continued*)

I start with basic employment and demographic data on me, and the children including birthdays, social security numbers, employers and duration of employment.

Banks require a detailing of all income. This includes direct income from your practice and, if married, your spouse's income, and indirect income such as interest, dividends, rental payments from real estate, etc. They also require knowledge of your taxes. The banks also want a listing of your monthly expenses. This includes amounts for debt service such as mortgage, car loan, investment loans, student loans, etc. and is detailed at the end of the statement. They also like a detailing of all other expenses including food, transportation, utility bills, vacations, and essentially everything. I find this onerous and would not take the time to list such things individually unless specifically requested. One number for your total monthly expenses is usually sufficient.

I have found the simplest way to supply the income and tax data is to provide the first two pages of last year's tax returns. If the bank asks for more data and details, just supply the entire return. Everything is there, it is accurate and is much easier than filling in all the blanks on the form. Remember, your time is worth $100–$200 an hour, don't waste it filling out forms.

Next, I list assets in retirement accounts. I then divide non-retirement assets into cash (or cash equivalents) and non-cash. The former includes liquid assets (*see* Chapter Fourteen), things that can be converted into cash very quickly, such a checking account, passbook savings, money market account, bonds, stock brokerage accounts and CDs.

I then list non-retirement, non-cash assets, things that are fairly illiquid. This would include limited partnerships, stocks of personal or closely held corporations, collectibles, art and anything else that has a significant value. When listing things such as collectibles, I have found it much easier to place an aggregate value on the collection rather than list each individually. Let me emphasize you must be very honest when placing a value on such assets. For example, you know to the penny what your checking account is worth or the value of your CDs, whereas many of the assets in this category are impossible to value precisely. Please be conservative. If the bank finds you placing wildly inflated, essentially bogus values on such assets they will be rightfully quite perturbed and you will lose credibility.

Being able to accurately value an asset is more than just an academic exercise. In the credit market mess that resulted in the collapse of many of the nations largest financial institutions in 2008, the presumed financial wizards of Wall Street were invested in all sorts of esoteric vehicles that were carried on their books at computer-estimated values (called Level 3 assets). When an attempt was made to mark the assets to market (determine the real value), they were essentially impossible to accurately value. No one will buy anything when they do not know what it is worth.

Remember also that although a collectible (and, in fact many assets) may be worth some particular amount, but after price negotiation and fees and commissions associated with a sale or auction, you will probably only realize 75–85% (at the absolute most) of this value. Then further subtract the taxes on the gains (if any) to estimate what you may realize.

I always list automobiles with an appropriate value, they are worth real money, but I never include the value of the autos in the final calculation of net worth. They only represent money in your pocket if sold, but then what will you drive?

I then list real estate, both my home and investment real estate, and life and disability insurance policies with policy numbers and amounts. The bank needs to know their investment is protected should something happen to you.

I then list in detail any indebtedness or other obligations or required payments with the amount of the monthly payment and the total loan amount.

At the end of the section on indebtedness, I then put the following line:

(**Note** – all credit cards and similar accounts are routinely paid in full every month).

If you can say this, your personal stock has just gone up ten points with anyone who reads your financial statement.

At the end I add up assets, subtract liabilities, and you have your net worth. The first time you do this it will take a good deal of time but the yearly updates rarely take much more than an hour.

SUMMARY OF CHAPTER TWELVE

- Keep a budget. It will save you money.
- Are you using something sufficiently to justify the expense?
- When you find what you are looking for, stop looking.
- Be a good record-keeper, it will protect you.
- All adults should have a will.
- Keep a personal financial statement and update it yearly.
- Be conservative when estimating the value of assets.
- You must be able to place a value on something to be able to buy or sell it.

REFERENCE

1. Orman S. The Road to Wealth: A Comprehensive Guide to Your Money. New York: Riverhead Books, 2008.

Chapter Thirteen

The Importance of Relationships: Goodwill, Friendship and Reciprocity

If you know people and have credibility with them, if you treat them nicely and with respect, they will not only give you the benefit of the doubt, but they will bend over backwards to help you. I am not referring to real personal friendships, rather I am talking about productive, long-term business acquaintances and relationships based on credibility.

. The following examples are anecdotal but illustrate my point.

I have lived in Columbia since 1982. In spite of being quite attentive to my personal financial affairs, 4 or 5 times I have bounced checks. All but once was my fault. These experiences bring up a personal observation. It has been my experience that front-line bank employees, such as tellers and the like, make more mistakes and provide more misinformation than you might think. If what you are told does not sound correct, question it.

The first time I bounced a check was after I had been in practice for about 10 years. I had done the vast majority of my banking and had my home loan, safe deposit box, and checking account at this bank since coming to town. One afternoon the executive vice-president of the bank called and said "Bob, your account is overdrawn. However, because we know you so well, we have paid the check (it was more than a thousand dollars) but would appreciate if you could come down this afternoon or tomorrow and take care of things." I did. This is service! I fully

R.M. Doroghazi, *The Physician's Guide to Investing,*
DOI 10.1007/978-1-60761-134-9_13,
© Humana Press, a part of Springer Science+Business Media, LLC 2005, 2009

appreciated it and realized what they did for me and told them so.

However, this bank was subsequently taken over by another bank, which was taken over by another bank that is now the largest in the country. About 10 years later, after all of the take-overs, and after this gentleman and the other officers I knew had left, I bounced another check. The treatment this time was much different. I only found out that I was overdrawn when I began to receive notices that a total of six checks were bounced – with a $20 fee for each = $120 in fees. I did not receive a personal phone call but was provided an 800 number to call to obtain more information.

To digress for a moment. I later read an article that this particular bank, and several others, made a tremendous amount of money on fees in this circumstance. Say there was $1,000 in your checking account and you wrote five checks – one for $1,100 and the other four for $20 each. They would post the $1,100 check first, thus making your account overdrawn, and then bounce the other checks so that they could generate over-drawn fees on each one. I consider such a practice preda-tory. Most banks post checks by number. The article also noted that these banks were willing to lose up to one-third of their accounts to generate more fees on the remainder.

Back to the subject. Was I wrong in my account being over-drawn? Absolutely. Did they have every legal right to do as they did? Of course. But as a practical matter, in hopes of generating some fees they lost the business of a good, and big, customer. Over the years I had taken out and paid back multiple loans which generated more than $100,000 in interest income for the bank. I ran thousands of dollars through my checking account monthly and I used other services of the bank. I went to the bank and had all of the fees removed from my account. Then over a reasonable period of time I took all of my business out of that bank. There are now about a dozen banks in Columbia, and they are one of only two with whom I do not have a deposit or an active account. If they had cut me just a little slack, as in the earlier episode, they would still have my business. In hopes of generating $120 of fees, they lost a big customer.

I have used the same insurance agent for 25 years – home, cars, watercraft, rental property, umbrella policy, everything. I just call him up, tell him what I need, and it's done. Several years ago, the statement on a policy for a rental property was not even mailed until the due date. As soon as I received the statement I called the agent. I mailed the check that day and he called the underwriters and told them it was their fault, not mine, that the payment would be late. This is service, and it is due to the credibility generated by long-term relationships.

One of the very basic messages of this book is to make every effort to minimize fees (*see* Chapter Twenty-Two). There are times though, when the extra personal service or superior advice is worth the additional cost. As all good physicians know, use your judgment.

It is not uncommon for things obtained on-line to be cheaper than those obtained in person at a bricks and mortar store. But if there are problems, and there are occasionally, then the small savings from ten transactions could be more than negated by the big problems with one transaction that is not adequately serviced. I prefer to deal with people. And if they know you, and you are a good customer who pays their bills on time, you will come out very far ahead in the long run.

Reciprocity is a basic rule in business. If a local hardware store has all of their accounts at one bank, the officers of that bank use that hardware store. In fact, whenever they go to the store they make sure the owner notices. The owner of an auto dealership has made generous financial contributions to a charity for many years. That charity will go to him or her first when they need to purchase a vehicle. A good number of people and firms with whom I do business subscribe to my newsletter (*see* www.thephysicianinvestor.com for a free, introductory four month subscription).

A physician is in business to see patients and make a living. If you are a reasonable physician and a reasonable person, you should expect that (other things being equal, such as you participating in their insurance plan or one of their family members are not already seeing another physician) the people you do business with reciprocate and see you when they need a physician. If you have purchased four Fords over the last ten years and the owner of the dealership chooses another physician instead of you, purchase your cars elsewhere. And the next time you see him at a party, be sure to mention how much you love your new Honda.

SUMMARY OF CHAPTER THIRTEEN

- If you are a long-term, solid customer who pays their bills on time, you have built up more credibility that you can imagine.
- Price is important, but service is important too.
- If you do business with someone, you should expect their business in return. If they do not reciprocate, take your business elsewhere.

Chapter Fourteen

Uncle George's Rule, or Why Cash is King: The Concept of Liquidity

My father and my Uncle George worked at General Steel Industries in Granite City, Illinois. The plant (formerly called the Commonwealth) was a foundry, making such things as castings, box car frames and tank hulls. My father was a foreman and Uncle George worked on the betatron, x-raying the castings for imperfections. When the plant closed in the early 1970s, my father, losing his job of 37 years, hired on at the School Board as a custodian, and continued to mow lawns for extra money. Uncle George, losing his job of 30 years, went to work at the May Co. (Famous Barr), in a clerical/stockroom position. My Uncle, always a little more free-spirited than my father, began to make the rounds of area pawn shops, buying or selling anything to make a few extra bucks.

Uncle George told me that whenever he had difficulty closing a deal, he would put the merchandise he wanted in one pile, put the cash he was willing to pay in another, and say simply to the owner of the pawn shop "which pile do you want"? Only once was he turned down. Although I do not frequent the pawn shops, I have used this principle in my personal financial dealings. "Which pile do you want"? People invariably take the money.

This little bit of family history is the introduction to a discussion of the concept of liquidity. Liquidity is the ease with which something can be sold. Cash is liquidity. As Yogi Berra (Berra

R.M. Doroghazi, *The Physician's Guide to Investing,*
DOI 10.1007/978-1-60761-134-9_14,
© Humana Press, a part of Springer Science+Business Media, LLC 2005, 2009

and Joe Garagiola are from "The Hill" in St. Louis. The Cardinals passed on Berra to sign Garagiola) says, it is just as good as money.

The weakness of cash is that over the long-term, i.e., years, its return is inferior to almost all asset classes. In an inflationary environment cash is continually losing purchasing power. But the shorter the time frame, the more powerful cash becomes. When talking now, cash is all-powerful. You can take it anywhere and buy anything. With cash, you can pick up things on the cheap. This is why Cash is King. It would appear possible to purchase something instantly with a credit card or check, but this can be quite difficult if the seller does not honor the credit card, or if you are over the credit limit, or if the check is not from a local institution. I am sure you have seen the sign "out of town checks not accepted". A passbook savings account can be converted to cash on demand. A cashier's check, money order or traveler's checks are cash. A checking account, if not overdrawn, can be converted to cash. A Certificate of Deposit (CD) can be converted to cash, but there is an interest penalty if redeemed before the date of maturity. Also note that converting a check, passbook or CD to cash presumes the bank has sufficient liquidity. Securities, such as the stocks or bonds of major corporations traded on the major exchanges, such as General Electric (GE) or International Business Machines (IBM), can be converted into cash within several business days. United States government debt, from savings bonds to Treasury notes, bills and bonds, are also highly liquid.

On an international scale, gold is highly liquid, it is money the world over (*see* Chapter Thirty-Eight). Diamonds are probably the easiest way to transport a concentrated amount of wealth. I discuss liquidity now for several reasons. Most physicians have no idea of the concept and why it is important. Their high salary (high cash flow), can disguise the fact that a good deal of their money is tied up in illiquid investments.

Secondly, in a crisis, the paramount issue is liquidity, quick access to your money. In the United States we have become terribly complacent. I suggest you read *The Black Swan* [1] and *Wealth War & Wisdom* [2] as a reminder that once or twice a century really catastrophic events do occur, almost always without warning (*see* Chapter Thirty-Nine).

We presumed our financial and banking system was so sophisticated and strong that the stories told by our grandparents about a "run on the bank" were just vestigial nightmares of the Great Depression, or the sort of thing that only happens in bananas republics. Considering the recent failures of Bear Stearns (BSC), Lehman Brothers (LEH), American International Group (AIG), Fannie Mae (FNM), Freddie Mac (FRE) and Washington Mutual (WM) requiring unprecedented government intervention to prevent the entire financial system from seizing up, and the possibility that the progressive decline of the once-mighty US dollar could at some time turn into a rout, it would be reasonable to discuss how to have quicker access to your money should the need arise.

It would not be uncommon for a physician in their mid-forty's to have built up $250K of equity in a $350K home, have $500K in retirement accounts, $75K in 529 or similar plans for the children's education, and a total of $20K in the check and money market accounts. This is certainly a good deal of wealth, but the liquidity is zilch. I think everyone is aware of the illiquidity of real estate. In this example, you may have a quarter million of equity in your home, but it is not one penny in your pocket. You cannot take your home to McDonalds to buy a hamburg. The money in the retirement and college accounts is also fairly illiquid. In a real pinch, the only money you could get your hands on quickly is the money in the checking and money market accounts.

One benefit of writing this book is that it has helped me with my personal investments. In preparing the first edition, I began to appreciate the importance of liquidity. As I neared retirement at the end of 2005, for a variety of reasons, not least of which is that my personality dictates that I have ready access to my money, I decided to sell the two illiquid positions in my portfolio.

Both were stock in local companies. One was a bank that kept a list of people interested in purchasing stock. The first person I called said yes and we closed in about one week (Note: Another reason I sold this position in 2006 was because of my concern that we could have a real estate/credit melt-down that would affect the banks, which did come to pass).

The second was a locally-based company with about three hundred shareholders, the perfect example of a closely-held corporation. They were and are a profitable business that even pays a small dividend. However, I was completely on my own in finding someone to purchase my shares. It took a year, and take my word, it and was a real pain in the rear. How do you know who is interested? Whether I was right or wrong, I finally sold at a loss just to get out.

Because of this experience, I have come to appreciate the function of "market makers", i.e., brokers, middle-men, dealers and agents. Although their fees often seem high, they do create a market and facilitate transactions. If you wish to sell your position in a public company trading millions of shares a day on the national exchanges, it can be done with the flick of a computer key or a phone call. If you wish to buy into a closely-held company or limited or general partnership of any kind, please recognize before you invest that it may be difficult, bordering on impossible, to liquidate your position at anything close to a reasonable approximation of its value in a time frame that fits your needs. This is just one more drawback of these kinds of investments, which I discuss in more detail in Chapter Thirty-Five.

The rougher the times, the greater the crisis, the more important the liquidity of your assets. In deflationary times, such as the Great Depression, debt becomes the number one issue. If you do not have sufficient cash or easily liquidated assets to service debt payments, you are in big trouble. You could even be forced into bankruptcy. Cash actually becomes the preferred investment, because it gains in purchasing power as prices fall.

Some years ago I did a treadmill on a retired professor with a German accent. I asked him why he came to this country. He was a German Jew, his father was a professional, and they lived a comfortable middle-class life. He said that one day "the Gestapo came to our home and my mother mouthed-off to them. When my father got home that evening and learned what she said, we packed our bags and were gone the next morning". They lost everything but the clothes on their backs – and their lives!! If they had a quantity of gold, jewelry or diamonds, their task of starting a new life in this country would have been far easier. Pray to God we are never in such dire straights.

The ultimate liquidity crisis results in a "run on the bank". This is exactly as the name implies. People lose confidence and become so concerned about their money that they literally "run to the bank" to withdraw their money before the bank goes under. The assets of the bank may be greater than their liabilities, but unless they have sufficient liquidity, i.e., cash or lines of credit from other banks, to meet the withdrawals, they could be forced to close. Another example of being solvent but illiquid is a farmer with $2M worth of land but insufficient cash to cover the $50K of notes that are due on his farm equipment.

Considering that over the last year multiple financial institutions have failed and more are expected to be relegated to history, I suggest you review your personal financial situation to insure you have sufficient liquidity to service debt and cover your personal needs. We seem to be at a time where CASH IS KING.

SUMMARY OF CHAPTER FOURTEEN

- Liquidity is the ease with which something can be sold.
- Cash is liquidity.
- Which pile do you want? People *always* take the cash.
- The shorter the time frame, the more powerful cash becomes.
- Cash loses value to inflation, but gains value during periods of deflation.
- Physicians may have significant assets but poor liquidity.
- In the current financial environment, it is essential to have a strong cash position.

REFERENCES

1. Taleb NN. The Black Swan: The Impact of the Highly Improbable. New York: Random House, 2007.
2. Biggs B. Wealth, War & Wisdom. Hoboken, NJ: John Wiley & Sons, 2008.

IV Attaining Specific Goals

Chapter Fifteen
Paying Daily Bills

The bottom line here is that you must have adequate funds available when bills are due. This is basic financial or money management, essentially the concept of cash flow.

One point before proceeding. If you are a physician making a six-figure income and are always having to scramble to come up with cash to pay daily bills, you are in big trouble. Contact a financial planner, banker or accountant immediately.

I have taken pains to keep this book focused on a physician's personal finances and investments, minimizing the discussion of the financial aspects of a physician's practice. However, I will make a point here. Over the years, my former associates displayed a great deal of cooperation and foresight and because of this, once a year we set our monthly salary. Thus, I knew that on the first day of each month I would receive a check for some specific amount. This makes paying bills so easy. More importantly, it makes you a better investor by knowing that you will have some particular amount of money available each month for income-averaging into your favorite mutual fund(s), mortgage payment(s) for your home or rental property or for other investments.

Contrast this to the situation where a physician receives a check on the fifth business day of each month dependent only upon the amount collected (not billed, but collected) in the proceeding month minus expenses. If you had a great month, took no days off and were very busy, the check could be for

R.M. Doroghazi, *The Physician's Guide to Investing*,
DOI 10.1007/978-1-60761-134-9_15,
© Humana Press, a part of Springer Science+Business Media, LLC 2005, 2009

thirty or forty thousand dollars, double or even more than your average check. But if you took a week off, and it was the beginning of the year, patients had not yet met their deductibles, you might even be negative. You return from your Florida vacation with great memories and a wonderful tan but owe three thousand dollars on the credit cards and must write a check to your practice to cover overhead – OUCH! If this describes your practice I suggest you and your associates be creative and determine some formula to even out the highs and lows, ideally being able to depend upon some minimum salary each month. It will make you a much more successful investor.

The first rule is to pay your bills in full and on time. If you have built up a nice record of being a prompt payer, people will "cut you some slack" when the occasional problem occurs. But if you are always slow in paying your bills, creditors have every right to not give you the benefit of the doubt.

Likewise, there is no reason to pay bills too early. The mortgage is due on the first and there is a penalty if paid after the 15th. Mail the check on the 10th. It is the 10th of the month and you receive the credit card bill due the 29th. Mail the check on the 22nd or 23rd. Renewal notices for magazines and journals often begin to arrive as much as four to six months before the subscription expires. Wait until the minimal time necessary to insure uninterrupted service to mail the check.

While money is in your possession it is working for you. When money is in someone else's possession, you do not receive interest. This is the essence of the phrase everyone has heard: "time is money." The goal is to keep the money in your pocket for as long as possible.

The total of all of your bills, including the mortgage payment, car payment, utility bills, credit card bills, etc. comes to $6,000 a month. By the timely payment of the bills, you are able to keep that six thousand dollars in your possession an extra ten days each month. This is a third of the month, taken over a year, this is a third of the year, or four months. Four months of standard investment return on six thousand dollars at 10% is $200.

You may be thinking: "All of this effort for $200. This guy needs to get a life." Writing a check on the 20th of the month as compared to the 10th of the month, what effort is this? It is such attention to detail magnified by all of your business transactions compounded over the course of many years that allows you to accumulate wealth and attain financial security. Details are important. The most successful people are the ones who pay the most attention to details. In finance, details represent money in your pocket.

Many banking transactions and bill paying can now be performed on-line. The records are as good or better and it saves stamps, envelopes and time in general. Likewise, make sure that your accounts and personal information are secure from identity theft (*see* Chapter Thirty-Seven). There is also the option of automatic bill paying, that is, giving someone such as your home mortgage lender direct access to your checking account to automatically withdraw the appropriate amount of money at the appropriate time to pay the bill. If you are a spendthrift and the only way to impose financial discipline is to never allow the money to touch your hands, then you may consider this. Otherwise, I prefer to pay my own bills on time and not allow others direct access to my money.

If I lose money on an investment because of a poor decision that was my fault I say so be it, try to learn from the loss and do better the next time. If I do not earn more money because I am not willing to see that extra patient or work that extra thirty minutes at the end of the day, that is my decision. But I will not lose a penny to paperwork. This is like seeing a $10 bill on the street and just bending over and picking it up. It is yours for the seemingly most miniscule of efforts.

SUMMARY OF CHAPTER FIFTEEN

- Attention to detail is money in your pocket.
- Pay all bills on time, but not too early.
- Time is money.
- Do not lose a penny to paperwork.

Chapter Sixteen
Your Home

COMMENTS FROM THE FIRST EDITION

One of my ex-partners favorite sayings was "even a blind pig can find an acorn sometimes". If there was one thing I nailed in the first edition (which went to press in early 2005) it was the unfolding housing bubble and sub-prime mortgage mess. To quote from the first edition:

1. "Professor Schiller of *Irrational Exuberance* [1], Alan Abelson of *Barron's*, and the author feel we are currently experiencing a real estate 'bubble'. ....Apparently in some 'hot' markets, when a home or property is listed the 'list' price serves as the 'base' price for the subsequent bidding war. Those who lack the perspective of time recognize that this is not the normal or routine state of affairs of any market . ... . Such things raise the concern of a 'blow-off' or 'speculative' top".

   I can take my own advice. I purchased a second condo at the Lake of the Ozarks in 2002 as a full-time rental. By 2005, I was worried about the market and considered selling. After a meeting of the owner's association in June, where the rules were changed to make renting more difficult, I immediately called the real estate agent to list the property. It sold quickly and I realized a nice gain (I sold too early, not too late, *see* Chapter Thirty).

2. I felt that lenders were irresponsible, and said "Today, collateral is often not required . ... . I feel banks are far too lenient in their lending practices. Part of this problem is that the bankers are often not lending their own money. They just

R.M. Doroghazi, *The Physician's Guide to Investing*,
DOI 10.1007/978-1-60761-134-9_16,
© Humana Press, a part of Springer Science+Business Media, LLC 2005, 2009

do the paperwork, sell the loan and take the fees. It is then someone else's problem if it cannot be repaid. Considering that a significant percentages of mortgages are sold to Fannie Mae (FNM) and Federal Home Loan Mortgage (FRE), the problem is actually now everyone's".

Fannie Mae, Freddie Mac and American International Group (AIG) failed and were taken over by the government. Bear Stearns (BSC), Lehman Brothers (LEH), Merrill Lynch (MER) and Wachovia (WB) are history, Washington Mutual (WM) and Countrywide Credit (CCR) have failed, and other banks and mortgage companies will join them.

3. Over the last several years, many people have lost their homes when their Adjustable Rate Mortgages (ARM) reset to a rate they could not afford. I said "One...caveat with an ARM: in the past it was not uncommon that the interest rate during the initial period was a 'teaser' rate, i.e., it is set slightly lower than it would otherwise be to 'tease' you to take the note".

The end result is that many people were teased into buying a home they could not afford and is now in foreclosure.

4. I said "To carry this concept of paying as little as possible on a loan to its illogical conclusion, consider an interest-only mortgage .... It would appear that both the borrower and the lender are assuming a terrible risk in such situations".

Hundreds of thousands of people have lost their homes to foreclosures and our banking system is imploding because of mortgage product that can only be considered insane.

5. I did not agree with the "standard teaching, almost gospel, that your home is your best investment".

The current real estate market, the worst since the Great Depression, with prices down almost 20% from the peak (and still dropping monthly), has completely destroyed the myth that real estate always goes up. All investments have risks.

CONTROL EGO

A physician's home may be a good investment for their heirs, but I contend it could be one of the poorest investments of a physician's life if the home is too expensive. There are many reasons for this. Chapter Four discusses the basic human failings of arrogance, ego, greed and envy. Chapter Twenty-One details the seductiveness and destructive power of debt. Chapter Three shows why compound interest is an investor's best friend. A home mortgage is compound interest in reverse, working against the borrower. Unless caution is exercised all of these factors have the potential of turning your place of residence into a life-long drain on your pocketbook.

Inability to control arrogance, ego, greed and envy can easily result in the purchase of a home that is far beyond what an impartial assessment of your financial situation would dictate. You may be a wonderfully skilled physician, possibly a specialist or even a sub-specialist. Prominent people, who can afford the best, demand to see only you. You are the best physician in town or your state or for that matter possibly anywhere. You must have a home that reflects this, that is commensurate with your status as a prominent physician. A humble nine or ten room 4,000 sq foot residence is not adequate. It is just not appropriate for such a prominent, important physician to live in a neighborhood next door to a bank vice president, or a two wage-earner family such as a nurse married to a college professor or a man whose family has owned a local clothing store for three generations.

Such a physician must live in an exclusive area where everyone is equally as prominent and as important, where the movers and shakers live. It is mandatory that such a physician own a million dollar, 10,000 sq foot home in the best neighborhood. The first place a physician can work on controlling arrogance, ego and envy, and thus achieving better control of their finances, is quite literally in the home.

Consider these practicalities. You own a million dollar home and for the sake of this discussion it is paid off. Your personal financial statement reads – home value – $1,000,000. The number may appear impressive on paper, but it is not one spendable penny in your pocket. Your family must live somewhere. The equity in a home, whether it is paid off or not, is just a number on paper.

It is, of course, possible to borrow against a home. Any bank would be delighted to extend a physician a home equity loan.

Home equity loans are unwise and dangerous. When I was growing up, home equity loans were called what they are; second mortgages, a term more descriptive of their oppressive nature.

I know a couple who purchased a home in 1982 with a $65 K mortgage. There was some serious family illness, but they also took out several large home equity loans for improvements and other things. Twenty six years later they now owe $95 K. As my friend says "there's something wrong with the picture here". That is what a second mortgage (aka home equity loan) will do to you. Your goal should be to pay your home off as quickly as possible rather than use it as a piggy bank or an ATM.

You may establish a home equity line of credit. This is exactly what it sounds like – a line of credit, i.e. – the bank has agreed in advance to loan up to some particular amount of money at predefined terms, backed up by the equity in your home. These do allow considerable financial flexibility. As this book goes to press, because of the credit crisis, some banks are freezing home equity lines of credit. Confirm that yours is still available before trying to use it.

I established a home equity line of credit some time ago and have used it three times. Several years ago we were involved in an automobile accident and our car was totaled. We needed a new car quickly but had only about one-half of the cash for the vehicle we hoped to purchase. I called the bank and because I had previously arranged the line of credit, a check was drawn up in less than thirty minutes. This saved me the hassle of applying for a car loan or selling an investment to raise cash. Being forced to liquidate an investment at an inopportune time can destroy otherwise well-laid plans.

Another example of when a home equity line of credit would be useful is when an opportunity arises with little or no notice and you do not have sufficient cash available to cover the purchase. You have been waiting for a particular collectible or antique. Auction catalogues for coins, stamps, baseball cards, autographs, etc., are often mailed only three to four weeks at most before the sale. Thus there is minimal notice. Or a dealer may call with a collectible you have been waiting for years to come on the market. You have twenty-four hours to make up your mind before it will be offered to someone else.

A friend and I had been looking for recreational property with a lake. When what we wanted finally came available, I took a home equity loan and paid it off over about six months as CDs matured and other money came in (i.e., I already "had" the money for the item, it was just not readily available at that moment). Opportunities such as this do not arise often and a home equity line of credit can allow you to take advantage of them. But remember, this must be used very sparingly and the situation must be very compelling, because you have just put your home on the line.

You could say it is possible to sell a home at anytime to realize the equity. In the real world, such as the current market, it is not that easy. If a buyer can truly afford a million dollar home, they are going to be a very successful, very particular person with specific tastes, desires, requirements and needs. Such buyers know exactly what they want and if a home does not meet these exact features, they will not buy it (unless the price has been discounted so significantly that they will consider it, essentially a distressed sale).The less expensive the home, the more marketable. The more expensive the home, the less marketable, a problem greatly magnified in a smaller community. There are very few buyers indeed at the million-dollar level. Remember also that you must pay a real estate commission unless the home is sold by the owner, something I would not suggest for the average physician (it is not as easy to adequately advertise and show a home as you might think). In the end, your dream home, the most amazing home on earth, worth a million dollars on paper, is really not worth a million dollars. In addition, if this is a forced sale, or the home is being sold into a weak market (such as now – ???), the amount received will be further compromised.

The following is a true story. A physician built a million dollar dream home. An additional two hundred thousand dollars was spent on furniture and another $100–200K on change orders because this or that just did not look quite right. After all, everything must be perfect in a dream home. In the end, he could not afford the home. The debt was just crushing. I later heard a perfect term to describe this situation – "golden hand-cuffs." It is both insightful and sublime.

Several years later (this was long before the housing bubble) the physician was forced to sell. Everyone wanted to look but there were no buyers. The home sat on the market for some time and finally sold for between sixty and seventy cents on the dollar. The physician not only lost all of his equity, but had to bring money to the table to complete the sale. He was forced to pay to sell his dream home! This is Pain with a capital P.

LIVE CLOSE TO WORK

I recommend you live as close to work as possible. I purchased my current home in February, 1987 through a closed bid process. An appraiser looked at the home and gave me his estimate of the value. He also said "Doc, you have to consider the intangible of how close this home is to the hospital (four and one-half minutes door-to-door). Twenty or thirty minutes every day for twenty years is a lot of time". It is some of the best advice I ever received, and I still consult this gentleman when I have a real estate question in his area of expertise.

If you work 12 hours a day, and sleep and basic toilette take 8 hours, you have only four hours of "marginal" time for every-thing else: meals, time with your children, exercising, reading, relaxing, everything. I believe buying a home with a 45 minute drive each way to work would be one of the worst strategic decisions of your life. One-third of your free time is completely wasted sitting in (frustratingly slow) traffic.

Instead of owning a big home with a big yard (which you hire someone else to maintain) in the suburbs, buy a smaller home or condo much closer to your work, and purchase a nice piece of recreational land within 1–2 hours drive where you go every other weekend. You will not only save on gas (energy *will* be an increasingly precious commodity) and depreciation of your car, but you will be happier because of the extra free time. If you live close enough to walk, you will also get in your exercise for the day.

DEALING WITH REAL ESTATE AGENTS

In the first edition, I proposed a somewhat whimsical, tongue-in-cheek example of what a real estate agent might say when you and your spouse are being shown a million dollar home. Just as it is a physician's job to care for patients, a real estate agent's job is to sell homes. The agent would say the same to potential buyers when selling your home. They could say, "Doctor, this is a very elegant home in a prestigious neighborhood. You better buy it now because it will sell quickly. We have three other people interested in this home. We think at least two of them will place a contract before the weekend. Look at that four-car garage. Isn't it heavenly? Now you can buy another Hummer. Creative financing (the folly of unconventional loans is now painfully obvious) is available for someone with your income. Your spouse will love the kitchen. This is in the best school district. The home is expensive, but it is worth it. This will be the best investment of your life. Somebody who works as hard as you deserves a home like this."

Now let me provide a real-life example of an exchange I had with an agent. In 2008, with home prices already off significantly and falling every month, a home in the neighborhood came on the market. I was interested, not only as an investment, but also so I could "control" who lived in the vicinity. The home was listed over the weekend. I contacted the agent on Tuesday to arrange to see the home on Thursday morning.

The reply: "Dr. Doroghazi. . .So far there has been a frenzy of activity, so if you find time in your schedule before Thursday, let me know".

My reply: "I am very surprised there has been such a frenzy of activity. Is the home already under contract? If so, I have no interest in seeing it. If it is sold by Thursday morning, then so be it. I have walked by several times on my daily walks, and have not seen anyone".

Within several hours the response came back "Considering our current (slow) market, I guess I got a little excited at the couple of showings we had in 24 hours and called it a frenzy. I'm sure that probably sounded a bit like a "real estate line" ".

Real estate agents play these sorts of games because they work. Remember, Jedi mind tricks only work on the weak mind, on droids and clones. Don't let this sort of jive (glib, deceptive or foolish talk, Webster's) fool you. Make it clear to the agent that it turns you off. As Sgt. Friday (Jack Webb) says in Dragnet "Just the facts, M'am".

In 1996, I decided to purchase a piece of recreational property at the Lake of the Ozarks. I talked to a local real estate friend, who referred me to one of the senior, most competent agents at the Lake. When I spoke with Nancy, I said (essentially) "I have every intention of making a purchase, just give me the facts, and I will make my own decision". She showed me 11 properties in one day, and I purchased one, which I still own. Tell the agent exactly what you want. If they persist with the smoke and mirrors routine, find another agent, because they clearly consider you "The Mark".

One last point: Real estate commissions are negotiable. If an agent tells you they are fixed and non-negotiable, that is not true. That does not mean you will receive a better rate, but it doesn't hurt to try, especially in the current market.

THE MORTGAGE

How much should you spend on a home? It is actually more instructive to begin with what should be avoided. I will start with an example of what may have been encountered with the irresponsible mortgage lending practices of 2005–2007, which allowed up to 33% (or even more) of your gross income to go toward mortgage payments. For ease of comparison, I presume throughout this book that our average physician makes $250 K per year and the interest rate on a loan is 7%.

Say you were unwise enough to borrow the limit and purchase a $1 M home with a 5% ($50 K) down payment. For a 30-year mortgage, this gives a monthly payment of about $6,500. Be sure to add the cost of homeowner's insurance, Private Mortgage Insurance (PMI) because you had less than a 20% down payment, and property taxes. You also may have other debt, such as auto or student loans, and you need money for other savings such as retirement and your children's education.

Even if it were possible to meet the monthly payment, consider the absolute amount of money. What if your income falls – more overhead because of increasing malpractice costs or more office help to complete paperwork, the federal and/or state government increase taxes, the economy worsens, physician re-imbursement continues to decline, you become ill, the payments for your employees' benefits continue to increase – then what was previously viewed as just a percentage of your income, is in absolute terms, a tremendous amount of money.

A mortgage payment of $6,500 for 12 months a year for 30 years = $2,340,000. After thirty years a million-dollar dream home costs 2.39 million dollars ($2,340,000 plus the $50,000 down payment). Ten years of your thirty years of practice just for mortgage payments. This does not include furnishings, maintenance and other expenses. The total cost is mind-boggling.

Here is my suggestion. The cost of a home should be such that the mortgage can be paid off by age 45. To accomplish this, there must be no pre-payment penalties on the mortgage. In fact, the physician investor should INSIST on no pre-payment penalties on all loans.

There is one situation that I do encourage you to purchase as much as you can afford. This concerns the amount of land around the home. I have spoken with several physicians who wished they had purchased more land around their home than they did originally or thought they could afford. This relates less to the investment aspects of the land and more to the ability to control the subsequent construction around the home. I have yet to hear a physician complain that they purchased too much land. If this were the case, you could just sell the land that appeared superfluous. Otherwise, purchase as much land around your home as you can afford (note I emphasize afford). It is not often that you can control your neighbors (or lack of neighbors).

I remember shaking my father's hand when he paid off the mortgage in 1959 (the home was purchased in 1956). If a foreman at a foundry can pay off their mortgage by age 42, surely a high-income physician can pay off their mortgage by age 45.

I paid off my mortgage when I was 41. Do not underestimate the feeling. It was spectacular. You and your family will always have a place to live. When the mortgage payments stop, which is similar to when your children have graduated from college and are self-sufficient, it is as if an armored car drops a bag of money on your doorstep each month, money that can be invested.

Now for the practical financial reasons of the early payoff of a home mortgage. A mortgage is compound interest in reverse, compound interest working against you, to the determinant of the borrower. A $312,500 home is purchased with a 20% down payment and a $250,000 mortgage at 7% interest. In my opinion, you cannot afford a home without a 20% down payment. Lenders agree and routinely require private mortgage insurance (PMI) with a down payment of less than 20% (*see* Chapter Eighteen).

Before moving on, let me say that several people have suggested my example of a $312,000 home is unrealistic. They note that the average home price in their area is significantly higher and/or the home they wish to purchase is significantly more expensive than my example. My response is that they must change their expectations, since it seems they cannot afford the average home in their area or the one they wish to buy.

Table 1 outlines the details of amortizing this mortgage over a period of ten, twenty, or thirty years. For merely $275 a month,

Table 1
$250,000 Mortgage Amortized Over Various Lengths of Time

	Monthly Payment	Principal/ interest	Principal paid in 10 years	Interest paid over life of loan
10 year payout	$2,902	$1,444/ $1,458	entire amount	$98,325
20 year payout	$1,938	$479/$1,458	$83,065	$215,179
30 year payout	$1,663	$204/$1,458	$35,496	$348,783

Data courtesy of Dan Scotten, Boone County National Bank, Columbia, MO.

two extra hours of work a month, 4 minutes a day, you can pay off the mortgage in 20 years rather than 30, saving more than $133,000 in interest alone. The difference in interest paid is money in your pocket. Also, remember to add ten percent per year to the interest saved because this is money available to invest. The final results are astounding.

THE EARLY PAYOFF OF A HOME MORTGAGE CAN BE THE EQUIVALENT OF AN ENTIRE LIFETIME OF SUCCESSFUL INVESTING

Please do not be concerned about losing the tax deduction on the interest. A dollar is spent on interest to save 35 or 40 cents on taxes. That is a loss of 60–65% on every dollar of interest paid. I do not consider this to be particularly astute investing. This mind-set underscores our country's infatuation with debt, which is encouraged by the government through the taxation of profits, thus discouraging investment, and the granting of deductions for interest payments, thus encouraging debt.

Because it appears that the two decade bull market in bonds is over and in the long term interest rates are headed higher, I strongly recommend you take a fixed-rate mortgage (with no pre-payment penalties) as compared to an adjustable-rate mortgage (ARM) even though the initial "teaser" rates on the latter may be lower. One exception would be if there were a good chance you will be moving in three to five years. For example, you are just beginning your training with every expectation that when finished you will be moving back to your hometown to join your father in practice. An ARM, or a balloon note, which does not adjust during the period that you plan to own the home would probably be a better choice.

Let me make a comment about reverse mortgages. It is not uncommon for the elderly, especially if they are from a more humble background, to have a good deal, or even all, of their wealth tied up in their homes. Like a farmer, they may be real estate rich but cash poor. Rather than discuss the pros and cons in detail, I will make the same comment I make about borrowing from your retirement account: As a gut feeling, I just do not like the concept. My recommendation: Sell the home to a relative (or an investor), sign a lease for the appropriate duration (with a clause that if you must go to a care facility/nursing home you are out of the lease), invest the money, and pay the rent from the return on your investment. This should be a slam-dunk for any investor – a physician, a solid renter, with a long-term lease.

OTHER IMPORTANT ISSUES

Please note that the above discussion is not to discourage you from purchasing a home. To the contrary, home ownership is part of the American dream and should be one of your basic lifetime goals. Rather it is to discourage you from purchasing a home that is too expensive with financing that is disadvantageous to the borrower. Instead of paying someone else rent, you are accumulating equity in your own home. If the home is held long enough there is also a good chance it will appreciate in value. One of the basic goals of an adult should be the purchase of a home that is financially within their budget at the earliest reasonable time.

There are several other points to remember when purchasing your first home. Establishing a new household requires thousands of dollars in addition to the mortgage, insurance and real estate taxes. There is furniture, kitchen utensils, yard equipment, and these cost thousands of dollars. Never borrow money to buy furniture (except appliances). Allow the rooms to sit vacant until there are sufficient funds to pay cash for the furniture (Do not let vacant rooms embarrass you. People who are careful with their money will realize you are careful with your money. I did not have all of the rooms of my home furnished until I had been in practice 7 years). Purchase quality. It is a terrible waste of resources to buy furniture merely to fill a room and then three or four years later buy all new furniture. Cheap furniture looks cheap and used cheap furniture has almost no resale value.

You must resist the temptation to buy a home as large as your parents or your senior associates. Remember these people worked twenty or thirty years to get where they are. A thirty-year-old should not expect to have as much as a sixty-year-old. Patience, patience, patience.

The majority of the above general comments regarding the purchase of a stand-alone home apply to the purchase of a condominium or townhouse as you principal residence. The concept of cooperatives is found in some large metropolitan areas, especially New York City. In co-ops, a corporation owns the building and then you purchase a share of the corporation. I admit I have no personal experience at all with a co-op, but I just do not like the idea of other people having so much say in my personal residence.

It is essential to limit the number of times you move. The average American family will have three homes over their adult lifetime. This fits nicely with the following scenario. Purchase your first home when you begin residency or fellowship. I dearly hope the down payment will not be borrowed from your parents. If you do not have the money for a 20% or more down payment, it means you cannot afford the home. More importantly, you are now in your late 20s or early 30s, and probably married. You are an educated adult, a medical doctor, a trained professional, a respected and privileged member of our society. It is time to start paying your own way in life. No one will develop an adequate sense of self-reliance if they must keep going to their parents for money. When will it ever end? The answer is never! In their book *The Millionaire Next Door* [2], Stanley and Danko have a pithy and medically-appropriate term for the above situation, which they refer to as "economic outpatient care (EOC)."

A twenty-eight-year-old has been a steelworker or teamster for ten years. They lived with their parents for several years after high school graduation and then rented a one bedroom apartment. They drive a seven-year-old car with 83,000 miles and have finally saved twenty-four thousand dollars for the 20% down payment on a $120,000 home. A thirty-one-year-old medical or surgical sub-specialty Fellow is loaned or given fifty thousand dollars by their parents for the down payment on a $240,000 home. Who is to be more proud of their achievement?

It may be possible to borrow the down payment for your home from your retirement savings. It is extremely unlikely that a physician at this time in their life will have any significant retirement savings but it could apply to your spouse. You must consult the plan administrator or your accountant to see if this option is available. My completely unscientific but visceral opinion is not to pursue this. Borrowing from yourself just does not seem logical. If things go badly I suppose you could stand in front of a mirror and berate the first person you see. I mention this for sake of completeness as this option is generally noted in books on financial planning.

Unless you practice in the same area where you performed your training, you will purchase your second home at the time you enter practice. Four to seven years later, after becoming a partner, you should be in a solid financial position and can purchase your final home.

A nice investment possibility is to keep the previous home as an investment. You know the area well and no one knows the home better. Staying in the area also makes it easy to keep a close watch on the property. Consider this possibility if the rent covers or nearly covers the mortgage. There is already a 6% gain by saving the real estate commission. On a $160 K home, this is a savings of almost $10 K. This all presumes that you have saved the 20% down payment for the next home. Looking back, I wish that I had done this. It now seems so easy and so obvious. I moved into my current home in 1987. If I had kept the previous home, the mortgage would have been paid off long ago and the home would be generating at least $1,500 a month in rental income. Four or five such investments could almost fund your retirement.

It is mandatory to resist the urge to move too often (this also applies to changing jobs too often, *see* Chapter Thirty-Nine). Choose your home wisely and stay there. With every move there are commissions and fees, not to mention the inevitable remodeling and other expenses such as new furniture. Do not be diverted from your ultimate goal, which is to have your home paid off as early as possible, hopefully by age 45. Each move delays this goal by two years or more.

Before concluding, let me discuss remodeling and additions. The most desirable way to pay for these is with cash. If you cannot pay cash, then consider you cannot afford the addition. If you do borrow, I suggest the second mortgage be amortized over a very short period of time, such as just one or two years. Remember, any such borrowing just delays one of the most important financial goals of your lifetime, that is, paying off your mortgage as early as possible.

When planning a major addition or remodeling, it is important to keep in mind not only what you like but what other people need and desire and find tasteful since all homes, sooner (often sooner than you think or plan) or later must be sold. The first point is that in only very rare circumstances will there be a dollar for dollar increase in the resale value of the home, a problem further accentuated by the current bear market in real estate. A more reasonable estimate is that a nicely-planned remodeling or addition may realize 50–75% of the cost as an increase in the resale value of the home.

Poorly planned additions or remodeling have the capacity to actually decrease the value of a home. Be sure that the workmanship and materials are as good as or better than the quality of the rest of your home. A cheap addition will look cheap. The addition must also fit both the style of your home and the neighborhood. If you live in a neighborhood built before the Great War, do not put on an addition that looks like a tribute to pop art. Not only will this decrease the value of your home, but you will also have some perturbed and upset neighbors.

Always use a general contractor. There are many reasons why not to try to supervise this yourself. I cannot imagine a physician has sufficient expertise to accomplish this. There are always codes that must be met and whenever there is structural work it is essential to know such things as if the wall being removed or moved is weight-bearing. As a practical matter, a physician has no "pull or influence" with the subcontractors. Your project will always be last on their list, to be done at their convenience and on their timetable, not yours. This is not an idle comment: a friend's addition sat unfinished for months while the contractors were off elsewhere.

SUMMARY OF CHAPTER SIXTEEN

- Owning your own home is part of the American Dream.
- The more expensive a home, the poorer the investment.
- Control ego when buying a home.
- Call a home equity loan what it is: a second mortgage.
- Real estate is illiquid.
- Live as close to work as possible.
- Real estate commissions are negotiable.
- If you do not have a 20% down payment that you have saved, you cannot afford a home.
- Take a ten (or at most fifteen) year, fixed-rate mortgage.
- Avoid a reverse mortgage.
- Own your home by age 45.
- Mortgages (and all loans) should always be considered in terms of the absolute amount of money.
- Each move delays your ultimate goal of owning your home free of a mortgage.
- Do not look upon your home as a piggy bank or ATM.
- Consider a home equity loan or line of credit only under very restricted circumstances.
- Insist on no pre-payment penalties.
- Avoid "creative financing."
- **The early payoff of a home can be the equivalent of a lifetime of successful investing**.
- Pay cash for remodeling or additions.
- A poorly planned addition can decrease the value of a home.

REFERENCES

1. Shiller R J. Irrational Exuberance. Princeton, NJ: Princeton University Press, 2000.
2. Stanley T J, Danko W D. The Millionaire Next Door: The Surprising Secrets of America's Wealthy. Marietta, GA: Longstreet Press, 1996.

Chapter Seventeen
Funding Your Children's Education

I feel the best and most desirable way to fund your children's education is for your children to work hard, save their money, and pay for as much of their own education as possible. The greater the contribution they make to their own education and to supporting themselves in life, the greater their sense of appreciation for what they have achieved. I paid my own way through college and medical school so it can be done.

However, considering that the total annual cost at a public four year college is about $16,000 and a private college or university is double that, and possibly the additional cost of graduate or professional school of another $100K or more, it is unlikely that even the most gifted, hard-working and thrifty young man or woman will be able to completely pay their own way.

If you do wish to pay all of your children's educational expenses, encourage them to pay their own living expenses. Another option would be to make it the children's responsibility to provide their own spending money when they turn 16 and can thus have a part-time job, and that they are responsible for some percentage of their educational expenses – such as a quarter or a third – after scholarships, but before loans and your contributions. They could also be responsible for a percentage of the down payment and upkeep, including insurance, of the car.

Children can earn money before they are sixteen. They can mow lawns, wash cars, have a paper route, do any sort of

R.M. Doroghazi, *The Physician's Guide to Investing,*
DOI 10.1007/978-1-60761-134-9_17,
© Humana Press, a part of Springer Science+Business Media, LLC 2005, 2009

errand, baby-sit (boys can baby-sit), or as several of my friends did, perform basic agricultural jobs such as hoe beans or canta-loupes. After turning sixteen, they can have after-school and weekend jobs. I worked between 30 and 38 hours a week at Graham's Book Store in Granite City during my junior and senior years in high school. There are the summers between college and many students also work during the college year.

(Because of liability issues, many people are turning to pro-fessional services and are increasingly hesitant to hire kids to mow their lawns. Bright, hard-working people from all over the world who wanted to get ahead used to come to the United States. If the system continues to stifle initiative, they will just go somewhere else).

FINANCIAL AID

Approximately two-thirds of college students receive finan-cial aid as grants, scholarships or loans. Thus assistance is available for the majority of students. Aid is available from almost every level of government, from the schools, private and public companies, institutions, fraternal and charitable organizations, foundations, and individuals. The unifying fac-tor for obtaining whatever aid is available appears to be persis-tence in pursuing all options.

Because of the credit crunch, more and more commercial banks are exiting the student loan business, and those that are still lending are often charging a higher rate of interest, more fees, and requiring a co-signer on the note (NEVER FORGET: You co-sign a note, you are liable). Even Sallie Mae (SLM, www.salliemae.com), the government-sponsored enterprise, is not immune to the problems.

The standard financial aid formula assumes that 5.6% of the parent's assets and annual income, excluding money in retire-ment accounts or representing equity in a home, may be spent to pay college expenses. This same formula assumes approxi-mately one-third, 35%, of the money held in the child's name can be used for college expenses.

The search for information on financial aid may begin at anytime, but the general applications for aid from the schools directly, the state, or private organizations, is usually in the fall of the year prior to beginning college.

As soon as possible after January 1st, but not before, in the year the child will attend college, the student may submit the Free Application for Federal Student Aid (FAFSA). Federal aid is awarded on a first-come, first-served basis so it is essential to submit all data and applications at the earliest possible time. This application will be used to determine eligibility for Pell and Supplemental Educational Opportunity Grants (SEOG), and loans such as Perkins Loans, Stafford Loans, Plus Loans and other federal and private loans. Pursue all reasonable options. Persistence is the key.

If your child is extremely bright, or has a gift or special talent in sports, music, the theater, or in fact, almost any extra-circular activity, significant, and sometimes even full, financial aid is available. Many colleges and universities often provide a significant discount or even full tuition if the parent is employed at or on the faculty of the school.

Approximately one-third of students do not qualify for any financial aid. If you make our average physician's salary of $250K per year and have been thrifty and invested wisely, you may join me as one of the privileged few to pay "full boat" tuition and fees.

Two additional factors must be considered in planning and saving for your children's college education. It has been standard to assume an undergraduate period of four years. However, barely one-third of first-time freshmen entering a four-year bachelor's program complete their degree within four years. Not surprisingly, the best schools have the highest four-year graduation rate.

There are factors that prolong the time in college, such as switching majors, taking a double major, transferring schools, or inability to enroll in a required course. Both of my boys finished in four years, but in my otherwise limited experience, a prolonged time in college is usually due to factors that *are* directly under the student's control, i.e., the student did not plan well or work as hard as they could have. Many schools are also increasing the number of requirements for graduation, thus necessitating more time in school. A good incentive to help your child remain focused on graduating in four years is to give them the responsibility of paying a higher percentage, or even all of their expenses – educational, living, rent, car, etc. – should their undergraduate education extend beyond the traditional four years (not including, of course, legitimate factors truly beyond their control).

For many years the cost of higher education has considerably outpaced the general increase in the cost of living in the United States. What seems like a grand and princely sum now will probably be inadequate in ten or fifteen years. Plan accordingly.

Every college and university has their own website. Just a few of the websites that can provide additional information include:

www.ed.gov
www.fastweb.com
www.simpletuition.com
www.nicep.com
http://www.nslds.ed.gov

Although this may sound elitist, I believe it is one of the ten best pieces of advice in this book: Send your children to the best school you can afford. It is worth every penny, and more. This is one of the real payoffs of working so hard. You will never, ever, be sorry that your children received the best education money can buy.

There are reasons besides the obvious superior education. Your child will make more and better contacts that will serve them well in both their professional and personal lives. And going to the best schools is something that can never be taken away from you. If you graduate with honors from one of the 10 best medical schools in the country and train at the best program in the world, and for personal reasons choose to settle in a small Midwestern town while someone who did not even apply to such programs because they knew they would never be accepted ends up in NYC or Boston or San Francisco, you, and they, will always know that when the competition was heads up, you came out on top.

SPECIFIC TAX-ADVANTAGED OPTIONS TO SAVE FOR YOUR CHILDREN'S EDUCATION

I said that Chapter Twelve (Documents Required for Financial Security) was the most boring. This topic is the most daunting, almost mind-boggling in its complexity. There are scores of issues to consider, and for each there are tax ramifications, a variety of nuances, the effect and inter-relation of one option on the other, the almost yearly changes in the rules, and the various eligibility requirements, qualifications, and exclusions. It is OK to feel a little overwhelmed when studying this topic. I believe I am relatively intelligent, but I must admit that at first I felt like a dumb rat in a really big maze. Before you put your first dollar into one of these plans or accounts, which is ideally before your child reaches their first birthday (so that compound interest can do as much of the heavy lifting as possible), it is *absolutely mandatory* to seek the assistance and advice of a financial planner, wealth advisor, or accountant, someone who is really expert on this subject. And before you see them, you must do your homework so that, with their advice, *you* can make an intelligent decision.

Excellent sources of information to assist you in saving for your children's education are Joseph Hurley's website www.savingforcollege.com. and his book *The Best Way to Save for College: Complete Guide to 529 Plans* [1]. Everyone gives Hurley's work their strongest recommendation.

These are the options available.

SERIES EE/E OR SERIES I U.S. SAVINGS BONDS

Do not overlook this option. Savings bonds are easy to understand. They are liquid, and are backed by the full-faith-and-credit of the U. S. Government. Bonds are available in denominations as small as $50 with all levels of increments up to $10,000. Series EE/E bonds are issued at half face value, the Series I bonds are issued at 100% face value.

The principle advantages of Savings Bonds are that the interest is not taxed until the bond is redeemed, and it is exempt from state and local, but not federal, taxes. This compares to a passbook savings account or CD, where the interest is taxed as it is received. There are also other factors to consider, including that the tax benefits may be limited by income and other conditions may apply.

Interest on savings bonds compounds twice a year, on May 1st and November 1st. The interest paid on Series EE/E bonds depends on when they were purchased. The interest on Series I bonds is indexed to inflation (I believe the government's official numbers significantly underestimate the true rate of inflation. This is just one more reason why). Since time is money, the best time to redeem a Savings Bond is the day after the interest is posted.

Savings Bonds may not be particularly glamorous but they can form a part of the savings for your children's education. The main weakness is that over the long term, even those indexed to inflation will not maintain their purchasing power.

UNIFORM GIFT TO MINORS (UGMA)/UNIFORM TRANSFER TO MINORS (UTMA)

The UGMA is the principal method I used to save for my sons' education. It was the easiest and best option available in the mid-to-late 1980s when I began putting money away for them. It is simple and does not require the advice of a professional.

The money is an irrevocable gift to the child, although the parent remains the custodian and thus supervises the investment of the money, until the child reaches the age of majority, which is eighteen to twenty-one years old, depending upon the state.

The principle advantage is that the money is taxed at a different marginal rate than the parents. Regardless of the child's age, the first $850 per year of unearned income is exempt from tax, and the next $850 is taxed at the minor's rate. If the unearned income is above $1,700 per year, if the child is younger than 18, the excess is taxed at the parent's rate, if they are above 18, it is taxed at their rate (remember that tax laws change frequently).

The UTMA is similar to the UGMA but the custodian can postpone the final distribution of the funds until the child reaches the age of 25. This variant may be advantageous if your child waits several years after high school before attending college or if they plan to attend graduate or professional school.

There are two significant shortcomings of the UGMA and the UTMA. First is that the gift is irrevocable. When the child reaches the age of majority (UGMA) or 25 (UTMA), the money is theirs, with no strings attached. If your child is destined to be a productive member of society, they will presumably use the money for continuing their education or otherwise wisely and appropriately. If your child should turn out to your disappointment, the money is theirs, to potentially waste as they see fit.

The other significant drawback of these accounts is that because the money is in the child's name, colleges expect them to use 35% of the assets per year, as compared to 5.6% of the parent's assets, decreasing their chances of qualifying for financial aid.

COVERDELL EDUCATIONAL SAVINGS ACCOUNT

Previously known as an Educational IRA, this allows a yearly non-deductible contribution of $2,000 for each child under 18. Suze Orman feels this should probably be your first choice to fund your children's education. She notes, however, that unless Congress extends them, some of the advantages of this program will expire in 2011. Unfortunately, as with so many of these options, eligibility is phased out at higher Modified Adjusted Gross Income (MAGI).

ROTH IRA

This is an excellent way to save for college that offers some features even more favorable than the Coverdell Account. Again though, eligibility is phased out in the income range of most physicians.

STUDENT LOAN INTEREST DEDUCTION

It is possible to deduct up to $2,500 annually of the interest paid on student loans, but the benefits are limited by income. For more on student loans, *see* http://studentaid.ed.gov/.

REPAYING STUDENT LOANS

It is often possible to delay the repayment of the principal and/or interest on student loans while you continue further schooling and training. Contact the lender, the holder of the note, for details and for the appropriate paperwork. Consider a deferment if it is advantageous for you. It may also be possible to consolidate your student loans. Again, consider this if it is advantageous to you, especially if you can refinance a variable-rate note into one with a fixed-rate.

Likewise, when it comes time to repay, you must pay. Some people consider student loans to somehow be different than other loans. They are not. You were leant money in good faith and it must be repaid. Wages can be garnished, you may be sued, and it will affect your credit rating if a student loan is not repaid. Even filing bankruptcy will not dismiss a student loan. When you repay your student loan you are making money available for other students to continue their education just as this money allowed you to continue your education.

STUDENT LOAN FORGIVENESS

This advice is for both practicing physicians and their children. The average medical student graduates with $140K of debt. When entering practice (or even if already in practice) make every effort to have your employer, or the group you are joining, or the hospital(s) at which you will practice, help with your student loans.

There is a physician shortage, and it will worsen. This allows the physician entering practice considerable leverage, especially if the hospital or group you are joining needs your specific services. There is an excellent chance they will assist with some percentage of your student loans for each year that you practice.

This work is devoted to a physician's personal investments and finances, not to the finances or economics of the practice of medicine. However, I will make one comment. If you are in the private practice of medicine, avoid being an employee of a hospital. On the surface it may appear appealing, but in the end it is rarely advantageous.

TAX DEDUCTION

It is possible for parents to deduct up to $4,000 of higher education expenses, but as with almost everything else, it is phased out at higher adjusted gross income.

HOPE SCHOLARSHIP (TAX CREDIT) AND LIFETIME LEARNING CREDIT

A tax credit is different than a tax deduction. A charitable gift is an example of a tax deduction. A deduction decreases your taxable income. For example: a charitable gift of $1,000 to the Boy Scouts decreases your taxable income by $1,000, thus saving approximately 40% of the deduction, depending on federal, state, and local tax rates. A tax credit is much more valuable. A tax credit does not decrease your taxable income, it decreases your taxes. A tax credit of $1,000 decreases your taxes by $1,000, essentially $1.00 of tax credit = $1.00 of savings.

With the Hope Scholarship, you can deduct as much as $1,650 a year from your taxes for every college freshman and sophomore in your family. With the Lifetime Learning Credit, you can deduct 20% of the first $10,000 paid for out-of-pocket qualified expenses up to a maximum credit of $2,000 per family per year. This credit is for students in their junior year and beyond.

Of course, benefits for both of these credits phase out at higher parental income.

SECTION 529 PLANS

Many advisors consider these plans the premier option of the tax-advantaged vehicles to save for a child's education. I will outline what I feel are the advantages and disadvantages of the 529 Plans.

There are two basic types of 529 Savings Plans.

COLLEGE SAVINGS PLANS

These state-run plans let you invest in a tax-deferred account to save for tuition *and* other legitimate college expenses such as room, board, and fees. Each state has their own 529 Plan and the details vary state by state.

ADVANTAGES OF STATE-SPONSORED 529 PLANS

1. EVERYONE IS ELIGIBLE. A major drawback of almost all of the other options is that they are limited by income.
2. The tax advantages are impressive. The money deposited is post-federal tax (similar to a Roth IRA). The earnings grow tax-free and all of the money withdrawn that is used for higher education expenses is federal tax-free. This tax treatment was set to expire in 2010, but Congress has acted to make it permanent.
3. Many states follow the federal tax-free treatment. As an incentive to encourage residents to use their home state plans, some provide further tax advantages.
4. It is possible to invest in other states' plans if you feel it is superior, but you must weigh this against the loss of the in-state breaks just mentioned.
5. The contribution limits are very high, in some cases more than $250,000 for a single beneficiary. This amount should fund your child's entire undergraduate education, even at the most expensive private schools. This should also be sufficient to fund at least some or possibly all of a postgraduate or professional education.
6. The plans are extremely flexible. The beneficiary can be changed. Suppose you have saved an equal amount for

two children. One child is lazy and barely finished high school. The other child is a star. The money can be transferred from one child to the other child's account.

7. The donor maintains control, as compared to the UGMA and UTMA.
8. As compared to pre-paid tuition plans (see below), the full value can be used at any accredited college of university in the country (and some foreign schools).
9. There are no age restrictions. If you would like to pursue further education, such as returning to school for an MBA or a JD, you may establish a plan for yourself.
10. The money may be used for any qualified higher educational expense, including room, board, books, and graduate education, as compared to the pre-paid plans, which can be used only for under-grad tuition and fees.
11. Because the money is in your name, it has much less of a detrimental effect on your child's eligibility to qualify for and receive financial aid. Only 5.6% of the parent's assets are considered available to be spent per year on college tuition, as compared to 35% of assets in the child's name.

Overall, the advantages of these plans are impressive and it is easy to see why they are so popular.

MY RESERVATIONS REGARDING 529 PLANS

1. These plans are very complex. I have listed only a fraction of the pros and cons. The rules vary from state to state. Expert advice is mandatory. I devote Chapter Nine and many further discussions throughout this book to the importance of understanding your investments.
2. Impartial advice is essential. If you receive advice from a broker/agent who recommends the options which generate commissions for them, there are sure to be fees that would otherwise be avoided.
3. Because this is a gift, it must comply with all gift tax rules. These should be detailed in the general rules and guidelines you will receive. If a grandparent is making a gift to a

grandchild, it must be within the guidelines of the Generation Skipping Taxes.

4. The state controls the investment, so it will lean far toward the risk-averse options such as cash and fixed-income. Over a long period of time, especially one of high inflation, your money will lose purchasing power.

5. When the government makes the rules, they can be changed at any time. This is my principal concern, not only here, but as it relates to almost all of your investments.

Let me provide examples of when the government has changed the rules to the detriment of the citizens. In the 1980s, everyone, regardless of income, could contribute to an IRA. It was an excellent way to save for retirement. So many restrictions have been added that the average physician no longer qualifies (*see* Chapter Nineteen, Funding Retirement).

Because money will be in these plans for many years, it is possible that economic or political conditions could change so significantly that the rules could be changed even on money already invested in the plans. The money would not be "grandfathered" but would be subjected to whatever changes were enacted.

Before 1933, gold circulated freely in the United States and the U.S. dollar was "as good as gold." (*see* Chapter Thirty-Three). Any citizen could exchange paper money at the Treasury for specie. In March of 1933, in the depths of the financial crisis of the Great Depression, among Roosevelt's first actions after taking office were to close the banks and call in the gold. The United States effectively repudiated the gold standard.

Also during the Depression the highest marginal income tax rate was raised to 90%. It is conceivable that should an economic crisis arise, the government could be sufficiently hard-pressed for revenues from any source that the current tax advantages of the 529 Plans could be significantly changed. Or the government could mandate that 529 Plans, or for that matter, any type of tax-deferred account (such as your retirement account), place some percentage of its assets in Treasury bonds to help finance the deficit.

In 1964 the United States repudiated the silver standard. Prior to that time, dimes, quarters, half-dollars, and dollars were silver and one-dollar bills were "Silver Certificates." Now our coins are base metal with minimal intrinsic value.

In the summer and fall of 2008, the government has shown it will intervene in the markets whenever it sees fit. The government will do whatever it wants whenever it wants, and if it hurts you that is too bad. Ronald Reagan said that the nine most dangerous words in the English language are "I'm from the government and I'm here to help".

6. As always, be aware of fees. There is no reason to purchase a 529 Plan through a broker or salesman because there will be fees. Let me also take this opportunity to again remind you there is never any reason to buy any mutual fund with a load.

PREPAID TUITION PLANS

These plans allow you to lock in future tuition costs at today's levels. The money is invested either as a lump sum or a series of payments (i.e. amortized) and the state guarantees to cover a specific number of tuition credits at a state school.

I would recommend the 529 Plan as compared to these plans because of greater flexibility. The weaknesses of Prepaid Tuition Plans in comparison to the 529 Plans include:

1. The money is invested by the state with the goal that the anticipated rate of return will match the projected tuition costs at the state's schools. Thus the performance often lags what you may earn in other investment vehicles.
2. If your child decides on an out-of-state public school or a private school, not only will the money invariably be inadequate to cover costs, but some plans do not allow the full benefit to be transferred.
3. These plans cover tuition. Other costs, which are significant, such as room, board, books, etc. are not covered.
4. Almost all programs require either the account owner or the beneficiary to meet state residency requirements.

There is a variant of these prepaid tuition plans for private colleges, known as the Independent 529 Plan, sponsored by about 250 private schools known as the consortium. This plan offers the same federal tax benefits as the state-sponsored 529 Plans. The program manager is TIAA-CREF and there are no fees (*see* www.independent529plan.com).

PAY FROM YOUR OWN FUNDS

The above discussion of all the advantages of the various options not withstanding, I believe you should keep some of the money for your children's education in your personal portfolio earmarked for this purpose.

1. There is no doubt who controls the funds.
2. You maintain flexibility by not having the funds tied up.
3. Should the government change the rules for any plan, it would have no effect on funds saved in this way. This is similar to my advice given elsewhere on the importance of having savings for retirement outside of defined retirement plans (see Chapter Nineteen).
4. The decrease in the tax rate on dividends and capital gains to 15% has made this option a little more competitive (Although remember that tax laws change frequently).
5. Sometimes one becomes so concerned, almost mesmerized, with potential tax advantages that they lose sight of the basic goal of investing, which is to maximize profits. This advice is similar to that given elsewhere regarding tax shelters (see Chapter Twenty-Five).

SUMMARY OF CHAPTER SEVENTEEN

- Send your children to the best school you can afford.
- Encourage your children to pay for as much of their education as possible.
- Take full advantage of all financial aid.

- The length of a college education is often longer than four years.
- The cost of a college education is rising faster than the general cost of living.
- There are many tax-advantaged options to fund your children's education. Unfortunately, many of these are not an option for most physicians.
- Expert advice is mandatory to help plan your strategy to fund your children's education.
- The government can and will change the rules at any time.
- Paying for college from your own investments is an option.

REFERENCE

1. Hurley J F. The Best Way to Save for College: A Complete Guide to 529 Plans. 8th Ed. North Palm Beach, FL: Bankrate Inc., 2008.

Chapter Eighteen
Insurance

Insurance works by determining and spreading risk. The amount of the premium is determined by an actuarial who calculates the likelihood an event will occur, and then the premium is set to adequately cover this possibility and provide a reasonable profit margin for the insurance company. Sometimes this is a fairly easy task, such as determining the life insurance premium on a group of 57-year-old, non-smoking, well-educated, ideal weight, normo-tensive men or women. Sometimes the insurance companies do not adequately handicap risk, as Warren Buffett admits following the terrorist attacks of September 11, 2001. When risk has been handicapped many people then pay a premium, such as 100 homeowners, to fund the large payout when one home burns.

The function of insurance is to manage risk. It is to protect against a loss that an individual cannot afford to sustain, such as the permanent loss of income (disability insurance), loss of life (life insurance), or home (homeowner's insurance).

Insurance is not an investment. It is not a viable vehicle to save money. This is such an important point, I will repeat it. *Insurance is not an investment.* If anyone says this, you know they are wrong. This statement is such a red flag that if an agent trying to sell you a policy says insurance is a good investment, I suggest you find another agent.

Insurance is also not meant to make your spouse or children and heirs rich. It is meant to supply and fund their basic needs,

R.M. Doroghazi, *The Physician's Guide to Investing,*
DOI 10.1007/978-1-60761-134-9_18,
© Humana Press, a part of Springer Science+Business Media, LLC 2005, 2009

to make sure they have a home and an education. To buy a ten million dollar life insurance policy for your spouse and children to live in luxury they never would have dreamed possible were you alive is not logical. This would be a terrible waste of resources. It is possible to be over-insured, and if you receive all of the advice on the insurance you "need" from an insurance agent, who makes their money from the commission by selling insurance, you could be.

DISABILITY INSURANCE

It is not adequately appreciated that disability insurance is the most important type of insurance a professional such as a physician must have. Your most valuable financial asset is not your home, your vacation condo, your car or any other piece of personal property. Your most valuable asset is your skill as a physician and the earnings generated. Two hundred and fifty thousand dollars a year for twenty-five years is $6,250,000. This is your most valuable financial asset, your capacity to work and produce income.

Becoming disabled occurs more commonly than you might appreciate. The average person is almost 5 times more likely to become disabled than have their home damaged by a fire. The average person is almost 6 times more likely to become disabled than to die prematurely.

There are general limits on the amount of disability coverage that may be purchased. Benefits are usually limited to approximately two-thirds of one's income. In addition, benefits are usually capped at $15,000 a month or less, depending on the policy. You can have multiple policies but I see no need for this. The reason benefits are capped is if they become too "sweet" too many people would find it "easier" to become disabled.

What is the definition of disability? Is it a general definition of being able to perform any kind of work, or does it relate to your particular specialty? In insurance language, this concept is referred to as "owner's occupation" as compared to "any occupation." The former definition means that one is disabled if they can no longer perform their current occupation. The later means that one is disabled only if they cannot perform any work at all. The following is true example. A right-handed cardiac surgeon suffers a small embolic cerebrovascular accident (CVA) from unrecognized intermittent atrial fibrillation. Occasional palpitations had been noted but were dismissed. The stroke results in just enough loss of the manual dexterity in the right hand that the surgeon can no longer adequately perform in the operating room. He can walk and talk without a deficit, perform a general history and physical examination, provide consultations, teach students and give talks, read studies such as EKG's, echocardiograms, or vascular studies, but can no longer perform surgery. Clearly a physician needs an "owner's occupation" policy.

The above situation also emphasizes the importance of "residual benefits." Should you still be able to perform some physician duties, but not your specific specialty, residual benefits guarantee a certain percentage of your previous income in comparison to the income of the new job.

Other important factors relating to disability insurance include:

1. The length of the elimination period (the equivalent of a deductible on automobile or homeowners insurance). The more quickly the policy provides benefits, such as one or two months, the more expensive the insurance. The longer the elimination period, such as six months, the lower the premiums. I recommend the longer elimination period. The average physician should have sufficient funds to cover the hiatus.
2. Disability insurance is expensive. If possible, purchase the policy through a group. The premiums will be lower than an individual purchasing the same amount of coverage.
3. Obtain a policy that is non-cancelable and with guaranteed renewal. If you pay your premiums on time, the policy cannot be cancelled and the premiums cannot be raised during the life of the policy.
4. Some policies offer a cost of living adjustment. If they do, take it. Even with inflation of only 2% per year, after twenty years the purchasing power of a dollar has dropped by

almost fifty percent. Since I believe inflation is greater than the government's official figures, and that it may accelerate in the future, a cost of living adjustment is essential. Choose the highest that is offered.

5. Be sure the policy is purchased with after-tax money. If the policy is purchased with pre-tax money, the benefits are taxable. If the policy is purchased with after-tax money, the benefits are considered after-tax and thus not taxed. You will be paying more on a small number (the premiums) to potentially save much more on a larger number (the benefits) should you become disabled.

6. Consider dropping the disability insurance when you reach your mid-to-late 50s, and have all or almost all of your major obligations funded, and/or are within a few years of retirement. You do not need to carry disability insurance right up to the day of retirement.

7. I believe a physician should be covered by disability insurance as soon as they complete medical school. It would be a crying shame to spend 4 years of college, four years of medical school, have a six-figure student loan debt (*see* Chapter One) with the big money just around the corner, and suffer a disabling injury. The only logical solution would be for the hospitals to purchase coverage for all physicians-in-training.

AUTOMOBILE INSURANCE

Everyone needs auto insurance, and make sure you have sufficient liability coverage.

Allow me to make a comment about AAA (Automobile Association of America). Being a member of AAA can provide many benefits aside from the obvious ones should your car break down. Discounts for many expenses, including travel, rental cars, hotels and even some parking facilities are offered. On a recent trip I obtained enough discounts in these areas to cover my AAA premiums for the year. This is an example of how good planning and attention to detail can result in money in your pocket.

HOMEOWNER'S INSURANCE

Everyone needs homeowner's insurance. Also keep the following in mind:

1. You may insure for a natural catastrophe not covered in standard policies, such as a flood or earthquake. The most powerful earthquake ever recorded in the continental United States was in New Madrid, in southeast Missouri, in 1811. Because there are still occasional tremors in the area, I have earthquake insurance. It is not as expensive as you may think. Terrorism insurance is also available.

   Some homes are in areas where there is a high probability of a natural disaster, such as a flood, landslide or hurricane. Appropriate additional insurance may be mandated and even if not may be a good idea to limit your potential loss. An even better option is not to buy a home in such an area in the first place.

2. The possessions of a home are typically insured for a standard percentage of the value of the home, usually fifty percent. If you have particularly valuable, and non-standard home items – such as art, collectables, valuable musical instruments, antique furniture, etc., be sure they are adequately insured.

   An excellent way to record all of your household belongings is to make a videotape inventory of every room in your home and keep the videotape in your safe deposit box. This provides documented proof of your personal possessions.

   The replacement value of the clothes and other items that you have accumulated over time can be much more than you would imagine. Ten men's suites ($750 each), ten dress shirts ($100 each) ten men's sweaters ($75 each), forty or fifty nice pieces of women's clothing, five or six formals and gowns, and several score of shoes will come to twenty to thirty thousand dollars. There is also the children's clothing, replacement linens for the bed, kitchen utensils, and supplies and just all of the "stuff" that accumulates. With a videotape you have the best chance to receive adequate re-imbursement. Some friends suffered a devastating house fire. It was terrible. What was previously an area kept spotless by weekly dusting, mopping and polishing became a foot-deep pile of cinders and rubble that was scooped up with a shovel and thrown out the hole in the wall that was previously the window. You must have an adequate inventory of your belongings in order to submit a complete list of items lost.

You should have a replacement cost policy as compared to an actual cost value policy. With the latter, the policyholder is reimbursed for the cost of the belongings minus depreciation. A nice living room couch purchased 10 years ago for $2,000 may now have a depreciated value of only $100.

3. If you have multiple insurance policies with the same company – auto, life, home, etc. – they will typically offer a discount, which can be very substantial. Be sure you are receiving all discounts you are due.

4. My home was built in 1939 and has many features of workmanship not present in most homes built today. The standard homeowner's policy is for replacement value, in general, at current levels of workmanship with standard products. If your home has special features of workmanship, request a special rider to replace things comparable to what was lost, not comparable to current construction practices. This will cost more, and will probably require a visit by an underwriter who specializes in this area, but is worth the added expense. Because of the workmanship in my home, it would cost 50% more to replace it than I could receive by selling it.

5. Be sure that the total amount of coverage has kept pace with inflation and with the appreciation in the value of your home.

LIFE INSURANCE

The first step is to determine what amount of insurance is required. Financial planning and insurance guides provide several formulas for suggested amounts, the most common being to have life insurance equal to seven years salary. I find this recommendation far too high and the use of such a formula too constraining. I will simplify things by posing this common sense question: what are your obligations?

You will often see recommendations that all adults should have life insurance. I disagree. If you are un-married and have no dependents, as is the case with many medical students and even some house staff, I do not think life insurance is required.

Or you have reached your golden years and things have gone well financially (possibly because you read this book). You are 57 years old, the children are self-sufficient, there are no personal debts, you have 2.9 million dollars of income-producing assets and a net worth of more than 4.5 million dollars. At this point you do not need life insurance. From the time you first start to look for life insurance, anticipate that coverage will not be required beyond age 60. The reason is that you should be set financially and premiums rise dramatically at this age because the risk of dying increases pari passu. This emphasizes one of the weaknesses of whole life. With whole life you have insurance for your whole life and there are clearly times that life insurance is not required.

If you own a home with an outstanding mortgage, are married and have children who are not yet self-supporting, then you have an amazing amount of obligations. I would suggest you have sufficient insurance to cover debts, such as the amount of your mortgage, car loans, student loans, and any other indebtedness. I also suggest sufficient insurance to cover loans on illiquid investments, such as limited partnerships or closely-held companies. Outstanding loans on assets that cannot be easily converted to cash could result in a cash crunch, necessitating further borrowing or a distressed sale of the asset. You also need sufficient insurance to fund your children's education and an amount to fund the daily expenses for your spouse and children. Subtract from this the amount already accumulated in savings.

I would also suggest life insurance on your spouse. There are always expenses and disruptions when a spouse dies. If you do not have children and your spouse works, your life-style, expenses, amount of debt (such as a mortgage) are probably predicated on two incomes, necessitating some amount of insurance.

Whether your spouse works or not, if they are the sole or principal care-giver for the children, their death will be associated with significant expenses and residual obligations. Your work will be disrupted for some time – weeks or more likely months – while you get your life back together. Your income will almost certainly drop significantly during this period. At this terrible time in your life your goal will be just to put one foot in front of the other, get through the day, and hold your family together. The further addition of monetary worries could make things unbearable, especially if you do not have family, such as parents, siblings, or in-laws, to help. Who will supply childcare, or go to the store and run errands? If you must pay for all of these it will be very expensive. A policy of $250–500 K on a non-bread winning spouse is reasonable.

Before describing the types of life insurance available, I will make several recommendations about when life insurance is not required.

If a homebuyer has less than the traditional twenty percent down payment, the lender will require Private Mortgage Insurance (PMI). The bank is doing this to protect their interests. Note also that PMI can be dropped when you accumulate twenty to twenty-two percent equity in your home (Depending on your adjusted gross income, the cost of PMI may be deductible).

However, if the bank "suggests" but does not require PMI, the answer is always no. In essence, you are buying an insurance policy for the bank. It is always a very poor investment for you, a good one for the bank. This does not negate my advice that you should personally have sufficient life insurance to cover major debts, where your heirs (and not the bank) are paid the benefits.

The loss of a child is incomparable and the pain must be unimaginable, but there is no reason to purchase life insurance on a child. When I was growing up it was not uncommon for parents to buy whole life policies on their children, in effect, as a way to save for their college educations. As previously mentioned, insurance is not a viable vehicle for investing.

One pitch often used to induce a parent to purchase life insurance on a child is that by doing so the child is assured of being able to purchase more insurance when they become an adult. This is a bogus argument. There is no need to purchase life insurance on a child.

The two principal types of life insurance policies are term and whole life.

Term life insurance provides a specific benefit to your heirs while the policy is in force, that is, during the term of the policy. The premiums are significantly lower than for whole life but there is no other cash or investment value to the policy itself.

Whole life provides lifetime death benefits to your heirs upon your death but also builds up a cash value as time goes on. The premiums on whole life are *significantly* higher than on term. Because whole life has a cash value, it is a real asset, and this does provide some options, such as the possibility to borrow against this cash value. Hopefully this option will never be required and should not be a factor when one considers purchasing life insurance.

I do not like whole life at all and strongly recommend against it (except as described below). What you are doing, as compared to a term life policy, is giving the insurance company your money to invest, and paying them an obscene fee to do it. The long-term return is rarely more than five percent. The average physician investor would be much better served buying a term life policy and investing the difference in premiums in a mutual fund.

The agent's commission on whole life insurance is amazing. Of the first year's premiums, 80–90% – Yes, Eighty to Ninety Percent – go to the selling agent as commission, leaving a dime and a few pennies to build up as the cash value of your policy. In addition, the agent receives residual commissions on subsequent premiums. Because of these commissions and further administrative fees it can take six or seven years for your whole life policy to build any positive cash value. The agent's commission is considerably less on term than on whole life. It is safe to say that this is why the agent always mentions whole life first and gives it their strongest recommendation.

I will relate two real-life examples of how terrible an "investment" whole life insurance can be. Some friends asked me to review their general financial situation and provide advice. She was 42 years old at the time and at age 24 purchased a whole life policy for $100,000. The monthly premium was $23.26. Exactly eighteen years later the cash value of the policy was $2,559.88. She had paid a total of $5,024 in premiums. This represents a return of negative 49%. Eighteen years and she is down 49%. Remember that it took our stock market 25 years (1954) to return to its 1929 pre-Depression peak just to break even. In this real-life example, a whole life insurance policy is worse than the financial equivalent of living through the Great Depression. If this $23.26 per month had been invested at the standard 10% return, my friend would have just less than $14,000.

I recommended she buy an appropriate amount of term life insurance, cash in her whole life policy and put the proceeds into a Roth IRA. When she supplied the insurance company the written notice, she was reminded that "we may defer this payment of net cash value for up to six months."

A physician friend asked me to evaluate his general financial situation. He had more assets than he thought and we also concluded he was over-insured. He spoke with the agent about dropping his $1 M whole life policy. The premiums are $5 K per quarter, and the policy has a "cash value" of $32,748. The cash surrender value is $12,275, i.e., it *does not* have a cash value of $32,748. He would have to pay the premiums for another 15 years to get his money without a penalty. I recommended he stop paying on the policy and apply the premiums to his mortgage. He sent an email "Wish I'd read your book sooner. Getting wiser".

This is how I would consider whole life: The only way to realize an adequate return is to die!!

Consider the above scenarios from another perspective. If I can help you avoid just one such situation, you have saved many times the cost of this book. That is an important point many do not understand. This book, no book, will give you advice that applies to everything. If I can help you do just one smart thing (be a regular saver) or avoid one dumb thing (such as not opening a restaurant), you have generated a return of greater than an order of magnitude on your investment in this book.

There are special situations that require a significant amount of cash be available upon one's death and if they are in their 60 s or 70 s or older, then a whole life policy is appropriate. An example would be a buy-sell agreement. However, this is an estate-planning question and should have been addressed by the lawyer who drew up the buy-sell agreement. A whole life policy can also be used as a way to make a charitable donation; you make the premium payments, and the charity is the beneficiary of the policy. Again, consult your estate lawyer.

Should you be in the unfortunate situation that you have already purchased a whole life policy, I recommend that you first purchase an appropriate amount of term life insurance. Then admit to yourself that you really goofed up (it will be difficult), swallow hard, cash out your whole life policy, learn from your mistake, don't look back, and give the same advice to your friends.

There is something called a life settlement, where a third party (investor) will buy your policy for more than the cash value but less than the death benefit. I mention this for completeness, I am not recommending it.

For the average physician investor, I recommend the purchase of an appropriate amount of term insurance for all of your life insurance needs. Do not even consider whole life.

LONG-TERM CARE INSURANCE (LTCI)

Because young people think they are indestructible, most have never given any thought to LTCI. But after a bad auto accident, I am more realistic.

It is essential to consult a tax professional before purchasing LTCI because if particular criteria established by the IRS are met, the benefits could be tax-free. For the self-employed, LTCI may be a deductible business expense.

There are several factors to consider when purchasing LTCI.

1. You must be sure you can still afford the premiums after retirement. It would be an unmitigated disaster to pay on a policy for 20 years, and then in your seventies, when your

need for the benefits may be imminent, be forced to drop the coverage because you cannot afford the premiums.

2. The best age to purchase a policy is in your mid-to-late 50 s, but before age 60. This will help minimize the payment of premiums during a time when the need for the benefits is unlikely, such as before age 55, but allow a policy to be purchased for a reasonable premium while you are still in good health.

3. Purchase a policy that reflects the cost of a skilled facility in your area. The policy must have a provision for inflation, provide home-health coverage and a four to six year (or even longer) period of benefits.

4. Since it may be decades before you may need the benefits, the company must still be in business forty or fifty years from now. This is clearly not a situation to go with a start-up company because the premium may be a little lower. Independent companies such as Moody's and Standard & Poors and others rate the financial position of insurance companies that offer long-term care policies. Consult these ratings and consider only companies with superior financial positions.

5. The benefits are not open-ended, the maximal lifetime benefit is defined when you purchase the policy. You pay so much in premiums, you can only realize so much in benefits.

Overall, I am neutral to slightly negative on LTCI. Some people just feel better having insurance. If you do, consider this: Rather than buying a policy with maximal lifetime benefits of say $150,000, just buy the same amount of TIPS (Treasury Inflation Protected Securities). The investment will reasonably track inflation, the money is available any time if you need it, and whatever is not spent will still be in your estate, to do with as you wish.

You do not need LTCI if you have more than $2 M of income-producing assets, because you are essentially "self-funded". A 5% return on $2 M is $274 per day, which is significantly more than you would realize from most LTCI policies.

I devoted Issue #12, March 19, 2007 of my newsletter to this topic. If you would like more details, the newsletter is posted on my website www.thephysicianinvestor.com

EXTENDED WARRANTY

Expensive mechanical products, such as a car, washer, dryer, etc., come with a standard manufacturer's warranty, guaranteeing parts and/or service over some specific period of time and some specific set of conditions (be sure to retain all warranty information). When the original warranty expires, you will usually receive an offer to extend the warranty. These should be evaluated on a case by case basis, but as a general rule, I recommend against them, they are rarely a good investment. The company selling the extended warranty (essentially an insurance policy) has set the cost of the product to both cover their costs and realize a profit (which is usually quite significant, and explains why they push extended warranties so hard). The latter is just a fee at your expense. Local appliance dealers will sometimes offer an extended warranty at a cost significantly lower than that offered by the company. Even though these are less expensive, they still represent a fee that can be avoided (the dealer may not even be in business in 5 years). You are better off buying a quality product from a reputable dealer, taking good care of it, not purchasing an extended warranty, and saying an occasional prayer to the Whirlpool god that your icebox does not break down.

(I must admit I am amused when I see an advertisement for a product with a 50-year or similar guarantee or warranty. I will not be around in 50 years and they may not be either. It is very easy to make a promise when there is almost no chance you will have to pay off).

The function of insurance is to cover a loss you cannot afford to sustain, such as your livelihood or home. Although washers, dryers, air conditioners, etc. are expensive, they do not need to be insured, which is what an extended warranty is. Remember that such appliances are routinely built to provide good service for 15–20 years or longer. If they are breaking down in four or five years, the time usually covered by the extended warranty, you have unfortunately purchased a poor product.

Always buy quality. This relates not only to performance but also to durability and dependability. I like to purchase the high end of the middle range of appliances, because I believe it provides the best combination of good quality and affordable price. With the top-of-the-line things, you are often paying more, sometimes much more, for the fancy bells and whistles which rarely add much to the basic function or to the durability or reliability.

The average busy physician has so little free time that when you want to use something such as a tractor, a piece of wood working machinery, or whatever, you want it to work. If it breaks down, you either do not have the mechanical skill and knowledge to perform the repairs yourself or you are forced to spend your free time repairing the machinery instead of having fun.

MEDICAL INSURANCE

Everyone must have medical insurance and I am confident that all readers of this book do.

If both you and your spouse work, or for whatever reason you both have health insurance, make sure you are not paying for overlapping (i.e. redundant and non-necessary) coverage. The savings could be substantial.

I suspect that even though medicine is your profession, you may not realize how expensive good medical coverage is. Any physician who draws a salary – academic medicine, private industry, employed by a hospital or large group or clinic, physician still in training – just receive this as a benefit and have little or no idea of the direct cost. Even physicians in a group practice, as I was in, only note the cost of the insurance as just another (albeit quite large) expense on their monthly overhead statement. The full cost of medical insurance will not be truly appreciated until you must pay the costs directly out of your pocket. I suspect that many physicians also do not appreciate that health insurance is the Number One issue when many working stiffs look for a job.

UMBRELLA POLICY

Unfortunately, sometimes it seems like everyone wants to get into your pocketbook. You need not only sufficient liability limits on all standard policies such as home, rental property, auto, etc., but you also should have an umbrella policy that provides additional liability coverage above and beyond that in the standard policies. Umbrella policies are not as expensive as you might think (they are for back-up, not your primary line of defense) and do provide a nice layer of protection between a plaintiff and your personal assets. Obtain these through the same company that writes your other policies and there will be even further cost savings.

SUMMARY OF CHAPTER EIGHTEEN

- The function of insurance is to manage and spread risk.
- You must insure things you cannot afford to lose.
- Insurance is not an investment.
- You could be over-insured if you receive all of the advice on your insurance needs from an insurance salesman.
- Your most valuable asset is your ability to work and generate income. Good disability insurance is mandatory.
- Disability insurance should be purchased with after-tax money.
- A physician's disability insurance must be "owner's occupation."
- The amount of life insurance required depends upon your obligations.
- There must be adequate life insurance on the spouse that provides child care.
- Avoid Private Mortgage Insurance
- There is no need to purchase life insurance on a child.
- TERMITE – Term for everything, invest the rest. Avoid whole life.
- The only way to realize an adequate return on whole life is to die!!
- No life insurance should be required after age 60.

- Consider long-term care insurance, but only from companies with a strong financial position.
- Everyone needs medical insurance.
- Avoid extended warranties.
- Consider an umbrella policy.

Chapter Nineteen
Funding Retirement

HOW SECURE IS SOCIAL SECURITY?

My first recommendation: Do not rely on the government for anything! Whatever the government gives it can take away. If Social Security and/or Medicare are still providing benefits when you retire, consider whatever you receive "gravy." If you expect either of these programs to provide a significant percentage of your retirement needs, you may be disappointed. The government is already ten trillion dollars in debt and has taken over Fannie Mae (FNM), Freddie Mac (FRE), American International Group (AIG), General Motors (GM) and has injected trillions of dollars more into many other companies and financial institutions. There just may not be anything left when you retire.

Some people still naively believe that all of the money they paid in to Social Security over the last 30 or 40 or 50 years is sitting in a bank account somewhere with their name on it. That is not how it works. Your money coming in immediately goes out to fund someone else's benefits. Whatever money you (may) receive in the future is from payroll taxes paid by people working at that time. The term for this is "unfunded liabilities".

There is currently a "surplus" in the Social Security Trust Fund, that is, more is coming in than is paid out in benefits. The Trust Fund sends this excess to the Treasury, which immediately spends the money to help fund the budget deficit. In return, the Trust

R.M. Doroghazi, *The Physician's Guide to Investing,*
DOI 10.1007/978-1-60761-134-9_19,
© Humana Press, a part of Springer Science+Business Media, LLC 2005, 2009

Fund receives an IOU from the Treasury (the government is borrowing from themselves, never a good practice). It is estimated that in 2018 or 2019 (or earlier), barely a decade away, Social Security will be in a deficit, paying out more than it takes in. So when it is time for you to receive benefits, the Trust Fund will send the paper IOUs back to the Treasury, the Treasury will send paper money to the Trust Fund, and the Trust Fund will send paper money to you. That paper money will be worth less, possibly much less, than it is now.

I have seen numerous recommendations regarding when you should start taking your Social Security benefits. I must caution you that my opinion is in the distinct minority, but I want my money as soon as I can get it. First of all, I have no idea how long I will live. Secondly, I do know that I can invest my money better than the government. Lastly, as the Social Security Trust Fund slips into deficit, and the government's fiscal situation continues to deteriorate, one way to decrease the payout will be to add a "means testing" to determine if you qualify for benefits, i.e., if you are worth so much your benefits will be decreased or eliminated. I certainly do not have as much as Bill Gates or Warren Buffett, but means testing would be the end of my benefits. When it comes to Social Security, I will turn a phrase from that savant Wimpy of the Popeye cartoons. "I will gladly get paid less today than hopefully get paid more on Tuesday".

I would also raise a significant caveat about pensions and other benefits, such as medical insurance coverage, from employers. This could apply to a physician working in industry or to your spouse if they are not a physician. It also could apply to some of your patients, especially if they were employed in the "smoke stack" or other industries with significant legacy costs. Ten years ago the people at Enron (and more recently Bear Stearns (BSC) and Lehman Brothers (LEH) probably thought they were "In like Flynn" (an expression referring to the handsome movie star of the 30s and 40s Errol Flynn) but now they have almost nothing. As a corollary, if you or your spouse are in private industry, do not have more than 10% of your retirement money in company stock. You already have a huge investment in the company (your job), so if they go out of business you will suffer a double loss.

There is a government agency known as the Pension Benefit Guaranty Corp. This agency currently pays benefits to more than one million Americans (mostly retired steelworkers and airline workers) and insures the private pensions of millions more. If current financial conditions persist, this agency will run out of money in about a decade. If it were a private agency it would already be considered insolvent.

The one person you can always depend on for your retirement, for anything, is you. Plan accordingly. And no matter what your age, start planning *today* to take every advantage of your greatest investment friend; compound interest.

You must have a defined strategy, these being your goals – when do you want to retire and how much money will you need? You can then define your tactics – the specific steps to be taken to achieve these goals.

I will mention but not discuss the general topic of estate planning. This is a subject in and of itself. Your age, your children's age, your financial situation, insurance, current tax laws, the state where you reside, what you would like to do with your money, your marital situation, how your will is structured, trusts, everything. All are important.

I recommend the input of a lawyer who specializes in estate planning. Many lawyers say they can provide help with estate planning but seek out the assistance of a specialist in this area. Accountants can provide tax advice, but this is an area that requires a grand, all-encompassing strategy or design, and this is best provided by a lawyer specializing in estate planning. You should always try to minimize fees, but there are times when you must pay-up to receive good advice. Do not try to save a few bucks on legal fees and end up with a poor estate plan.

ANTICIPATED AGE OF RETIREMENT

Many non-medical people retire from their primary livelihood and then take a part-time job either in their previous area of employment or in a completely different field to supplement income. This is rarely an option for a physician in private practice. Because so much of a physician's overhead is fixed, such as office space, personnel, equipment and malpractice insurance, part-time work as a physician is generally not a financially viable option. Because medicine is a profession, mental and procedural skills are best maintained by constant use and practice.

As a practical matter, there are not many jobs that you can just walk into with no training that pay the $100–$200 per hour that a physician can obtain for their time. A physician's skills are so specialized that they really do not lend themselves to many other types of work. I feel that, expect in special circumstances, a physician must practice full-time until they retire, and then just walk away. From both a financial and professional point of view, there are few other options for the physician in private practice.

Some physicians say they will never retire, although people do change their mind (sometimes involuntarily). Many physicians aim for the current standard retirement age of sixty-five, some earlier, and some later. Whatever the age at which you hope to retire is your personal choice.

There are several important issues. The first is that if you do not make adequate financial plans, you may be working longer than hoped because you are forced to. This is not a desirable situation for you or your patients.

The second relates directly to being a professional. No professional is the same at age 75 as they were at age 35 or 40. This has been dictated by nature. The person who was the best neurosurgeon or best oncologist in the world at age 40 may still be an absolutely outstanding physician at age 70 or 75 or 80, but they are not what they were at age 40.

I attended my first professional baseball game in 1958 at "old, old" Busch Stadium (previously called Sportsman's Park) at the corners of Grand, Dodier, Sullivan and Spring in North St. Louis. None of the superb athletes playing major league baseball in 1958 have played in a major league game for more than three decades. Many of the stars of that time – Ted Williams, Mickey Mantle, Warren Spahn, Eddie Matthews, Roger Maris, Don Drysdale and Ken Boyer – have died.

Mental and physical skills decrease with age. You should not allow your personal financial situation to dictate how long you practice. These comments are not a criticism of elderly physicians and should not be considered as such. There are physicians in their 70s, 80s and even 90s who are better physicians than I ever dreamed of being. The point is that you must manage your personal finances such that you are not forced to practice for financial reason when your skills may no longer be adequate.

HAVE ALL MAJOR OBLIGATIONS FUNDED

Hopefully this was obvious. Do not retire until you are debt-free or near debt-free. If something goes wrong, there is no income stream to fall back on. You should own your home outright with no mortgage, the same for a vacation home or recreational property. Do not retire with two ten-year-old automobiles that each have 120,000 miles. Have new vehicles purchased free and clear before retirement.

Every ten or twenty years, all homes require major repairs and maintenance, such as a new roof, painting, replacement of windows and frames, outside wood, gutters, and major plumbing, electrical and heating and cooling system work. Furniture wears out. Such major projects often cost ten or twenty thousand dollars or more. The same for a major redecoration project or addition. Have these completed and paid for before retirement.

You can be a little more lenient in this circumstance with debt as it relates to investments. I would not be overly concerned if you have one or several pieces of rental property that have built up significant equity and a strong cash flow that easily covers the note. I would be quite concerned with a highly leveraged investment where the absolute amount of debt represents a significant percentage of your net worth. If the investment failed, it could take you down. You could have the opportunity to become re-acquainted with all of your old patients when you hire on as a greeter at your local Wal-Mart.

The other principal obligation to be either completed or have funded is your children's education (*see* Chapter Seventeen). Most likely they will be out of school and self-supporting by the time you reach retirement age. If not, be sure there are adequate funds specifically targeted to their education, including graduate or professional school if this is being considered.

HOW MUCH MONEY IS REQUIRED TO RETIRE AND LIVE COMFORTABLY?

One way to look at the money you have saved – retirement plan and non-retirement plan savings – in the same way a college or university uses their endowment. They spend a particular amount each year, but do not touch the principal and retain enough of the earnings so that the corpus of the endowment at least keeps pace with or preferably outpaces inflation. An investment that does not at least keep pace with inflation is a loss. Consider inflation a hidden, insidious, and cruel tax.

I would suggest you have enough *income-producing assets* to be able to live off an amount equal to *at most* 5% of the total value of the assets per year. Five percent of $2M is $100,000. If you do not have a mortgage or educational bills, could you live off $100K per year?

If you did not understand this concept, consider the inverse. Five percent equals one-twentieth of the whole. To determine what amount of income-producing assets are needed to retire, determine what yearly income you feel will be required to live the style you desire, and take that number times twenty. If you would like a yearly income of $100,000, twenty times $100K = $2M.

I have seen several articles that suggest the closer this number is to 3%, the better. If you can live off an amount equal to 3% of your income-producing assets per year, the chance of running out of money before you die is almost zero. But this means you need almost $3M of assets to generate $100K of yearly income. If you are not good with managing money, I would suggest you use the 3% in your calculations. It may require you working a year or two longer, but the peace of mind is worth it. If you are better with money, use the 4–5% number.

If you are retired, try to keep at least three years of living expenses in completely risk-free, cash-equivalent investments, such as a money market, passbook, CDs, short-term T-Bills, etc. In this way, should there be a bear market in stocks, you know that your living expenses for the next several years are well-funded and you will not forced to liquidate investments at a bad time.

I do have one encouraging piece of information. Many retired physicians, including me, say their financial needs are just not as great as they originally estimated. Much less for clothes; I used to buy 2 new suits a year, now one is quite sufficient. I wore a starched cotton shirt to work every day. My laundry bill is cut by more than half. No drive or commute to and from work – I used to put 12K miles per year on my car, now it is 5K. It may even be possible to get by with one less vehicle. No practice-related expenses, and the children are now self-sufficient (they now treat me to supper when I visit). Almost all retired physicians I have spoken with have fewer expenses than originally anticipated. There does appear to be some hope.

Likewise, you must also re-evaluate your situation from time to time, and be realistic should there be a material change. These are all real-life situations. What if a child and their spouse both die in a boating (or auto) accident, and you must raise the children? What if your child's spouse goes wacko, is a drug addict, squanders all of their money, and does everything they can to make your child's and grandchildren's life hell-on-earth, with 6-figure legal bills that, in the end, you must pay? What if investments you had every right to feel were solid end up worthless, and your net worth is cut in half? What if you are in your late 60s, retired, and your spouse of 38 years decides they don't love you anymore, and gets half of the money in the divorce? You better realize pretty quickly that some things you considered "necessities" are actually luxuries and adjust your spending accordingly.

I emphasize income-producing assets. Your home is certainly an asset but not an income producer. The same applies to recreational or vacation property, unless you are willing to rent or sell them, and collectables, art, and antiques. These may have significant value but produce no income unless you are willing to sell them. Many people do not need or want as large a home after they retire. Many move to smaller homes or condos or even sell their home and then rent (to your children and rent it back from them, *see* Chapter Thirty-Two). In this way the equity of the home can be converted into liquid assets. (I have already discussed in Chapter Sixteen why you should avoid a reverse mortgage as a way to cash out on your home).

Several people I have spoken with have lost the passion to collect as they grow older. They would rather use the money to help their grandchildren, travel or very often donate the proceeds to charity. In some people, altruism does increase with age.

Many people do not realize that a dollar in a traditional IRA, 401(k) and all similar pre-tax plans is not a dollar. Money in these vehicles has grown tax-free but the entire amount will be taxed when withdrawn. One dollar in such plans minus taxes is the money in your pocket. It would be more appropriate to consider money in these plans as future income rather than savings. I suggest you consider $1.00 in these plans to be worth about 70 cents or even less. If you do not understand this point, discuss it with your accountant or lawyer. It would be terrible to retire and only then realize that you have twenty, thirty or forty percent less than originally thought.

The election of 2008 will take place while this book goes to press. Whoever is elected will inherit such a mess that they will be forced to raise taxes. In one day, your retirement account could lose 10–15% or maybe even more of its value.

I recommend you read as much as possible and discuss with your accountant the Alternative Minimum Tax (AMT). This was enacted by Congress in the 1960s because at the time several hundred taxpayers with multi-million dollar incomes were able to avoid paying any income tax. Congress rarely repeals tax laws once they are on the books. Because of the inflation of the last four decades, many millions of Americans are now stung by the AMT. At the time of your retirement you will become well acquainted with the AMT (if you have not already).

Because of us and our research colleges, we are living longer, healthier lives. The person that lives to age 65 in the U.S. can look forward, on average, to living about another 15 years. This will hopefully continue to increase, although average life expectancy could start to drop due to the obesity epidemic. There is a good chance that the average physician could live twenty or twenty-five years, or even longer, after retirement. Take this into consideration. It would be terrible to run out of money at the most vulnerable time of your life.

SPECIFIC VEHICLES FOR RETIREMENT SAVINGS

It has been standard teaching that around the time of retirement you should change your asset allocation from "riskier, more aggressive" investments such as growth stocks or real estate to "more conservative, less risky" interest and dividend producing investments such as cash and money markets, CD's, bonds and high dividend stocks such as those of utilities. I will discuss in Chapter Thirty One why I feel terms such as aggressive, conservative, more risky or less risky do not appropriately characterize how you should evaluate an investment. All investments have risk.

I do agree you need to make some adjustments around the time of retirement and beyond toward more cash-like investments. There are two reasons. The first is that judgment, general mental capacity, stamina and desire decrease with age. You just may not have the mental or physical capabilities to follow your investments as closely as in your younger years. Everyone's personal circumstances are different, but when this situation arises, it would be reasonable, and advisable, to cut back on investments that require closer monitoring and input, such as a position in a specific stock, in favor of investments that do not require as much attention, such as an index mutual fund or a CD. The larger mutual fund/money managers offer target-date funds that automatically change the asset allocation as you approach retirement.

The other reason to consider increasing fixed-income investments at this time is because of volatility; the increase or decrease in value that occurs with all investments from time to time. In a bear market, the average stock drops 20 or 30% or more. It could take several years, or even a decade or more, to recoup the losses. When your investment time frame is ten years or less, you need more cash. If it is two years or less, you should be completely in cash. An 80- or 85-year-old does not have the luxury of time and could have a major health event – illness or hospitalization – when the value of their assets is at its nadir. I have avoided giving specific percentages for a change in the asset allocation of your portfolio at this time because everyone's situation is different, making specific recommendations difficult or impossible. However, I do remind you of my comments above that after retirement you should keep at least three years of living expenses in cash and cash-equivalent investments.

Although some change in asset allocation at this time is warranted, a major or especially an abrupt change is probably not desirable. Most fixed-rate investments do not keep pace with inflation. If you could find quality fixed-income investments that yield 10%, it would be possible to live off 5% and re-invest the other 5%. But such investments do not exist. Rather, your return will be 5%, which is your goal for living expenses, but there will be nothing left over to re-invest. Every year you will lose to inflation, and if you should live another 20 or more years the relative value of your investment portfolio will be only a fraction of what it was earlier. Many do not realize this weakness of the "income-producing strategy" emphasized by many of the general works on financial planning for retirement. You must always maintain some equity-real estate exposure in your portfolio to generate growth.

Another reason to not significantly or precipitously change asset mix is because whatever you have done so far has been successful, you know it, understand it, and are comfortable with it. And it will hopefully allow you to maintain the purchasing power of your portfolio.

If there are not many direct income-producing assets what is the source of money to meet the daily expenses of life? Say a retiree has a $2M portfolio with $1M (50%) in an S&P 500 Index mutual fund, $400K (20%) in fixed-income investments, $400K (20%) in real estate, as 2 properties of $200K, each generating a rental income of 7–8% per year, and $200K (10%) in hard assets.

Just sell something. For 30 years you have income-averaged into the S&P 500 Index Fund. Now just income-average out. Rather than send them a check each month, direct them send you a check for $5K every month. Add the income from the rental properties and the dividends from the income-producing assets and you have $100K a year. Or at the appropriate time, sell a piece of real estate. The $200K will provide your living expenses for the next 2 or more years, during which time you do not need to withdraw anything from the stocks or fixed-income investments. Thus you could generate the 5% for living expenses and may at least keep pace with inflation.

You should, ABSOLUTELY MUST, have significant savings outside of your retirement plans. If your average yearly salary while working was $100K, then probably most of the income-producing assets you will have at age 65 are in your retirement account. If you made an average of $500K per year, so much money was generated above that which can be contributed into retirement plans that non-retirement assets will probably be greater than assets in tax-advantaged retirement plans. As John D. Rockefeller said: "Save as much as you can." For the average physician making $250K per year, the amounts in retirement and non-retirement assets will probably be fairly close.

Remember, a dollar in a traditional retirement plan is not really a dollar. In addition, if almost all of your assets are in retirement plans, they are not only relatively illiquid, but you are a "hostage" to the tax laws. By the time you retire, the rules governing retirement plans will have changed, possibly significantly, and almost certainly to the detriment of those who have worked hard and been thrifty and saved as much as they could. It is extremely important to have significant assets outside of traditional retirement plans.

Websites that can help with retirement information include Social Security Online www.ssa.gov and nonprofit investment advisor BetterInvesting www.betterinvesting.org. The websites of almost every major broker also offer retirement calculators.

TAX-FAVORED RETIREMENT ACCOUNTS

I have already mentioned Suze Orman's book *The Road to Wealth* [1]. Her works are so popular because they are of the highest quality. And her general message is the same as mine: work hard, save your money, the less debt the better, and don't do stupid things. I again recommend you purchase this book. Some of the general points made here are from her work, and her book provides further details that are far beyond the scope of this book.

Four pieces of advice:

1. Contribute the maximum amount.
2. Invest as early in the year as possible.
3. Take full advantage of any matching contributions by your employer. This is free money. You will not be afforded such opportunities often.
4. Once you get money in a retirement plan, you must resist any temptation to withdraw it early. I suggest you look at money in a retirement account as a farmer looks at his seed corn: You must be desperate to break into your retirement account. An especially vulnerable time is when you switch jobs and roll money from one plan to another. Some plans even offer 401(k) debit cards (I believe this is a breach of fiduciary responsibility).

By investing as early in the year as possible, your earnings are tax-sheltered for longer. Say you contribute $5,000 on January 1, 2009. Now say you procrastinate (this applies only to others, not you) and do not make the deposit until April 14, 2010. You have lost 15 months of tax-sheltering of your earnings. Compare our standard 10% return (untaxed) to a 10% return that is taxed, thus netting proceeds of approximately 6%. A 40% difference in return. Do this for 30 years and you have made, or lost, an absolute fortune.

Consider another example. Suppose you invest $5,000 at the end of each year in a tax-deferred account at our goal of a 10% annual return. You begin your contributions at age 35 (after finishing your training). Thirty years later (at age 65), you will have accumulated $822,470. Not bad. However, had you made the contribution at the beginning of the year instead of at the end, you would have amassed $904,717! This is a difference of more than $82 K, and you did it without any more work and without contributing one additional red cent! ATTENTION TO SIMPLE DETAILS CAN PROVIDE FINANCIAL SECURITY.

There are several general points of importance, but be aware that there are even exceptions to some of these.

1. Continue to contribute to tax-deferred plans for as long as possible, literally up to the time of retirement.
2. You may begin to withdraw money from such plans at age fifty-nine and one-half.
3. You must begin to withdraw money from such plans – except Roth IRAs, where mandatory withdrawals are not required – by April 1 the year after you turn 70 ½.
4. It is the government's desire for you to have all money withdrawn from tax-deferred accounts by the time of your death.
5. Standard teaching is that when there is an option, use money from non-retirement savings first, since taxes have already been paid on these funds. This allows money in the tax-favored accounts to continue to grow tax-deferred. However, see my comment above regarding the importance of also maximizing non-retirement plan savings.
6. Because there are so many options, expert advice is mandatory.

The basic dividing line between all tax-favored retirement plans is whether you are contributing pre-tax or after-tax money.

INDIVIDUAL RETIREMENT ACCOUNTS (IRA), 401 (k), 404(b), 457 PLAN, DEFINED BENEFIT PLAN, DEFINED CONTRIBUTION PLAN, PROFIT SHARING PLAN, MONEY PURCHASE PLAN, AND KEOUGH PLAN

The general concept of all of these plans is similar. Pre-tax money is contributed, the investment grows tax-deferred and most or all of the money, both the initial amount contributed (because it was not taxed at that time), and the earnings, are partially, or more typically, fully taxable when the money is withdrawn. There are a myriad of details and exceptions regarding who qualifies, how much can be contributed, etc., with each one of these plans and they may change every year.

I remind you of one point: Seek other people's advice, but this is your retirement money and thus your responsibility to make sure it is handled and invested properly.

ROTH IRAs

The other major type of tax-favored retirement plan is to contribute non-deductible, post-tax money that then grows tax-deferred.

1. The advantage of these plans is that all of the money – initial contribution (already taxed before contribution) plus accumulated earnings – is tax-free at the time of withdrawal. You are not a "hostage" to future tax laws and whims of the politicians. This contrasts to the plans described above, where there is a deduction at the time of the contribution but all the proceeds are taxed when withdrawn.
2. There are no mandatory withdrawals, i.e. – you do not have to begin withdrawals at age 70½. Money should be withdrawn from these last, if at all, to take full advantage of continued tax-free compounding. These also have advantages when inherited by your heirs.
3. There are other advantages (with accompanying exceptions) to Roth IRAs. See Orman's book for details.

The problem, as it relates to the physician investor, is that most physician's income is far too high to allow you, or your spouse, to participate in a Roth IRA.

However, once your children start to work, they can have their own Roth IRA. One of the best ideas I ever had to encourage my children to save was to open a Roth IRA and make them the following offer: I will match dollar for dollar whatever you contribute. Your children are encouraged to save, you are helping them, and they are learning more about investing. And you have also introduced them to their greatest investment friend, compound interest.

ANNUITIES

The short story on annuities is:

1. Do not purchase an annuity.
2. They are very complicated. In Chapter Thirty-Eight, I quote Peter Lynch's Principle #3 – "Never invest in any idea that you can't illustrate with a crayon." Apply this rule to annuities.
3. The fees and commissions are terribly high. An annuity is profitable for the agent and the company. They are rarely as profitable for the investor.

Now for the long story on annuities:

Do not purchase an annuity.

Webster's defines annuity as "an amount payable yearly or at regular intervals." Annuities arose in bygone times, centuries before Social Security, company pensions and IRAs, Keoghs, defined benefit and money purchase plans, before any type of formal retirement plans. The Knights Templar financed annuities in the Middle Ages.

Say in 1922, at age 62, a man sells his Pierce Arrow automobile dealership for $9,000. He takes this lump sum to a large insurance company and purchases an annuity. The man and/or his wife will receive a particular amount of money every year or every month until they die. They have just purchased their pension and funded their retirement.

But almost a century later, there are IRAs, Keoghs, 401-K plans, employer pensions and a variety of other options for everyone including the self-employed. There are also many types of annuities and they are extremely complicated. Remember, annuities do not provide a death benefit, and are thus not a life insurance policy.

Annuities are usually purchased with a lump-sum payment. They are not similar to a CD purchased at your local bank and thus are not federally insured. A single-premium deferred annuity could possibly be considered if you desire income in your retirement years but do not wish to take any market risk and do not wish to pay taxes now but anticipate (remember the AMT, and remember that tax laws change) you will be in a lower tax bracket after retirement. The price of lower risk is inferior return, further accentuated by the high commissions and fees of annuities. The payout of an annuity can be fixed or variable. There are also index annuities and split annuities, in addition to immediate, also called income annuities. These are complex!

When you annuitize your investment, you receive a fixed monthly income from the insurance company for life. The most common type of annuitization option is "life only." This is essentially a bet on how long you will live. If you are 65 and purchase an annuity, the amount you pay in premiums and receive in monthly payout is determined by the insurance company's data on the expected life span for a person similar to you. You will receive this amount every month until you die. If you die in one month, the payments stop. Too bad. If you live to 106, the purchase of the annuity was the best investment of your life.

When Einstein was asked about Werner Heisenberg's Uncertainty Principle, he said, "God does not play dice with the world" [2]. Warren Buffett detests risk. Einstein does not believe in uncertainty. Take their advice.

My general advice on annuities is similar to that on whole life insurance. The *only* time I would consider an annuity is when recommended by an estate lawyer or as a charitable gift. For example, many universities and large charities will annuitize your gift. You donate the money, so you not only receive credit for the gift while you are alive (*see* Chapter Forty, the Importance of Charity), but you will receive annuity payments until you die, a pretty good deal for both sides.

Otherwise, I do not recommend annuities. If you should even consider one, obtain impartial advice from someone besides the salesman, broker or agent selling the product. You will almost always be much better served by income-averaging into an S&P 500 Index Fund.

If you already have an annuity, I give advice similar to that regarding whole life insurance i.e., obtain impartial advice to determine if you should and how best to extricate yourself from the situation. Good luck, because you will need it.

MEDICAL BILLS

One of the best ways to maintain your wealth is to maintain your health. There is little doubt that the most expensive part of everyone's retirement will be medical bills. Not travel, your vacation home, your clothes or your automobile, food or your utility bills, but your medial expenses. Your doctor bills, your medications and your hospital bills. Because of current government regulations, physicians often do not receive professional courtesy. You will no longer be able to go to the medicine cabinet for samples or sign for stock bottles that end up being for your personal use. Medical bills will be the greatest expense of your retirement.

Current estimates are that the average 65-year-old couple will pay $225,000 for out-of-pocket medical charges over the next 15 years. This is not total medical bills, but out-of-pocket charges. Considering that a physician desires the best medical care, what are your options?

1. Stay healthy. Don't smoke, exercise your body and mind daily, monitor your blood pressure, watch your diet, maintain ideal weight, keep your LDL less than 100 (preferably 60–70), have a colonoscopy performed at appropriate intervals, buckle your seat belt, don't drink and drive a car or watercraft or use any type of power machinery or shoot a gun, use sun screen, wear polarized sun glasses when outdoors, obtain appropriate female and male tests and examinations, keep your vaccinations up to date, brush your teeth and floss as instructed by your dentist, etc.
2. I came to the conclusion long ago that the two principle factors determining whether the last years of your life will be golden or really rough are family and money. If you have

both, you are blessed. Even if you have just one, you will probably be OK. Save as much money as you can and plan to spend it on your health.

HEALTH SAVINGS ACCOUNTS (HSAs)

With a HSA, you contribute pre-tax money (similar to a traditional IRA) and use the money later for medical expenses. Only those with a high deductible general health insurance are eligible. They can be opened at any time, and dollars not used in any given year can be rolled over into the future. *See* www.irs. ustreas.gov and search for Publication 969, "Medical Savings Accounts" for more information.

Contributing pre-tax money that grows tax-free with tax-free withdrawals is now a unique way to save but was the standard of personal finance in our country prior to ratification of the XVI Amendment to the Constitution allowing the direct taxation of incomes.

SUMMARY OF CHAPTER NINETEEN

- The one person you can count on for your retirement is you.
- Hopefully Social Security and Medicare will be around when you retire.
- A means test for Social Security could decrease or negate your benefits.
- You could live thirty years after retirement, plan accordingly.
- Have all major obligations funded before retirement.
- An investment that does not match inflation is a loss.
- Have sufficient savings such that you can live off 3–5% of your assets per year.
- After retirement, keep at least 3 years living expenses in cash-equivalent, risk-free investments.
- Living expenses after retirement are often less than planned.

- Make full use of every tax-advantaged retirement plan and contribute the maximum.
- Make retirement plan contributions as early in the year as possible.
- Take full advantage of any matching contributions by your employer.
- Beware of the Alternative Minimum Tax.
- A dollar in a traditional retirement account is not really a dollar.
- Continue to contribute to tax-deferred plans right up to the time of retirement.
- Plan to have significant savings outside of your retirement accounts.
- Money in pre-tax retirement accounts is "hostage" to future tax laws.
- Help your children open a Roth IRA.
- Do not purchase an annuity.
- Medical bills will be the greatest expense during your retirement.

REFERENCES

1. Orman S. The Road to Wealth: A Comprehensive Guide to Your Money. New York: Riverhead Books, 2008.
2. Clark R W. Einstein: The Life and Times. New York: World Publishing, 1971.

V Pitfalls in the Quest for Your Financial Goals

Chapter Twenty
Who Can You Trust? How to Spot a Con Man

WHO CAN YOU TRUST?

Some will consider this chapter insightful, some of you may find it overly cynical, some will find it realistic and pragmatic. I hope it is all of these.

I will first discuss who I think can most likely be trusted, and then discuss people and circumstances where you are better served being skeptical and cynical.

The people that can be most trusted are your *blood* family. I grew up with a boy who owns a business that generates large amounts of cash. Do you know who counts the money at the end of the day and makes the bank deposits? His 85-year-old mother. Why trust anyone else when your mother can handle the money. At least 50% of doctors' offices are victims of embezzlement (*see* Chapter Thirty-Nine). Just look at your local newspaper. Robbery and stealing occur every day. I think my friend is a genius.

Politicians will often have family members, or people who were their friends when they were young, before they rose to positions of importance, as their closest advisors and confidants. To quote Nelson Mandela "There is little favorable to be said about poverty, but it was often an incubator of true friendship. Many people will appear to befriend you when you are wealthy, but precious few will do the same when you are poor. If wealth is a magnet, poverty is a kind of repellent" [1].

R.M. Doroghazi, *The Physician's Guide to Investing*,
DOI 10.1007/978-1-60761-134-9_20,
© Humana Press, a part of Springer Science+Business Media, LLC 2005, 2009

As a reminder, one of the main goals of this book is to instill a sense of healthy skepticism, to help you avoid mistakes. Everyone is happy when things go well. Hopefully with the lessons learned here, you will be protected and can avoid some ugly situations.

The people that can be most trusted are your blood relatives; your parents, grandparents, brothers, sisters, children and grandchildren. Aunts, uncles, nieces and nephews are one degree removed, but usually past muster. If you cannot trust your blood relatives, you are in tough shape.

How about this for a cynical and provocative but realistic comment: Can you trust your spouse? Fifty percent of marriages end in divorce (*see* Chapter Twenty-Three). Half of those who remain married are unhappy. Infidelity occurs all the time. You should probably also avoid investing with in-laws. As a practical matter, if your marriage should end in divorce, they are no longer your relatives at all and will not side with you in any dispute.

Investing with relatives refers only to worthy investments. Presumably you can trust your children, but when should you invest or loan them money? My general reply is that if your children are destined to succeed, they should be able to do it on their own. If a son or daughter has shown that they are worthy, that they are careful with their money and industrious, that they have noted a niche, have investigated it thoroughly, and present a detailed business plan, then evaluate it as you would any investment.

If an investment is made with a relative, everything must be absolutely business-like. The IRS has a variety of rules that apply when doing business with a relative, including forbidding any deduction for a loss on a guarantee made as a favor. Detailed papers and loan agreements must be drawn up and signed, and must be followed. Everything must be conducted at arms length.

Do not invest just because they are your children, to "help" them. The worst thing you can do is to support a child in a business venture that is unworthy. You are not only hurting yourself financially, you are hurting *all* of your children. If things go wrong they may/will expect you to bail them out rather than looking for other ways to salvage the business venture. In a formal business situation, there are managers and employees. It is difficult to discipline and essentially impossible to "fire" a child. This *will* affect your relationship with all of the children, and between the children. By helping one child, you are by definition showing favoritism. If things go badly, the more you assert your legal rights, the more you alienate your family. Talk about a lose/lose situation. See Issue #29 of my newsletter at www.thephysicianinvestor.com for a real-life example of how helping one child in business destroyed a family.

How many people outside of your family can you completely trust? During the Great Depression, some Hungarian friends were in a legal tussle and signed their home over to my grandparents until things blew over, when it was returned to them. Ask yourself that question: How many people would I trust enough to sign over my home? If there are more than ten people on earth, *inside and outside* of your family that you can trust with anything, you are either (1) a saint of a person, with powers and abilities far beyond those of mortal men (2) terribly naïve or (3) you come from a big, and good, family with a lot of brothers and sisters.

A person that can be trusted with anything is worth more than gold. Never lose that person as a friend. Is there anything in business, or in life, worth more than complete trust? No!!!

You cannot be a physician without trusting your patients. From the first day of training we are taught to trust our patients, their families, and our colleagues, and in fact everyone we deal with. Only in this way can we ask our patients to trust us to be their advocate, to do what is best for them. Not what is best for us, or for anyone else, but what is best for them. It is a prerequisite for being a physician.

This blind trust that serves us so well as a physician can lead to disaster in the real, financial, legal, non-medical world. Our training and goals as physicians must not change. Instead, we must be able to somehow turn off, to segregate, this unquestioning trust when we venture outside medicine.

Let me make an analogy to a prizefighter. Inside the ring, it is the boxer's goal to dominate his opponent mentally and physically. To intimidate him, to terrify him, to beat him as savagely, ruthlessly and relentlessly as possible around the head, neck and chest as to cause him to lose consciousness. These skills inside the ring can led to fame and fortune. Outside the ring, such behavior is not socially acceptable and does not serve a boxer well. It is the same with a physician. Trust is mandatory in the practice of medicine. Outside of medicine, implicit trust can and does lead to disaster. A physician's training to implicitly trust everything they are told is one of the basic flaws that afflicts physicians in their financial life.

Who should not be trusted? A flippant answer would be everyone else. The practical answer is that you must always be very careful. In "Rambo, First Blood, Part Two", Sylvester Stallone, as he is about to board the helicopter that will take him on his mission, leans over to Richard Crenna, his old commander in Vietnam, and says "You are the only one I trust". Rambo's judgment was as insightful and accurate as his fighting prowess was super-human. Make people earn your respect and trust.

There is one situation where you should be dogmatic, unyielding and just plain hardheaded. If a person has a past criminal record, disciplinary actions by regulatory agencies, such as the SEC (Securities and Exchange Commission), or any history of shady dealings, anything more serious than a traffic violation, under no circumstance should you even talk to him. There are so many honest people that there is really no reason to take any chance on a shady character.

A less compelling circumstance where I would be hesitant to invest with someone is when I have invested with them before and lost money. The problem here is presumably not one of integrity, but rather they may not be a good businessperson. Why take the chance?

I have seen several articles which shows how truly devious some people can be, and why it is wise not to invest with someone who has lost money, whether honestly or dishonestly. In general, when someone has been the victim of a scam, they look for assistance and advice to gain restitution. These articles provide examples of crooks who were principals in the initial scam and who set up a second scam to contact the victims to ostensibly provide them help and advice to get their money back. The fleecers knew these people were gullible and with the ruse were able to fleece them a second time. There are some very nasty people out there. As they say on CNBC, "Some people will do anything for money". Please be careful.

When investing with anyone, it is essential to determine their motives. How will they profit from the investment? Are their interests the same as yours? Will they make money when you make money or more importantly, can they make money even if you lose money?

Be cautious with salesman. Of course I am not suggesting they are dishonest, but rather they may make money from the commission on the sale, not from the return on your investment. Their motives are not the same as yours.

HOW TO SPOT A CON MAN

1. Greed is the con man's greatest ally (*see* Chapter Four), and I believe it can be numerically defined. If someone promises you, guarantees you, that an investment will generate a 20% or greater return, they are either (A) a well-known, Warren Buffett-class investor, (B) they could be the "next" Warren Buffett (one in a million chance), (C) they may be legitimate, but their results are over only a short period of time (50% chance this was due to luck), or (D) they are a con man. As a general rule, the higher the potential return above 20% – "double your money in three months" – the more likely they are to be bogus.
2. Charming and Slick. You are a 57-year-old man who looks, acts and talks like Archie Bunker. A drop-dead gorgeous young lady starts to hit on you. There are 3 possibilities: (A) You drop to your knees and say "Hallelujah, there is a God". (B) She is stoned, or (C) She just wants your money.

   Everything I have ever heard or read about con men includes descriptions such as charming, slick, I just felt I could trust him, etc. How else could they peddle something that is really just junk without being charming? I prefer people who are direct and have a few rough edges, if for no other reason than they are a little more like me.

3. Flash, Glitz and Throws Money Around. "He throws a hell of a party" (I have personally heard that). Con men routinely use hot cars, flashy jewelry, and jet planes (I know of one rented for just this purpose) to impress potential victims. As a practical matter, would you want someone who is supposed to be concerned with every 0.01% return on your account spending hundreds or thousands of dollars to impress a potential new client? Sam Walton drove a pickup truck and Warren Buffett treats potential business associates to hamburgers, cherry Cokes and ice cream sundaes (BRK owns Dairy Queen and a large position in Coca Cola (KO). The real winners in life impress people with their character and their accomplishments rather than bling-bling.

4. Religion, Race, Color or Creed. Many mainstream, legitimate organizations, from religious to fraternal or ethnic, offer members financial products, such as insurance, at a discount rate. Immigrants routinely do business with people of a similar background and language. My grandfather collected insurance premiums for the Verhovay Aid Assoc. (now the Wm. Penn Fraternal Assoc.) during the Great Depression from other Hungarian immigrants.

   Beware if someone brings up religion, race or ethnicity on a personal basis to gain your trust. "You're a Christian, I'm a Christian, you can trust me" or "African-Americans need to stick together". Also be concerned if all of the investors are of the same religious or ethnic group. Scams that target people of similar backgrounds are called "affinity" cases. There is no reason for these subjects to enter any discussion concerning investments. When they do, you better start to pray.

5. Secrecy. I have read of several scams where investors were instructed to keep things a secret. The perps didn't want to get outed by the pigeons talking too much.

6. If you cannot understand how an investment will make money, either because it sounds complicated, or just stupid (such as burning dirt, a real-life example), your concerns are probably well-founded.

7. Inconsistencies. Financial institutions do occasionally make mistakes. In my experience, it is usually clear they are mistakes and easy to track down the problem. But you were told one thing and it was something else, or you were supposed to get a check or paperwork and it did not come. Things just don't add up. Never let anyone blow you off when you notice an inconsistency.

Since this work is meant mostly for physicians, let me conclude this chapter with a medically-related example of the factors you should consider, the mental checklist you should complete, to determine whom you can or cannot trust.

When you or a family member were ill, how did you determine who would be the physician allowed to provide the care? How did you choose the person with whom you would trust your life? Their reputation was important, their credentials were important, you probably asked several colleagues and you may have even spoken with other patients. If you saw someone locally, you probably knew them for many years, saw them day in and day out, in the Emergency Ward, on the hospital floors, in casual conversation, in the doctor's lounge, at parties, at the grocery store, at the ballgame, or at your children's school. Only after all of these factors were taken into consideration were they chosen to be your physician or the physician for a family member. Before investing with anyone, complete the same mental process you would to choose your physician.

SUMMARY OF CHAPTER TWENTY

- The people you can trust most are your blood family.
- A person you can trust with anything is worth more than gold.
- Loaning money to a family member only to "help" them is actually doing them and you a dis-service, and may alienate the rest of the family.
- Our training as a physician to implicitly trust everyone does not serve us well when investing.

- Never invest with anyone with a criminal record or any history of shady deals.
- Be hesitant to invest with someone who has already lost you money.
- Be on the lookout for con men.
- What are the "motives" of the person with whom you are investing?
- Choose the person with whom you invest the same way you choose your physician.

REFERENCE

1. Mandela N R. Long Walk to Freedom: The Autobiography of Nelson Mandela. New York: Little Brown and Co, 1994.

Chapter Twenty-One
The Malevolence of Debt

Let me begin with this statement: No debt, no bankruptcy. You may not have much, you may not even have anything, but if there is no debt, you cannot go bankrupt. When you own something "free and clear" of debt, it is yours.

There are multiple problems with debt. The first is seductiveness. Debt is the financial equivalent of the dark side of the force. It is like the song of the Sirens, ready to entice the unwary onto the rocks of financial destruction. Even the bravest man should not be ashamed to admit they are afraid of debt.

Everything is driven by basic forces. The more insight and understanding you can gain into these basic forces, the easier it is to comprehend the concept and to profit, or to take steps to prevent problems or mistakes. The fact that money must be borrowed to make a purchase indicates that you cannot afford it in the first place. To make a medical analogy, debt is a negative feedback. The fact that you must borrow money tells you that you are circumventing a natural control mechanism. If we were required to pay cash for every purchase or investment, we would make significantly less mistakes.

It is impractical to buy some things with cash, especially your first home. Many people borrow to purchase their first car, although when I began driving in 1967 my father and I each paid $100 for a 1956 Chevrolet. The car broke down in eight months but did get me to my evening job. We then put up $400

R.M. Doroghazi, *The Physician's Guide to Investing*,
DOI 10.1007/978-1-60761-134-9_21,
© Humana Press, a part of Springer Science+Business Media, LLC 2005, 2009

each for a 1964 Plymouth Belvedere (with the push-button gears on the left side of the dash) that gave good service for 3 years.

If a loan is made to purchase a car, keep the term of the note as short as possible. A five-year car loan is a terrible drain on resources. Apparently there are now six-year car loans – I have heard they come with a ball and chain. Leasing a car is even more undesirable. You may be enticed into leasing to be able to drive a more expensive vehicle than you could otherwise afford to purchase. Leasing a car is literally throwing money away. It is infinitely better to purchase a less expensive car that you can afford than to lease. At the end of the lease you have nothing.

GENERAL GUIDELINES FOR BORROWING

This is one of the most difficult areas of money management and investment advice: What is an appropriate amount of debt? Before providing a detailed discussion with many examples, I will make two general, easy to remember points:

BORROW ONLY FOR YOUR EDUCATION AND YOUR HOME
THE LESS DEBT, THE BETTER

When you become a self-supporting adult, one of the first things you (and your spouse) should do is promise yourself you will not borrow for anything besides your education and your home. If you can do this, you have taken your first step toward a life of financial security.

Whenever buying anything, consider the item being purchased. Is it a depreciating asset or an income-producing asset? The former relates to consumption and taking on debt for such a purchase is to be strongly discouraged. You will never accumulate real wealth buying depreciating assets on credit. A car or boat is a perfect example. Unless you have terrible motion sickness, boats are cool, truly a blast. But every day that goes by, every time the key is turned on, the boat is worth less. I suggest that depreciating assets be purchased with cash (if purchased at all).

Several years ago, at the top of the credit bubble, I saw an advertisement in a Lake of the Ozarks real estate/boating circular freebee. It said that with proper credit, you could obtain financing for a new or used watercraft at a low interest rate with up to two hundred and forty months to repay. Two hundred and forty months = TWENTY YEARS.

Consider the math. You purchase a boat for $250 K (This is not expensive. In many places you would still be in the low-rent district). There is a down payment of 20% with the standard interest rate of 7%. The note is amortized over seven thousand two hundred days (240 months times 30 days a month). The total is about $422 K of principal plus (non-tax deductible) interest (I would never be in such a situation because I would have worried myself to death). How many cars are still running after twenty years? The floorboards are rotted out by then. If the boat is still sea-worthy, it is now worth just pennies on the dollar. You do not need many such purchases to live a life of never-ending debt and financial instability. I have heard two appropriately cryptic phrases to describe such a situation: "A nickel down and a nickel a month", and "A dollar now, the rest when you catch me".

Examples of income-producing assets include the farmer's purchase of a tractor or a physician's purchase of a piece of practice-related equipment, such as an EKG machine for the office. Successful businesses operate by the purchase of income-producing assets with a manageable amount of debt. The strategic use of debt can result in significant profit.

What is an appropriate amount of debt for you? There are a variety of formulas and recommendations that relate amount of debt to income or net worth. At the height of the real estate bubble, lending institutions used the following guidelines: Up to twenty-eight percent of gross income could be used for mortgage payments. Some lenders even stretched this to thirty-two percent of gross income (I have seen some numbers even higher). The other standard figure was that no more than thirty-six percent of gross monthly income could be used for total debt service (mortgage plus car plus credit cards plus student loans, etc.). I viewed these formulas with significant caution as they define the absolute maximum amount of debt that can be carried. Subsequent events confirmed my concerns. Should you wish to use guidelines, I suggest that the maximum amount of debt allowed be reduced by at least fifty percent. I suggest that no more than 15% of gross income go to mortgage payments and no more than 20% of gross income go to total debt service. As the current credit crisis unwinds, lenders are returning to more traditional, i.e. tighter, more responsible, lending standards (and as often happens, they very well may tighten too far, resulting in a credit crunch). Remember, the less debt the better.

Let me make some practical suggestions. If "everything must go perfectly" to service debt, it will not. If your income drops by fifty percent, could you still service the debt? This happens all-to- often in two wage-earning families when one person loses their job (unemployment is on the rise). If the debt was to be serviced from the anticipated income stream from the investment, could the debt still be repaid if the investment failed completely? Remember that debt mandates caution, natural control mechanisms are being circumvented.

Borrowing money is easy, far too easy. You just sign you name. Fifty thousand dollars, one hundred thousand dollars or even more. The amount seems like an abstract, just numbers on the page, blips in a computer memory.

Until recently, banks only loaned money to people with a solid down payment and other assets for collateral. Since local banks were loaning money to local people, the character and integrity of the borrower was also an important issue. The banks, quite appropriately, only loaned money to those they felt would pay it back. As the (now) old saying goes, banks only loaned money to people who did not need it. We are in trouble because banks abrogated their responsibility and started to loan money to people who really did need it (and not surprisingly, could not repay).

Many years ago, when a bank made a loan, it was usually directly from their deposits and their capital, money right out of their depositor's and the bank president's pocket. And he or she had no intention of loaning money if it could not be repaid. Now, debt is just too easy to obtain.

Here is the problem that confronts physicians. Because of their high income and cash flow, banks are delighted to loan money to physicians, and often in large amounts. One hundred thousand dollars, a quarter-million dollars or more. All that is required is a signature.

The first concern with any investment is not how much you can make (this encourages greed) but rather how much can be lost. If a $50,000 investment is made with cash on hand and it fails, that is of course terrible. Fifty thousand dollars is a lot of money, essentially a full year's savings for the average physician. But put it behind you, learn from the experience, and move on. Do not attempt to "make it up" on the next investment, as this will only compound the errors. This is no different than a gambler who is losing doubling their bet after each loss in an attempt to get even. It is inevitable that you will run out of money before getting even. And if you should happen to get even, it is very unlikely you will stop.

But if a $50 K investment made with borrowed money fails, you still owe the money. What if you are unable to repay? The bank can, and will, use any means at its disposal to collect. You should be working for yourself and your family, not the bank. (*See* Chapter Twenty-Seven on Dealing With Bankers).

The US Government has four options to repay its debts. It can print more money, and the presses are smoking. The government (at least now) can also re-finance, or rollover, the debt indefinitely. But a private citizen has only two options: you either pay off the debt, or you renege and declare bankruptcy. ALL DEBT MUST EVENTUALLY BE REPAID.

Let me make a comment about bankruptcy. The sanctity of contracts and protection of private property are cornerstones of our democracy. Hayek noted that economic and political freedom are inseparable [1]. Countries where private property is confiscated are called communists. Borrowing money is a contract. If you should loan someone money you certainly expect to be repaid. When you borrow money you are expected to repay it. To declare bankruptcy is to break your word. The most desirable way to avoid this is to never allow yourself to be in a position where it could happen.

THE PROBLEMS WITH LEVERAGE

Another word for debt is leverage, and it works both ways. If the benefits are doubled, the risk is doubled. Actually the risk is more than doubled. Consider as an example the purchase of a publicly-traded security. A $10K position in the NASDAQ Index 100 Trust (QQQQ) is purchased with cash. A 10% increase in the value of the security represents a gain of 10%. A 10% drop in the value results in a 10% loss.

But you borrow to increase the potential gain. Twenty thousand dollars of the QQQQs are purchased, $10 K with cash and $10K on margin borrowed from the brokerage. A ten percent increase in value of the QQQQs now represents a $2,000 profit (minus interest charges and commissions), which is a 20% return on $10K. Just by signing your name the return has doubled.

But what if the QQQQs drop 20% in price? This represents a 40% loss. Just as a gain is doubled, a loss is also doubled. Not only can you lose more with debt (leverage or margin), but the investment itself is less secure, less well capitalized. If the price of QQQQs drops by another 5% (or a total of 25%), because of the leverage the investment is now down 50%. At this point you receive a margin call from the broker. Either more money or securities must be deposited in the account (today!!) or the position must be liquidated, at, of course, the worst possible time. (The Federal Reserve sets the general margin requirements. Each specific exchange and brokerage house can set further margin requirements. These may change at any time. The brokerage house must, and will, liquidate some or all of your position if the margin call is not met). Now you have lost 50% and your position. As Warren Buffett notes, it is easy to put leverage on, it is not as easy to take it off. Buffett also says "The only way a smart person can go broke is through borrowing".

As a general rule, you should not meet a margin call with more capital. The margin call is telling you that the trade is going so badly that you must exit and cut your losses. The average physician investor has no business buying stock on margin anyway. If things go badly, do not blame the brokerage firm, blame yourself. In general, when things go wrong you are much better served blaming yourself than others. You cannot change other people, but you can change yourself.

Let me give an example of leverage (debt) involving real estate. A piece of rental property is purchased for $200 K with a 30% down payment, the remainder is borrowed. The value of the property drops 10%. Because of the solid down payment there is still a nice equity cushion, and the rental payments of $1,500 more than cover the monthly mortgage payment of $1,000. If the rental receipts drop by 10% to $1,350 a month, there is still a strong positive cash flow.

Now consider the same property with only a 10% down payment. If the value falls 10% there is no equity and if sold at this time, the 6–7% real estate commission and other charges come straight out of the seller's pocket. Because more money was borrowed, the monthly mortgage payment is higher at $1,350. If rental receipts drop 10%, there is now only enough to cover the monthly payment. Should there be any additional expenses, and there always are, the difference will come directly out of the owner's pocket. Should rental receipts drop further, cash will be required every month just to cover mortgage payments. Now consider this example with no down payment: it would be called a foreclosure.

An excessive amount of debt can destroy an otherwise completely solid investment. Under-capitalization is one of the most common causes of business failure. Say you invest in three limited partnerships or buy stock in start-up companies. Each position is $100 K, you put down $10 K on each and borrow the remainder. With only $30 K it is possible to make more than a quarter of a million dollars of investments. The total rate of return, if initial projections are correct, is 25% or 30%, or even more, a year (Beware of projected returns, they are no more than someone's guess. They always seem to go up so nicely. They are sometimes correct, usually far too optimistic, never too low).

What if everything does not go as planned, the economy softens, or it was a poor business plan. More ominously, what if all three investments fold and have no residual value (this has happened)? The dreams of riches have been replaced by the reality that you still owe the bank $270K, or as with the physicians described in Chapter Four, three to ten million dollars.

The amount of debt is often considered as a percentage of the entire investment. This is quite reasonable in the situation with which most people are familiar, namely, their home mortgage. Even if things go badly, there is still residual value.

However, you must *never* lose sight of the absolute amount of debt. Say that $300K cash is invested and $700 K is borrowed to participate in a limited partnership, or any kind of business. What if the investment goes bankrupt and there is no residual value or residual assets? What if the whole thing is a scam? Not only have you lost $300K, but you still owe $700,000. That is a lot of money! Our average physician makes $250 K per year. Before this investment, there was a solid net worth of 1.2 million dollars – Two hundred thousand of equity in a $325 K home, $100K of equity in a $200K vacation condo, $700 K in retirement accounts and $200K of non-retirement investments. Now you wiped out. Never lose sight of the absolute amount of debt. It is real money that at sometime must be repaid. There is little reason for the average physician investor to take on a large absolute amount of debt, no matter how apparently solid the business or investment. You are safer to embrace Dracula at midnight by the light of a full moon in Transylvania than take on such amounts of debt.

THE EARLY REPAYMENT OF DEBT

I will now change the focus from taking on debt to the question of paying off debt ahead of schedule. You can rarely make a better investment than the early repayment of debt.

For purposes of continuity in this book, I propose that the average physician makes $250K a year, has purchased a $312,500 home on which was made a 20% down payment resulting in a $250K mortgage at 7% interest. The average anticipated return on investments is 10% per year.

What is the return by accelerating debt payments? Seven percent? Ten percent? No, it is 17% (7 + 10). Just look at the numbers. At the end of a year, one dollar minus seven percent interest = 93 cents. At the end of a year one dollar plus a ten percent return = $1.10. A slam-dunk 17%. And your general financial position is also more secure because of less debt.

This is also an appropriate time to make a suggestion regarding the investment of an unexpected lump sum of cash, such as an inheritance, tax refund, bonus, or distribution from an investment. Pay off debt. An extra $10 K placed on a mortgage represents essentially one year of principal payments.

If such a windfall is viewed as a chance to splurge, to buy something that would not have otherwise been purchased, you can stop reading this book right now and save yourself the time since you will be exceedingly unlikely to follow any of the other common sense suggestions that I make.

If you are paying on several notes each month, which should be paid off first? Consider this:

1. This is probably most important. If one loan is significantly smaller, pay it off first. Suppose there are two notes, one for $100 K (home) the other for $10 K (automobile). The monthly payments are $1,000 on each note. Ninety-five thousand dollars can be paid on the mortgage yet there are still two monthly payments of $1,000. If ten thousand dollars is placed on the second note, it is paid off, cutting monthly debt service in half.
2. What are the rates of interest? If one is ten percent and the other six percent, pay off the note with the higher rate of interest first.
3. Does one note have a variable rate, especially a rate that can fluctuate frequently and by a large amount, such as a note tied to the prime rate? Pay this off first.
4. Is the interest tax deductible? Pay off the note with non-deductible interest first.
5. Student loans are one debt you may not wish to pay off early. There are several reasons. The time that you start paying on student loans is usually when you have finished training and started practice, the same time that you need cash to buy a home, start a family, and build reserves. The rate of interest on student loans may also be quite low. Likewise, if you really are doing well with extra cash, go ahead and accelerate your payments to help make more money available to other needy students.

CREDIT CARDS

I would be remiss if I did not finish a discussion of debt without mentioning credit cards. Depending on how they are used, credit cards can be either very good or very, very bad. Credit cards are extremely convenient, and are a must when traveling. A credit card is required to rent a car. There is always a receipt. And if the balance is paid off in full, every month, then you actually have the use of someone else's money for a period fifteen to forty five days, depending on the billing cycle. I believe 2 or 3 credit cards are enough for everyone.

Many credit cards also possess advantages, such as the accumulation of credits towards subsequent purchases, such as airline miles, discounts, etc. The critical point is the fine print. Are the rewards really as great as they initially appear or are they negated, or even more than negated, by other restrictions, fees, a higher interest rate, or any other type of requirement?

I had not used travel agents for some time, but with all of the recent flight cancellations, surcharges, and the other things going on, I have again started to use them selectively to navigate the landscape. The travel agent told me the airlines are offering less and less seats to redeem your frequent flier miles, and adding more restrictions. When given a choice between cash and almost any other benefit, take the cash. For further information on the best reward cards, I refer you to www.CardRatings.com.

But just as in medicine, everything is associated with risks and benefits. Credit cards make it so easy to spend money. You would spend less if required to pay cash for all purchases rather than just opening your wallet and "flipping some plastic." Except for special circumstances, if a physician making $250K a year cannot repay credit card debt, in full, each month, there is a serious lack of financial discipline. No matter where you are in your life, if you have credit card debt, you are in big trouble.

One comment about gift cards: I recommend you avoid them. There are often fees and charges and all sorts of restrictions. Many are never redeemed. If you want to give money, give money. It may not be imaginative, but there will be no complaints.

SUMMARY OF CHAPTER TWENTY-ONE

- Debt is seductive – it can ruin your life.
- Debt has a message – you cannot afford what you are buying.
- THE LESS DEBT, THE BETTER.
- ALL DEBT MUST EVENTUALY BE REPAID.
- Do not lease a car.
- Borrow only for your education and your home.
- Avoid the use of debt for the purchase of depreciating assets.
- Current guidelines for allowable amounts of debt are far too high and should be reduced by at least 50%.
- Debt can make solid investments unstable.
- The physician investor should not purchase stock on margin.
- The longer the repayment period, the greater the burden of debt.
- Never lose sight of the absolute amount of debt.
- Use unanticipated financial windfalls to pay off debt.
- There are few better investments than the early repayment of debt.
- The best credit card reward is cash.
- If you have credit card debt, you are in trouble.
- Avoid gift cards.

REFERENCE

1. Hayek F A. The Road to Serfdom. Chicago: University of Chicago Press, 1944.

Chapter Twenty-Two
The Perniciousness of Fees

I will make a medical analogy. Fees are like a parasite. They are not virulent enough to destroy the host but over the course of your lifetime fees can (will) make the difference between a vibrant, healthy personal financial situation and just limping along, with a significant amount of the fruits of your labor ending up in someone else's pocket.

John Bogle pioneered the S&P 500 Index Fund at the Vanguard Group. His principle thesis was that the average actively-managed mutual fund does not beat the general market averages, mostly because of fees. Fees diminish the profit in funds with superior stock selection (the minority) and further aggravate the problem in funds with inferior stock selection (the majority). Bogle is correct. Actively-managed funds under-perform the passive index funds by an amount essentially identical to their fees and extra trading costs. Minimizing fees is so important that I devote this chapter and multiple other discussions throughout the book to the topic.

Bogle spoke here in Columbia about six years ago. He used as an example what a small, seemingly innocuous 1% fee (essentially equivalent to the difference in fees between actively-managed and passive index funds), when magnified over time by compound interest, can make in your ability to accumulate wealth. Say you make partner at age 35, and save 20% of your $250K salary=$50,000. Examine Table 1, where the money is

R.M. Doroghazi, *The Physician's Guide to Investing*,
DOI 10.1007/978-1-60761-134-9_22,
© Humana Press, a part of Springer Science+Business Media, LLC 2005, 2009

Table 1
Fifty Thousand Dollars

	Compounded at 9% annual rate	Compounded at 10% annual rate	Difference %	Total Amount
10 years	$118,368	$129,687	+9.5	$11,319
20 years	$280,220	$336,374	+20.0	$56,154
30 years	$663,382	$872,469	+31.5	$209,087

compounded at the standard 10% return, and then because of a one-percent difference in fees, is compounded at a 9%.

In 30 years, at age 65, a mere 1% difference per year means a 31.5% difference in the total. If you live another ten or twenty or more years, the difference just continues to widen. Or look at it this way: Over thirty years, a 1% annual difference in fees is the equivalent of almost three years return on your money. What seems like a small, innocuous, almost insignificant fee is magnified by compound interest (when working against you it is your enemy), over the course of your lifetime into a fortune. It can mean the difference between retiring several years earlier, or between a golden, or not so comfortable, retirement.

Fees are typically described as a percentage of the total amount of money invested. This is a specious (having a false look of truth or genuineness-Webster's) argument, and greatly camouflages the true significance of the fees. I suggest you look at fees in comparison to the profit, not in comparison to the total amount of money invested. A ten percent return as compared to a nine percent return is a 1% difference when compared to the total amount invested, but is a ten percent difference in the fee and thus your profit!! Ten percent. This is how you must look at fees. There is no fee small enough to ignore.

I will discuss fees in two contexts. The first is directly related to investments, the second is as it applies to almost everything.

MUTUAL FUNDS

The majority of mutual funds, and the vast majority of mutual funds in which you should invest, are open-ended funds. There is no limit to the number of shares the fund may sell. Money can be deposited, or withdrawn, any day, with the price, or net asset value (NAV) of the shares determined at the close of trading each day. In a closed-end mutual fund, the number of shares is established at the outset and the shares are traded on the exchanges like a stock. The problem with closed-end funds is that sometimes the share price trades at a premium, sometimes at a discount, to the value of the underlying holdings. Because it can be difficult to accurately determine the true value of the assets, and because this difference between the price and the value of the asset can persist for a long period of time, you should probably avoid closed-ended mutual funds and stick with the more familiar open-ended funds. The remainder of the discussion regards only the latter.

I will tell you straightaway the main point of the following discussion:

THERE IS NEVER A REASON TO BUY A MUTUAL FUND WITH A LOAD OR EXTRA FEE OF ANY KIND

Some time ago I attended a conference where the lunchtime speaker was a memory expert. He said that if you repeated something eight times a day for five days, you would remember it forever. "Now I lay me down to sleep", or "I pledge allegiance to the flag", etc. As an example, he said there were commercials that had not aired for years, but if he started it, we could finish it. The one for my age group was "Winston tastes good like a cigarette should, Winston tastes good like a . . .xx xx. . .cigarette should".

So you will never forget, I suggest that eight times a day for the next five days, you repeat: "There is never a reason to buy a mutual fund with a load or extra fee of any kind".

Open-ended mutual funds are either load or no-load. In the former, a commission, or load, is taken off the top. This can be as high (obscene) as 8%, i.e. as little as 92 cents is invested for each dollar contributed. You have lost most of your first year's return before getting started. In a fund with no front-end load, the entire amount is invested.

Funds with any sort of load or extra fees under-perform no-load funds by an amount essentially equal to the extra fees.

Don't be stupid. When there is a load of any kind, you are just giving the mutual fund company your money and receiving nothing in return.

A front-end load may not be the only fee. There may also be an exit fee or surrender charge, which means that unless the fund is held for a specific period of time you may be charged to redeem or sell the shares. These are often around 5% and graduate downward with time, such as the full 5% the first year, 4% the second year and so on. Some funds charge redemption fees no matter how long the fund is held. There is no reason to invest in any fund that charges such fees.

Many no-load funds can be purchased through the broker directly into your account. However, there may be a redemption fee if the fund is not held a particular period of time, such as 6 months. These restrictions are typically spelled out clearly when purchasing the fund. The easiest way to avoid them is not to go through a broker and invest in the fund directly.

Some genuine no-load funds will charge fees if you trade in or out more than so many times per year. This is usually spelled out clearly and I consider them legitimate. The fund does have paperwork and trading expenses when shares are bought and sold. Likewise, there are no-load funds which are structured specifically for investors who try to "time" the market. If you are trying to time the market, Exchange Traded Funds (ETFs) are a far superior vehicle compared to mutual funds, because you can trade at any time during the day, rather than only obtain the NAV at the end of the day. In fact, as I will discuss elsewhere, ETFs are in some ways making the concept of mutual funds obsolete.

Another type of fee applies to many "no-load" funds sold through brokerage firms and insurance agents. When brokers and agents sell a load fund, it is obvious they receive the load as a sales commission. But when they sell you a "no-load" fund, they still receive a commission! The mutual fund company pays the broker a "12b-1 fee" that is taken directly from the assets of the fund. In the end, these fees are simply another extra cost paid by the investors.

The typical 12b-1 fee is ¼ of 1% and is paid *each and every year*. If at age 25, you invest $100 per month in a true no-load fund returning 10% per year, at age 65 you would have $46,000 more than if you had invested in a similar fund with a 12b-1 fee that reduced the return to 9 3/4%! My advice is to stay away from funds with 12b-1 fees; there are plenty of true no-load funds to choose from. In fact, as a general rule, there are always equivalent no-load alternatives to any fund with a load.

Mutual funds must charge some management fee to cover their legitimate expenses such as rent, personnel, advertising, and trading costs, and make a profit. Unfortunately, this desire for profit has so perverted the mutual fund industry that Swensen (*see* Chapter Thirty-Eight) says "The mutual fund industry fails America's individual investors". The Motley Fool (www.fool.com) shares Swensen's opinions. More information on the mutual fund families is free at www.finra.org the website of the Financial Industry Regulatory Authority, a non-governmental oversight group.

There are two general types of no-load funds, index (or passively-managed) funds and actively-managed funds. Passive funds mirror an index, the best known being the S&P 500. These funds are commodities. There are no decisions on what to buy or sell, the fund just stays balanced to the index. As an illustration, the expense ratio of the Vanguard S&P 500 Index is approximately 0.15%. The average S&P 500 Index Fund has an expense ratio of 0.4%. These are the benchmarks against which the fees of all mutual funds should be measured.

The management fees at legitimately run actively-managed mutual funds are usually around 1%. However, studies have shown that, over a long period of time, only about 20% of actively-managed mutual funds out-perform the Vanguard S&P 500 Index Fund. As recommended by John Bogle, Warren Buffett, David Swensen and Burton Malkiel, the core stock position in your portfolio should be the Vanguard S&P 500 Index Fund.

One to several times a year, the principal financial publications, such as the *Wall Street Journal*, *Barron's*, and *Forbes*, publish rankings of the mutual funds. There are actively-managed funds that do, usually over a short period of time, out-perform the index funds. Half of the time this is due to just plain luck.

And if there is a fund manager who is a star and consistently beats the market, they are often hired away by private money managers where they can make 10 or more times as much. Stick with the index funds.

Morningstar publishes mutual fund ratings which Swensen calls "backward looking and naïve". See my profile on David Swensen in Chapter Thirty-Eight and his book *Unconventional Success* [1] for a sober, eye-opening look at our mutual fund industry, and from which many of these points are taken.

Some funds unfortunately charge "management" fees that are even higher. It can be difficult or impossible to determine the exact amounts, even after reading the prospectus. These higher management fees do not result in superior performance.

Fees obviously count a great deal when buying a mutual fund, or for that matter, anything. What seems like a tiny number, when magnified over the course of your investing lifetime, can result in a significant amount of money in your pocket – or in someone else's.

STOCKBROKERS

When choosing the stockbroker that best fits your needs, first determine if you want someone's advice and recommendations, or if you make your own decisions. With a full-service broker, you work with your broker, just as you are someone's physician. The stockbroker can give suggestions based upon his or her expertise and judgment and provide research to which they have access. The commissions (fees) at a full-service broker are *very significantly* higher than with a discount broker. If you make your own decisions and just need a broker to execute the trade, you should use a discount broker.

Before discussing discount as compared to full-service brokers, I must warn you of something. *Never*, under any circumstance, purchase a stock or any investment from a "cold call", someone who calls and wants your business, no matter how legitimate they or their firm may sound. I suggest you read *Born to Steal: When the Mafia Hit Wall Street* [2] to see what can happen in such situations.

There is never any reason to buy anything from a telemarketer's "cold call." The first reason relates to the above scenario. The overwhelming majority of telemarketers are legitimate. Some may not be. Why take a chance? If you passed someone on the street who you thought could even remotely be a crook would you stop and talk to them, much less consider buying something from them?

The other reason never to deal with any cold caller is based on logic. Someone who knows nothing about you is telling you what you need, what is best for you. If I need a new pair of shoes I go out and buy them. Imagine a cold-caller saying "Robert, you should buy some new shoes today." Now substitute the name of a stock or a real estate investment or a limited partnership for a pair of shoes. Buying anything from a cold-call telemarketer is illogical.

I feel the *vast* majority of people are adequately served by a discount broker (*see* Chapter Thirty-Seven for a further discussion of the factors involved in choosing a broker). There is a spectrum in the quality of stockbrokers just as there is a spectrum in the quality of physicians. I make my own decision and do not require their service. In fact, I will relate why I do not use a full-service broker. As mentioned previously, I collect baseball cards and sport memorabilia. In the late 1980 s, Topps (TOPP), the largest baseball card company, went public. I was convinced the stock would do well. This was the exact time that the baseball card hobby was absolutely exploding. I called my full-service broker three times over the course of several months. Three times he talked me out of buying the stock. Over the course of the next four years the stock went up four to five times. Ten thousand dollars would have grown to $50,000. I could have made forty thousand dollars on baseball cards! I said to myself, "forget full-service brokers." I decided if I was going to make or lose money, I would do it by my own decisions, rather than paying a "professional" to do it for me.

It is not an exaggeration to say that this was one of the two or three most important events of my investing career. It was the realization that I know as much, or more, than an "expert." I am an expert on baseball cards and I clearly knew more about this subject than this Wall Street "pseudo-expert." Burton Malkiel's first recommendation in *The Random Walk Guide to Investing* (*see* Chapter Thirty-Eight) is "Fire your investment advisor" [3]. As the Internet bubble, housing bubble, sub-prime mess, Bear Stearns, Lehman Brothers, AIG, Fannie Mae, Freddie Mac meltdown has shown, just because someone works on Wall Street, or at a brokerage house or investment bank or hedge fund, does not mean they are a genius or will make you money or give you good advice. For the significant majority of investors, you will make more money in the long run, in fact, significantly more money, investing in a no-load index fund (such as S&P 500, Wilshire 5000, etc.) than trying to beat the market with the advice from a full-service broker.

When you use a stockbroker you must decide if you want to speak to someone directly or if you will trade on-line yourself. If you make your own decisions, all that matters is an adequate execution of the trade at the lowest possible commission. I will discuss on-line brokers in more detail in Chapter Thirty-Seven. My recommendation is if you wish to buy specific stocks make your own decisions and execute your trades on-line. Otherwise, income-average into an index fund with the lowest fees. Avoid full-service brokers. To again quote Swensen "The incremental fees paid for broker-assisted transactions purchases only a human voice".

OTHER FEES

There are fees and commissions for everything. Fees are a financial four-letter word. I have already provided multiple examples of how seemingly miniscule fees make a real difference in your ability to accumulate wealth. Everyone wants a piece of your hide. The word fee should immediately alert you that someone wishes to separate you from your money. Many things may not be called fees but are fees none-the-less. In general, anything added to the basic cost of an item is in one way or another a fee. You must be ever vigilant. Question all charges on a bill, not only because it may be a fee but because honest mistakes can be made. It may have an impressive sounding name, but it is often just a fee. A fee is either money in your pocket or someone else's. Which would you prefer?

Let me provide an example of how ubiquitous fees are in everyday life. In 2004 my younger son Michael purchased a cellular phone. Fee to initiate the service – $50. It does cost the company something to initiate the service, but this is still a fee (I always wonder why so many fees are a round number such as $50. The true fee could have been $31.87 rounded up to $50. You can be sure it was not $57.18 rounded down to $50). Michael had never taken out or paid on a loan or credit card and thus had no credit history. Because of this, an additional $150 deposit was required. The customer service rep told Michael that only two of the 31 people who purchased a cellular phone that day did not require a deposit. (It would be interesting to know the exact criteria for a deposit). I said in the first edition that "The deposit will be returned after one year (*hopefully*)". I got that one right. It is 2008 and my son still has not gotten his money back, and I assure you he has tried. There are people who do not honor their contract, and they are presumably the genesis of the security deposit. Likewise, it seems that the company has quite liberal criteria (favoring them) for requiring a deposit. Whatever the reason, the "fees" on this phone contract represented the equivalent of three days pay on his summer job. Or consider this: If my son had gotten the $150 fee back on schedule and deposited it into an IRA with a compounded annual return of 10%, this would grow to $11,000 by age 65. Minimize fees whenever you can.

The above example is similar to an escrow. Escrow is when a third party holds money that will eventually be paid to whom it is owed, essentially for safe keeping. The average physician will most likely encounter an escrow as it relates to paying expenses on a home, such as insurance or real estate taxes. For example, the real estate tax of $2,400 is due in December. The bank will require the person they loaned money for a mortgage pay $200 to the bank every month with their mortgage payment. The bank will keep the money in an escrow account (some are interest bearing, but most are not) so that by December sufficient money ($200 × 12 months = $2,400) has accumulated to cover the bill for the property tax.

For the average physician who makes the average physician's salary and pays their bills on time, there is no reason to make escrow payments. The reason is not only that you do not have control of your money, but you lose the interest, dividends and capital gains (i.e. – average 10% annual return) the money would have generated. Another real problem with escrow accounts is that examples have occurred where the lender has collected the money but failed to make the payout, resulting in the lapsing of the homeowners insurance or non-payment of property taxes. In the current credit crisis, there have been reports of firms holding funds in escrow going broke. Money presumed to be safe has disappeared. If an escrow account is suggested, say NO! A bank should not require an escrow account for a preferred customer such as a physician. If the bank says it is required (it is not), take your business elsewhere. An escrow account is no more than a fee.

There are occasional situations where an escrow account is appropriate. When entering into an investment, where your commitment is required now (say April 1st) but the partnership does not officially start until June 1st, the money (say $100K) will be held in escrow until that date. Assuming the standard 10% return, each day $100,000 is out of your possession, not working for you, is a loss of more than $27. Make the commitment whenever it is required, but do not deposit the money until the last possible day. Attention to such detail is money in your pocket.

Remember this simple rule: ALL FEES ARE NEGOTIABLE. This could save you money every time you walk into a bank and a good deal of the time when you conduct any business. A physician has financial clout. Use it! Banks and businesses want your business. You are not a 16-year-old part-time hamburg-flipper who comes to the bank, hat in hand, in hopes of obtaining a car loan. You are a physician, a respected member of the community, making a six-figure salary and hopefully with a very solid financial position. Use this clout to minimize fees, to obtain lower interest rates on loans, to obtain any perk or extra you can.

Some banks give "points or rewards" for the total amount of business with that bank. For example, if you have a particular amount of points the bank will add 0.1% to the interest rate on a CD. This is free money, take full advantage of it. Likewise, make sure this does represent real value. If this bank offers a 4.0% interest rate on a 5 year CD and with your points the rate is increased to 4.1%, yet a bank next door offers a rate of interest of 4.25% on the same CD, then it may not be the bargain that it appears (make sure that the CD is insured by the FDIC or FSLIC).

Insist on lower fees and you will receive them. The average physician should have enough clout to potentially negotiate away points on a mortgage. When applying for a mortgage loan, the loan officer will often tell the physician, especially new physicians in town, that they must open a checking account or accounts at the bank to receive the loan. This is just hype, it is not required. If you do wish to open further accounts, use it as leverage. If you do not, just say no. If you do not receive what you want, take your business elsewhere, where you will receive lower fees. The end point of every business deal is whether you do it or not, whether you say yes or no (*see* Chapter Twenty-Six). If you do not receive the terms you wish, the lower fees, the better interest rate, say no and take your business elsewhere. If you get up and start to walk away, the bank president will tackle you before you get to the door. You are a preferred customer.

If you are in private practice you may have further influence with banks, lawyers, accountants, and almost any business that your practice does business with. Use this as leverage to your advantage.

Never be afraid or embarrassed to ask. The worst that can happen is someone says no. It is more likely you will receive what you want, and even more. Even if they say no, they will respect you more for asking. In fact, they will realize you are not "The Mark" but rather a physician with some business savvy and guts.

One dollar here, five dollars there, fifty dollars. Fees are everywhere and if they can be minimized you can save money every day. Over the years the power of compound interest will magnify by many times every penny saved on commissions and fees. The great Benjamin Franklin was almost right. A penny saved is more than a penny earned (For more financial advice by Franklin, see reference [4].

SUMMARY OF CHAPTER TWENTY-TWO

- Fees are like a parasite. They can drain you of your financial health.
- Even apparently "tiny fees" can represent large amounts of money over time.
- Look at fees in comparison to the profit, not to the total amount invested.
- AVOID ALL MUTUAL FUNDS WITH A LOAD.
- Many "no-load" mutual funds have considerable fees. Read the fine print.
- Stay with open-ended mutual funds. Avoid closed-end funds.
- Core investment positions for all investors should include index funds with the lowest fees.
- Full-service brokers rarely justify their higher fees.
- If you make you own investment decisions, execute your trades as cheaply as possible.
- Fees are everywhere. They must be minimized.
- Anything added to the basic cost of an item is a fee.
- ALL FEES ARE NEGOTIABLE.
- There is never any reason to buy anything from a cold-call telemarketer.
- Avoid placing money in escrow whenever possible.
- Physicians are preferred customers. Use this to minimize fees and obtain perks.
- Fees are either money in your pocket or in someone else's.
- Just ask and you will be amazed how much you can receive.

REFERENCES

1. Swensen D F. Unconventional Success: A Fundamental Approach to Personal Investment. New York: Free Press, 2005.

2. Weiss G. Born to Steal: When the Mafia Hit Wall Street. New York: Warner Books, 2003.
3. Malkiel B G. The Random Walk Guide to Investing: Ten Rules for Financial Success. New York: W W Norton, 2003.
4. Benjamin F. The Way to Wealth, and Other Writings on Finance. Edited by Isaacson W. New York: Sterling, 2006.

Chapter Twenty-Three
Divorce: Beware of Gold-Diggers

Because of my interest in financial matters, and because I protect people's confidence, they share things with me that can be personally embarrassing, providing me with many of the quotes, scenarios and insights in this Chapter. Also let it be noted at the outset that I am divorced. Nothing here should be considered applicable to my personal situation.

I have heard that one way to get rich is to keep your first home, your first job, and your first spouse. Although terribly trite, it is quite true. One-half of marriages end in divorce, and one-half of those that do not are unhappy. The implication is that if the opportunity arose, the unhappy spouse could split.

If there is no prenuptial agreement, in general, the property accumulated during the marriage is split evenly. But your net worth is cut by more than half. In addition to the legal expenses, there may be an essentially forced liquidation of your home, vacation property or other investments to raise cash for the settlement, plus the lost opportunity of more profitable uses of your capital while your money sits in limbo awaiting the final judgment. I know of one physician forced to keep almost a million dollars in a money market account for almost two years during the bull market of the late 90 s, foregoing a half-million dollars of gains.

At a 10% annual compounded rate of return, money doubles in slightly more than 7 years. Since your net worth is cut by more than half, a divorce from your first spouse will cost you *at least* 7–10 years of your investment life. Divorce is like dropping a nuclear bomb in your investment portfolio, not to mention your family and emotional life.

R.M. Doroghazi, *The Physician's Guide to Investing*,
DOI 10.1007/978-1-60761-134-9_23,
© Humana Press, a part of Springer Science+Business Media, LLC 2005, 2009

A prenuptial agreement is your best protection. But you must understand it is not foolproof. Even a million word, 2-foot-high contract will not completely protect you when the other party will not, or can not, live up to the agreement. Since most physicians have not accumulated significant assets at the time of their first marriage (and, in fact, are often in debt from student loans, *see* Chapter One), a prenuptial agreement is usually not executed. Of course, if you do have significant assets, it is mandatory.

A prenuptial agreement is MANDATORY for a second, or later, marriage. You have probably been in practice for some time, with a solid six-figure income, and a significant personal net worth. Do not allow love and passion, no matter how intense, to overwhelm your sanity.

You also must understand that at this time you have become the target of the army of crass opportunists appropriately called gold-diggers. Leprechauns, mermaids and unicorns are make-believe. Gold-diggers are real, and you are now their mark. They could not care less about a 28- or 30-year-old house officer or fellow working 90 or more hours a week (at least it was that long in the good old days) and making less than a truck driver. They want big game. The cross-hairs of their scope are on the bull's eye over (of) your heart. They want the luxuries and social prominence your money and position can bring. They want to live in a big house, drive a cool car, wear lots of diamond-studded bling-bling, and go to exclusive parties, expensive fundraisers, and exotic vacation destinations. They want you.

Seven centuries ago Dante Alighieri wrote *The Divine Comedy*, arguably the greatest poem of the Middle Ages. In the Inferno and Purgatorio, Dante is guided by his hero, the Roman poet Virgil (author of *The Aeneid*). He is shown through Paradiso by Beatrice, and ultimately, St. Bernard is Dante's last guide in the after-life. In the Inferno, there are nine Circles of Hell, the greater the sin, the lower the Circle. Money grubbers are in the 4th Circle, murderers the 7th Circle, and procurers and seducers the 8th Circle. Dante would banish gold-diggers to Caina, the first zone of the 9th Circle, in the Pit of Cocytes, reserved for those treacherous to family and relatives, within site of the three-headed Lucifer, (paradoxically) frozen in ice at the center of the earth, inflicting eternal pain by gnawing on Judas, Cassius and Brutus, the greatest traitors to humanity.

What should suggest someone is more interested in your wallet than who you are? When a person you know is on your side, who has your best interest at heart, such as a sib, cousin, or close, dear friend of many years, tells you you are being manipulated, being played for a patsy, please heed their advice.

It seems that in high school the really popular members of the opposite sex rarely gave the hard-working, goal-oriented, average-looking guys much notice. One has to wonder what has changed in the intervening 20 or 30 years to make you so appealing. Have they finally come to appreciate your intellect, honesty and character, or do "money glasses" have the magical power to turn a sow's ear into a silk purse?

A prenuptial agreement is near worthless unless faithfully and meticulously implemented. Your lawyer must provide you with detailed instructions before the marriage so you have the appropriate accounts, trusts, etc., in place before tying the knot. The basic premise is that you must keep what is yours strictly segregated into accounts in your name only. If money that is yours by agreement is deposited in an account with their name, it will be argued that it has become marital property. Your well-laid plans and your position have been compromised.

The problem that may arise is that you are a good person, you wish to show trust in your new spouse, to welcome them into your family as an equal member. Your sincere, good-faith intentions are laudatory and are to be commended, but please do not do it. Think of a prenup as an insurance policy. If you end up living happily ever after, it makes no difference. But if things go sour, or if your spouse starts saying things like "you're putting my name on that, aren't you? You're including me and my family in your will, aren't you? Why don't you give me your power of attorney?" you will be happy as a clam that you have a strong prenuptial agreement and that you faithfully stuck to it.

Want to hear one that will curl your hair (or what is left of it)? A physician had planned for several years to retire and wound down his practice. He planned that living expenses would be covered by the return on his investments and her salary. The very week he retired, the week the really big money stopped, she was gone. It was only because he was a good investor and had a good prenup that he did not have to go back to work. As they used to say on Hill Street Blues "please be careful out there". Have a prenup and stick to it.

Consider the flip side of a prenup, i.e., if you are marrying someone with significantly more money than you. I would insist on a strong prenup and make sure it was strictly executed. I worked hard for what I have, and I could not stand if anyone accused me of being a gold-digger.

If your marriage is going badly, do not hope that expensive gifts will smooth things over. First of all, they will not. As it relates to this discussion, gifts are the property of those who receive them. I have heard of several times where the person made sure to say "now this is a gift isn't it (almost as if a court reporter were there)"? Also, beware of things that are not gifts, such as a piece of art purchased for the home, but they allege it is a gift so they can get it. These things can get terribly nasty.

Stories I have heard about gold-diggers remind me of a comment about dealing with Stalinist Russia. "What's mine is mine, what's your's is negotiable."

The term "amicable divorce" is second only to "pleasantly demented" as possibly the stupidest comment I have ever heard. By definition, someone asking for a divorce is telling you they do not love you, they want at least half of the money you have worked so hard to accumulate, and they want future compensation (alimony) for the rest of their lives. The soon-to-be ex may even wish to deny you access to your children. What is amicable about this?

Divorce is a war, the fight of your life. To those who have not had first hand experience with divorce, this will seem so over-the-top as to compromise my credibility. If you have been through a contentious divorce you will be nodding your head in agreement. Even if you have been involved in a medical malpractice suit that has gone to trial, the pain and anguish are an order of magnitude less, it does not even compare to that of a divorce.

At the very first sign of marital discord, you, *on your own*, see an attorney. If things eventually work out, nothing has been lost. If things do go bad, you have laid the groundwork to put yourself in the strongest possible position when things do fall apart.

How do you choose an attorney? If you have been in practice for some time, you have a personal attorney and you almost certainly have worked with other attorneys and firms through your practice or other business dealings. In addition to emphasizing the importance of a prenuptial agreement, I believe this is the most important advice in this chapter:

GET THE BEST LAWYER AVAILABLE

This will almost certainly mandate you do not use your personal attorney, or for that matter, any local talent. Go to the nearest large city and get the best divorce lawyer. Although they may seem (and usually are) expensive, you must remember that you are in a conflict that will affect the rest of your life. This sounds terribly cold and mercenary, but do not allow friendship and loyalty to your personal attorney, or other local attorneys, prevent you from securing the best talent. Do not feel guilty, (and do not let them make you feel guilty) you *must* do what is best for you. To make a medical analogy: Your local cardiac surgeon, a solid physician, good person and good friend, has never operated on a case like yours before. Wouldn't you rather have your surgery at the Massachusetts General Hospital, the Cleveland Clinic, or the Mayo Brothers (as some around mid-Missouri still call it), where they deal with this problem all the time?

Look at it this way. If you are in a dog fight and bring your toy poodle, what if the other guy shows up with a junk yard dog, the roughest, toughest, nastiest pit bull on earth? It's like bringing a knife to a gun fight. This is the battle of your life. Unless you have the absolute best legal talent available, you will lose, and lose big-time.

A good attorney should have a new will and other related documents drawn up and ready to be signed immediately after the divorce is finalized. I cannot imagine a more deplorable situation than going through a nasty divorce and dying the next day without having changed your will. And a new will is not enough. The way an asset is titled can even trump a will. For example; if you changed your will so that various assets in your estate go to charity, or your children or your sibs, but your bank account or brokerage account or IRA are still titled "payable on death" to your ex, your ex will get it.

SUMMARY OF CHAPTER TWENTY-THREE

- Get rich by keeping your first home, your first job, and your first spouse.
- Divorce will cut your net worth by more than half and cost you 10 years of your financial life.
- A prenuptial agreement is your best protection.
- Prenups must be faithfully and meticulously implemented.
- Leprechauns, mermaids and unicorns are make-believe. Gold-diggers are real.
- If you marry wealth, have a prenup so you cannot be accused of being a gold-digger.
- The gold-digger's creed: What's mine is mine, what's yours is negotiable.
- A divorce will be the battle of your life.
- Do not feel guilty if you do not retain your personal attorney to handle your divorce.
- Have a new will and similar documents ready to be signed as soon as the divorce is finalized.

GET THE BEST LAWYER AVAILABLE.

- Have a new will and similar documents ready to be signed as soon as the divorce is finalized.

Chapter Twenty-Four

Tips: Real Opportunities or Useless Information

The best way to illustrate how to differentiate a worthless tip from a real opportunity is to describe four situations. In the first three, I dismissed advice that was, in fact, a significant opportunity. The factor common to each was that the person was giving advice in their area of expertise. In the last situation, at the time I could have kicked myself for not taking the advice. Thirty years later it makes a perfect example for this book.

The first involved the president of a local bank, then and now a very good friend. His bank was owned by a holding company that also owned several other banks around the state. Over the course of several years he suggested that I buy stock in the holding company. His approach was very low key. The only time he directly mentioned this to me was when he told me of it initially. Over the next several years I was sent quarterly statements and other financial data. I looked at several, but I am very sorry to admit, just discarded the rest and did not take action.

This was at the beginning of the consolidation in the local/regional/super regional banking industry. This holding company was taken over by another bank and this bank was taken over by another bank. My investment would have grown from five to ten times over. This man knew what he was talking about. Banking was, and is, his business.

R.M. Doroghazi, *The Physician's Guide to Investing*,
DOI 10.1007/978-1-60761-134-9_24,
© Humana Press, a part of Springer Science+Business Media, LLC 2005, 2009

The second involved a patient. I took care of his father and I took care of him until I retired. He was a medical device salesman for more than twenty years. He once told me that a privately-held medical instrument maker was soon to come public. He already carried the product of a competitor, but thought they were a well-run company and that their product would do extremely well. (There are very few stronger recommendations than praise for a competitor). After the IPO in the bull market of the early 1990s, I proceeded to watch the stock go straight up. I finally bought and made some money but missed a good part of the move. The advice was from a good friend in his area of expertise.

The third opportunity involved a local businessman who inherited a building. I know this man and his family well, I had a previous investment with him, and he is still a very good and dear friend. His business is real estate and I still rely on his advice when considering a real estate investment. He asked me if I would go in with him for half of the building. I thought it was a great opportunity but I let someone dissuade me from investing (this is the second to last time I have gone against my own judgment). I have lost track of how much this building has increased in value. I would have made some very serious money.

All three of these were not tips but actual, real opportunities that I missed. All three were from reputable people dealing in their area of expertise.

When I was in medical school and during my training, I had several relatives who liked to play the ponies, so when I visited we often went to the track. We even saw the dogs run a couple of times. Once, at Roosevelt on Long Island (my cousin preferred the trotters), I was standing by this kind of sleazy-looking young man (looking back, he was actually about my age) who was checking out the horses through binoculars. He said "they took the blanket off number seven too fast, he won't win. Bet on number four". Of course I did not bet on four, who won easily. The next three races, same thing. He says why so-and-so would win, I bet on another horse, and so-and-so wins. I finally catch on that he might know what he was talking about, but then he was gone.

The point: He very well may have known what he was talking about, but in situations like this, it is still good to be skeptical of the source. At least now I am smart enough that I do not play the ponies or the pooches and I certainly would not listen to this fellow.

SUMMARY OF CHAPTER TWENTY-FOUR

- Real opportunity or worthless tip – consider the source.

Chapter Twenty-Five

Areas Where Caution is Essential or that Should be Completely Avoided

I will discuss this from two points of view, the first psychological, the second practical. Remember all advice in this section is in the context of invest only in what you know.

A simple rule – the more chic, the more glamorous an investment, the greater the chance for loss. The more an investment plays to ego, the more caution is mandated. Remember the doctor's lounge/cocktail party rule – do not invest to impress others. The goal of investing is to make money. For some people the glamour of an investment seems to be more important than the return on the investment. I would prefer a sheep farm or a concrete plant or a necktie factory that generates a 15% annual return, an investment that will double my money in five years, to a syndicate buying a thoroughbred horse that "might" be a Kentucky Derby winner, or that is producing a play on Broadway.

Another simple suggestion: I consider "traditional" investments to be cash, such as a passbook savings account or money market, a CD, the stock or bond of a major corporation, a mutual fund offered by a major reputable firm or a piece of real estate that you own directly. The majority of people should understand such investments. The further you get away from such "traditional" investments, the greater the chance of loss.

The following terms and phrases should immediately make you cautious.

R.M. Doroghazi, *The Physician's Guide to Investing*,
DOI 10.1007/978-1-60761-134-9_25,
© Humana Press, a part of Springer Science+Business Media, LLC 2005, 2009

1. Limited Partnership. In a limited partnership, the general
   partner makes the business decisions and conducts the affairs
   of the business. They may or may not have invested their own
   money. The profits are divided between the general and limited partners by whatever formula is agreed upon when the
   partnership is established. The general partner has unlimited
   liability whereas the limited partner is liable only for the
   amount they have invested or have signed in notes (thus the
   term limited partnership). An investment structured as a
   limited partnership is a completely legitimate way to conduct
   business. However, I believe more physicians have lost more
   money in limited partnerships than through any other type of
   investment. I admit I have lost money in limited partnerships
   but I have learned. A detailed discussion is warranted because
   the potential for disaster is great.

   a. It is the non-core, non-traditional investments that are
      usually packaged as limited partnerships. They are often
      more complex, more esoteric, and much more likely to
      fail.
         In *Gulliver's Travels*, after visiting Lilliput, Brobdingnag,
      and several lands in-between, Swift spoofs the British
      Royal Society when Gulliver tours the Royal Academy
      of Lagado in Balnibarbi. He describes the distinguished
      professors conducting experiments to extract sunbeams
      from cucumbers, to remove the gall, saliva and odor from
      human excrement to reduce it to its original food, to build
      houses from the roof down to the foundation, to have a
      blind man mix the colors for painters, and to feed spiders
      colored flies so they can weave silk of various hues. These
      are the exact sorts of things that in the twenty-first century
      would be packaged as a limited partnership and sold to
      physicians.
   b. Making money requires knowledge and hard work. Doc-
      tors should know this because they work hard. A limited
      partnership requires no work from the limited partner,
      aside from the initial evaluation of the investment itself,
      so the returns may be limited. I suggest that every word
      of the partnership agreement be read and fully

understood. I would also suggest that an attorney be routinely consulted before signing any partnership documents or contracts. In fact, as a general rule, if you sign any contract that you *and* your attorney have not read, you are headed for trouble. Do not be afraid to ask questions, it's your money. If you are currently an investor in a limited partnership, did you read the entire prospectus before investing?

c. OPM: Other People's Money. Many limited partnerships are structured such that the general partner personally does not invest any of their own money, all the money for the investment comes from the limited partners. Watch out here. The general partner's interests are not exactly the same as yours, and if things get tough, they could conceivably abandon the investment and just walk away. I was in a limited partnership many years ago where this occurred. When the general partner has some serious money invested, their interest is very similar to the investors. You both make money for the same reasons.

This brings up a general concept that applies to all investments. Have the general partners and executives invested their own money, do they have "some skin in the game"? Seek out such investments. These people want the investment or company to succeed as much, or usually more, than you. You can sleep a little better at night because you know they are staying up at night to make sure things go well.

d. You must understand how the profits are divided. Does the general partner receive a disproportionate percentage of the initial profits or does their share remain the same no matter how great the profit? Or do the limited partners receive a disproportionate share of the initial profits with the general partner receiving a greater percentage as the profits rise? The latter variant may be "safer" for the limited partner but will serve to cap the possible gain should the partnership be extremely profitable.

Another variant on this theme is where dividends, short-term capital gains, long-term capital gains and deductions, depreciation or tax credits are distributed on whatever particular formula has been agreed upon. Whatever the formula, be sure you understand it, and that it is equitable and not "stacked" in the favor of the general partner.

e. Completely avoid all limited partnerships sold by a salesman, broker or agent. The salesmen make their money at the time of sale from the commission, which is typically 8 to 10%. I have been unwise enough to make two such investments and both were 100% loses. A full year's standard return on investment is gone before the game has even begun. Whether the investor makes money is of no consequence to the salesman who has already made their commission. The mere fact that the investment must be sold through a salesman indicates that the general partner did not have sufficient personal funds or was not able to raise the money from knowledgeable insiders or by borrowing from banks.

Without exception, do not invest in any limited partnership sold through a salesman or broker or where the general partner makes their money through an up-front fee. You will be infinitely better served buying a CD at your local bank.

f. I devote Chapter Fourteen to the concept and importance of liquidity. In a limited partnership, your money is tied up for years; three years, five years, ten years or even longer. Limited partnerships are almost completely unliquid (i.e., cannot be sold at all, there is no market for shares in a limited partnership), much more so than real estate, which is illiquid. Even if a piece of real estate cannot be sold quickly, it may be possible to borrow against the property if there is sufficient equity. It would be much more difficult to borrow against a position in a limited partnership.

g. There is often a graduated buy-in, such as one-third at the time of the investment, one-third in one year, one-third in two years. This can be seductive because you may receive the full benefits of the investment but do not have to put up the entire amount of cash up front. Notes are signed for the amounts due at the later time and thus represent borrowing, leverage. I have seen investments fold in less than a year, but the notes that were signed are valid and the payments are still due. It is discouraging, indeed, a real bummer, to owe $25,000 on an investment that has already gone bust.

h. There is often the exclusivity angle. Because of the large buy-in – $25 K, $50 K or more – very few are eligible to invest. The investment itself often has an aura of glamour, such as a prominent piece of real estate, the purchase of an artwork or some other collectible or a venture in a foreign land. These factors are all tailor-made for a high earning but naïve physician to be separated from their money.

The above not-withstanding, you may still consider investing in a limited partnership but it is essential to know the investment and the general partner. Many legitimate and profitable deals are structured as limited partnerships. But remember my initial statement – I feel that more physicians have lost more money through limited partnerships than through any other type of investment. I remind you of the story in Chapter Four regarding the South American partnership that cost each participant between three and ten million dollars. Please be careful.

2. Tax Shelters – There are three problems with investments structured only to avoid taxes.

a. There is no such thing as a true tax shelter. There are ways to delay taxes and to minimize and decrease taxes but there is no way to truly avoid taxes. You make money, you owe taxes. You make money on Mars (and try to bring it back to the US), you owe taxes. No matter how see-mingly reputable the source, never believe anyone who claims to have anything that will allow you to avoid taxes. Accounting firm KPMG has paid $456 million (yes, million) in fines, penalties and restitution, and the indivi-duals they advised have repaid billions to the IRS over the last decade, on tax shelters sold by the firm. And if you do take some bad advice, it will be very difficult for someone with a physician-level education to plead ignorance to the IRS and the courts.

b. They are illogical. An investment should be structured to make money. If there are favorable tax consequences, such as legitimate depreciation or tax credits, all-the-better. But if an investment is structured only to generate losses, motives are misdirected. As a result the business tends to be flimsy at best.

c. Congress and the IRS are making a very concerted, and successful, effort to crack down on shelters they consider abusive. The more egregious, the more abusive the tax shelter, the more upset the IRS. Shelters meant only to evade taxes are a red flag. You could be exposing yourself not only to interest and penalties, but to detailed auditing of your entire return, back auditing and future audits. If you have any questions, *see* www.irs.gov and search for "tax shelters" to see what the IRS considers abusive. If you are participating in one of these, consult a tax lawyer immediately! If you fess up to the IRS, you have a better chance to limit damage. If they find you first, and they are looking, you will feel their full power and fury. I would rather be standing at the bar next to an inebriated, thoroughly upset heavy-weight-boxing champ than have the IRS on my case (At least you could offer to buy the champ another drink). I suggest you invest with a goal to make money and pay the taxes from the profits.

3. Restaurant. Dilettante rhymes with restaurant. Webster's defines a dilettante as a "person who cultivates an art or branch of knowledge as a pastime, especially sporadically or superficially, for synonym see amateur."

Restaurateurs readily admit they cannot perform brain surgery, so why do you think you can run a restaurant? It sounds glamorous but the time commitment is prodigious. What do you do if you are performing a mitral valve replacement and the restaurant pages because a customer is upset. It is essential to hire good help and keep them. Who cooks, who goes to market to buy the fresh food and vegetables? Who keeps the books? Who cleans the dishes, the floors, the tables and the toilets? It is very difficult to operate a profitable restaurant, just as it is very difficult to be a good physician. Forget about owning a restaurant.

This also applies to any type of storefront business. Examples would be a bed and breakfast, an antique shop, a knick-knack store, anything that requires time and knowledge. If your spouse wishes to open a business, are they a dilettante or a serious businessperson? After considering leases, construction costs, furniture, inventory etc., it often cost $100,000 or more to start a business. If your spouse is business-minded and has investigated all aspects of the business venture and has the time and skill to manage the business, then it may be a good investment. Maybe your spouse will hire you after you retire.

Viewed from a different perspective, it is very unlikely that any business you might imagine will be as profitable as your primary business, i.e. – your practice. If you really wish to increase your wealth, spend at least one hour every week studying your investments and forget about opening a restaurant or any other business (except as a potential transition in your post-medical retirement).

4. International investing. This does not refer to a mutual fund managed by one of the large companies – such as Vanguard or Fidelity – that invests outside the United States, either in a general international fund, or in specific areas or countries, such as Europe, Asia, Japan, China, etc. This also does not refer to a legitimate money manager who trades in foreign securities, currencies, or businesses. It also does not refer to the stocks of large foreign companies that may be purchased on our stock exchanges as ADRs (American Depository Receipts), such as GlaxoSmithKline (GSK), Novartis (NVS), etc.

Rather, I refer to a direct investment in a company or venture in a foreign land. This may sound thrilling or even enchanting but is fraught with hazard.

a. A foreign country can change the rules at any time and often does. Many countries have a long and sordid history of the repudiation of sovereign debt. The assets could even be nationalized and there is absolutely no recourse. The big oil companies, infinitely richer and more powerful than you, have suffered the confiscation of billions of dollars of facilities. If the President did not call out the Marines for them, he will not for you.

b. Our financial markets and institutions are in general the most efficient in the world. Other countries may be much different. It may be difficult to get money into the country and difficult or impossible to get it out. There may not be adequate banking services to conduct the business appropriately and you may not even be able to sell your business.

c. Contracts must be drawn up. They will be long, detailed – and correspondingly expensive. The legal fees could easily be $100,000 or more.

d. Do you speak the language? This is a perfect example of investing in what you know, or more likely, what you do not know. Have you ever traveled to the country? What if something goes wrong? How could you find out anything about anything? Do not invest in a gold mine in China if you cannot speak Chinese. The mine might not even be there. The purchase of a duplex down the street is more likely to be profitable than a direct venture in a foreign land.

e. Just traveling to the country could be hazardous to your health. Americans are beginning to realize that the freedoms we take for granted are not the norm in many parts of the world. Graft, corruption, bribery and intimidation are the standards of business in many countries.

5. Special Purpose Acquisition Companies (SPACs). Also known as "blank check" IPOs, they are shells that raise money through an IPO to eventually acquire an operating business. Even if these involve otherwise stellar and prominent names, considering how adept even the most prominent investment banks, brokerages and hedge funds on Wall

Street have been in losing money in the recent sub-prime, credit mess, I would avoid them

6. All the potential investors are physicians. This is a guaranteed loser. This is probably one of the ten best take home points of this book. When all the potential investors in the room are physicians, the investment is a guaranteed loser. Run the other way as fast as possible. Several other physician friends who are solid investors and careful with their money have also made this observation. Whenever I make this point in one of my talks, the reaction is always the same – a somewhat sheepish laugh accompanied by a head nod indicating agreement. If there is only one physician (you) and the other potential investors are solid successful businessmen or women, then consider investing (*see* Chapter Thirty-Nine for my comments on Angel Investor Groups).

7. Penny stocks. As the name implies, these stocks sell for less than or close to a dollar, sometimes for pennies. The usual reason the stock is so cheap is that the company is in trouble. In general, when the price of a stock or the total capitalization of the company drops below some minimum value it is "delisted" off the major exchanges. Likewise, the company may never have been large enough to have gained a listing. Such penny stocks typically trade in the "pink sheets" or Over the Counter (OTC) market and have a five-letter ticker symbol. You would be wise to steer clear of penny stocks.

Penny stocks are typically the ones hyped by promoters. It is safe to say that a "pump and dump" promoter will not call to suggest the purchase of Berkshire Hathaway (BRK), currently selling at about $130 K per share. Rather they will recommend, no, strongly recommend, Acme Computers and Software, trading at 9¢ per share. "Doc, if it goes up just 10 cents, which is my minimal target in the next 2 or 3 months, you'll double your money". Ninety thousand dollars could purchase almost one million shares of Acme. Wouldn't it be impressive to own one million shares of a company?

The only time I would consider buying a penny stock is if you have a very intimate knowledge of the company, such as if you work there, or it is a local company and you can see the business and talk to the people first hand. Otherwise, it is best to avoid stocks that sell for close to or less than a dollar, for pennies.

This is an appropriate time to discuss stock splits. If a company's stock has performed well, the Board of Directors may decide to split the stock (BRK is so high because Buffett has refused to split the stock). There seems to be almost a mystique associated with stock splits, but it does not represent any more money in your pocket. One hundred shares of a stock that sells for $100 = $10 K worth of stock. The company splits the stock 2 for 1 (it may be any multiple, 3 for 2, etc.). You now own 200 shares at $50 per share = $10 K worth of stock. Voilà. Just more paperwork.

I mention stock splits under the general heading of penny stocks because of a maneuver called a "reverse stock split." This only occurs when a company is doing poorly. The price of a stock falls to 50¢ per share and the company's board declares a "reverse stock split" of 1 for 20. Instead of owning 100 shares of a stock that trades at 50¢ = $50 worth of stock, you now own 5 shares (100/20) of a stock priced at $10 = $50 worth of stock. A reverse split can camouflage a company's poor performance because, without knowing some history, it may be tough to recognize that it has occurred.

8. How about this? If something sounds bogus, it is bogus. I am not referring to poor investments that fail, I am referring to out and out scams. A great many of the scams that I have read about and heard of, and a few of which I have personal knowledge, are generally based on such a flimsy assumption they should appear obviously bogus to even the casual observer (see the mention of *Gulliver's Travels* above). If you wonder how you could make money on something, your concern and skepticism are warranted.

9. Getting in on the ground floor. Everyone would like to invest in the "next" Microsoft (MSFT) or Wal-Mart (WMT). There is the further allure of exclusivity, being in something unavailable to a regular Joe Fireman or Jane Fifth Grade Teacher. The earlier you invest in the history of a business, the greater the

chance of failure. Trying to get in on the ground floor will *significantly* increase your mistakes. Waiting for the winners to become apparent is much more profitable. A medically-related example is biotech. Purchasing a position in all of the biotech companies that came public would have resulted in significant losses, whereas waiting for the winners to emerge, such as Amgen (AMGN) and Genentech (DNA), would greatly increase the chance for profit.

a. Initial Public Offerings (IPO). Let the company prove itself first. If you do buy an IPO, I strongly recommend a limit price be placed on your order. I know a physician who bought in to Netscape, the mother of the IPO/Internet mania of the late 90's. He purchased at the opening price, which was three times what he had anticipated.

b. Closely-Held Company. Not only are these smaller, with less of a track record, but there is rarely a pre-established market. These can be very illiquid, making it extremely difficult to sell your position (*see* Chapter Fourteen).

c. Venture Capital. Unless you are in a group such as the Centennial Investors here in Columbia, which I will discuss in more detail in Chapter Thirty-Nine, I suggest you avoid trying to be a (ad)venture capitalist.

SUMMARY OF CHAPTER TWENTY-FIVE

- The more glamorous an investment, the more caution required.
- Avoid limited partnerships sold by a broker or salesman or where the general partner has not invested any of his own money.
- Avoid tax shelters.
- Forget about owning a restaurant or any storefront business.
- There is almost no business as profitable as your primary business, i.e., being a physician.
- Avoid direct foreign investments.

- Avoid penny stocks.
- An investment that sounds bogus probably is.
- Do not be concerned about "getting in on the ground floor."
- Completely avoid anything where all the potential investors are physicians.

Chapter Twenty-Six
Yes or No

There are three components to all business deals. The second and third are the final agreed upon price and details, the terms. Everything in the final agreement is important, but there is something even more important than the price or the terms, and that is whether you do the deal or not, whether you say yes or no. The price and terms are immaterial if the deal is never consummated. The best way to avoid an investment with inferior terms and/or price is to say no, to not invest.

I devote this short chapter to this point because businessmen understand this concept very well but physicians have little insight into the power of being able to say no, to just walk away from the table. This inability not only affects physician's personal investments but also is important in their professional life when they deal with businessmen in a variety of situations, such as in negotiations with insurance companies or hospital administrators.

A basic element that characterizes a physician's poor business ability is they do not realize they have an alternative. They will negotiate, in fact, often barely negotiate or not negotiate at all, and think they have obtained acceptable price and terms, but the real problem is that they should not have done the deal for any terms or any price.

Let me provide an analogy. You have a vegetable garden full of weeds. A physician will spend hours of their valuable time meticulously picking the weeds from between the vegetables.

R.M. Doroghazi, *The Physician's Guide to Investing*,
DOI 10.1007/978-1-60761-134-9_26,
© Humana Press, a part of Springer Science+Business Media, LLC 2005, 2009

After several days of hard work the final product is still inadequate, and in fact, may never be adequate, no matter how much time and effort are expended. Sometimes the best or only reasonable course is to just plow things under and start over.

Good businessmen, if they do not receive acceptable terms and/or an acceptable price, will walk away. They will consider alternatives. This takes a lot of gumption, extra time and effort, and a lot of willpower, but they will walk away.

I am not sure why this poses so much difficulty for physicians. At least part of the problem is that physicians receive no instruction on negotiating, investing and business matters (*see* Chapter One). They are almost defenseless against sharp businessmen. Another part of the problem relates to the time pressures on a physician. A physician works sixty or sixty-five hours or more a week. They have spent every spare hour of the last two weeks, time away from their family, looking into purchasing a local rental property. They feel they must complete the purchase now because the next month is completely booked with call and other time commitments. The purchase is made for a price and terms that seem reasonable but the real problem is that the purchase should not have been made in the first place.

The goal of a businessman is to make money honestly. They will put in whatever time and effort are required to make a good product or service, and thus generate a profit. A physician practicing medicine will expend whatever time and effort required to take good care of a patient. For a physician and his investments, often as little time as possible is devoted to the task. Being a successful businessman requires time and effort. Being a successful physician requires time and effort. Being a successful investor requires time and effort. A physician will work sixty hours a week for a year to generate $50,000 of investment capital and then not spend one hour studying how to invest that money. This is just plain stupid.

Sometimes when I am considering a purchase, if I do not get what I want, I say to myself "Bob, you have survived for 57 years without this, you can make it a little while longer". It makes it much easier to walk away.

Take your time. Do not be afraid to say no. In business, "No" can be much more powerful than "Yes". Remember, real opportunities occur once or twice a year or less. Unless something is begging you to go ahead, just forget it. Wait. Even after all of the time and effort, if the terms and price are not acceptable, you must be willing to say no and walk away. There are alternatives, but it takes time and effort to pursue them. Businessmen understand this, physicians often do not.

SUMMARY OF CHAPTER TWENTY-SIX

- There are alternatives: It is far better to say no than to enter into an inferior agreement.
- Being a successful investor requires time and effort.
- The goal of a businessman is to make money honestly.

Chapter Twenty-Seven
Dealing with Bankers

I began Chapter Three with a quote from Einstein. I will start this chapter with a quote from the great American writer, wit and social and political commentator Mark Twain. He said "A banker is a fellow who lends you his umbrella when the sun is shining and wants it back the minute it starts to rain." This was more than an idle comment by Twain since later in his life, in 1894, his personal financial problems became so acute that he declared bankruptcy, affording him considerable experience in dealing with creditors.

In the first edition, I was in general cynical of bankers and encouraged you to be skeptical in your dealings with them. My impression has changed considerably over this last four years. My greatest enlightenment has been to understand the constraints and regulations under which lenders operate. Likewise, I believe bankers deserve all the criticism and punishment they are currently receiving for the credit crisis, for creating new mortgage products that were so irresponsible as to threaten the foundations of our entire financial system, for abrogating their responsibility as the ones who were supposed to maintain discipline, by creating novel financial derivatives just to generate fees that even they obviously did not understand, and by taking on leverage (40 or 50 or more to 1) that can only be considered insane.

My first point is to stress the importance of having a solid, long-term relationship with multiple bankers that is based upon communication, mutual trust and respect. Just as there

R.M. Doroghazi, *The Physician's Guide to Investing*,
DOI 10.1007/978-1-60761-134-9_27,
© Humana Press, a part of Springer Science+Business Media, LLC 2005, 2009

are several times in a patient's life when they really need a doctor, there will be several times in your life when you will be in a fix and really need the assistance of a banker. The critical point is that the relationship must be on your terms, not theirs. You must realize this in order to protect yourself from potential problems.

Just as a physician understands medicine, bankers understand money, especially the power of money. If you have money, you have influence with creditors. When you have money, you will be amazed how much you can receive from a banker. When you do not have money, or when you are in debt, they have the upper hand. If you drive to the bank in your leased sports car, already in hock up to your eyeballs to borrow more money for an airplane or to open a restaurant, the lender will be in the dominant position. But if debt is kept to a minimum, if you have a Fort Knox personal balance sheet, it is possible to deal with creditors on your terms, not theirs. It is an interesting feeling indeed to be able to say "NO" to a banker. In fact, they will want your business and respect you even more. Banks very much want your deposits, this is how they have money to loan, and they know if they should loan you money they are likely to be repaid in full.

To best appreciate the potential dark side of dealing with lenders on their terms, I suggest you *personally* speak with someone who has suffered a foreclosure. Until recently you would have had to seek out a farmer who has lost his land, or your grandparents, or a friend of your grandparents, who witnessed first hand the foreclosures of the Great Depression. Considering the current mortgage/credit crisis, probably just walking down the street and visiting with one of your (soon to be ex) neighbors will be sufficient.

I am not criticizing creditors for wishing to be repaid after making a loan. I have already clearly stated that the sanctity of private property and contracts and the repayment of debt is a cornerstone of our democracy. Be assured that if I loan someone money I expect to be repaid in full and on time. If I were a banker, I would do everything they do, everything honest and within the law, to protect my interests.

Note the word bankruptcy. To be bankrupt, you must be in debt, and it is the bank that has loaned the money to allow this to occur. Banks make money by charging fees for various services and by loaning money and charging interest. Auto dealers sell cars. Grocery stores sell food. Banks "sell" money. In the first edition I said "banks have been far too lenient and aggressive in 'selling money' and encouraging debt". There are times when you wish your predictions had not come true.

In 2005, I gave a talk and said "banks should be spanked for their current lending practices". Afterwards, an officer from a very responsible bank came up and said "Bob, to maintain our profits and market share, we are loaning money to people that we would not have 5 years ago".

I responded "and in 5 years you will wish you hadn't loaned them the money". I was wrong; it only took 2 years.

Banks are delighted to loan money to high cash-flow generators such as physicians. Just as a salesman cultivates and courts a client, bankers will cultivate and court physicians in hopes of loaning them money. Over the years, I have heard several bank officers say it is the general policy of their bank that when a physician comes in, loan them whatever they want. I believe this is irresponsible, and has made it too easy for some physicians to get into trouble. This is like a surgeon saying that all a patient needs to do is show up at their office and they will operate, no matter what.

You will be charmed. Charmed into borrowing money, often in large amounts, often more than is prudent. You will be invited to dinners, parties, and receptions. You will receive free tickets and favors. You will be treated with deference to the point of punctiliousness (marked by precise exact accordance with the details of codes or conventions-Webster's). You will never be called by your first name. Instead, you will always be addressed as "Doctor," even by the president or chairman of the board of the largest banks. Three or four short years before you were a resident taking call every second or third night (you can tell how long ago I trained) vacationing only at a relative's home to avoid a hotel bill, and now you and your spouse are at the opera seated next to a bank president.

Bankers will play to your ego. Do not be seduced. Do not be charmed into more debt than is prudent. You should be working for yourself and your family, not for the bank.

The charm and deference with which you were treated when borrowing money belies the treatment if you are unable to repay. If bankers looked more like *Australopithecus afarensis* than *Homo sapiens* and it was known from the outset that you and your entire family line would disappear from the face of the earth were you unable to repay your debt, then there would be no misconceptions and you could prepare and protect yourself accordingly. Do not be charmed into complacency. I assure you that the banker who took you to the ballgame or the opera, who introduced you at a private reception at their home to your United States Senator or the Governor of your state, will use absolutely every means under the law to get their money back, including forcing you into bankruptcy. Please, do not forget this.

Every word counts when signing a loan document. Logic suggests that anything there is there for a reason. Do not allow any question to be brushed aside with a response such as "oh, that's not important" or "that almost never happens" because it is important and it can happen. Do not sign the note and find a new banker.

Some of the terms that may be included in a loan document include various requirements for collateral and the possibility that the bank can "call in" the note. Some time ago I was a partner in a group that refinanced the note on a building. A clause in the note stated that even after a partner had sold their interest back to the partnership, their name would still be on the note and thus liable for repayment. I insisted that the clause be removed and it was. I have since sold my interest and my name is no longer on the note.

NEVER sign a note that can be "called in." This refers to the bank having the option to DEMAND "accelerated repayment" of the note. Upon written notice the bank can demand payment of the entire loan balance, usually within 30 days. What if $150 K is owed on an investment and the bank "calls" the note? Even if you are in a solid financial position and the investment is going well, how is it possible to raise $150 K cash in one month? In general loans are not called in when things are going well. Instead they are called when the situation is dire, when the borrower is not doing well or when the economy is collapsing, such as during the Great Depression, or when banks need to de-leverage their balance sheets and raise capital, such as right now, today. It could very well be impossible to repay and the borrower could be forced into bankruptcy. There are few financial situations that require more caution than a note that can be "called in."

I will share a personal experience that explains my previous cynicism, and use this to provide insights on the lender-client relationship, especially my different appreciation of the lender's perspective. Some years ago I was in an investment that went bad. It was the last time I made an investment on other's advice against my better judgment and the last time I had to talk myself into something. It was also the last time I really did not know all of the details of the investment. The whole project was a terrible mess and everyone involved lost a good deal of money.

Shortly thereafter I spoke with the bank officer who was supervising the loan on the project. I said, "Did you know there were problems with this project?" He replied, "We knew the project was considerably over budget and we had our concerns." I was so incensed I felt like punching him in the nose. This banker, and his bank, knew all of the investors, had dealt with us for years, and yet did not voice their concern and therefore we ended up taking a significant loss.

It had previously been my impression that a bank loaned money because they thought the investment for which the money was being borrowed was sound. No! A bank loans money because they think the money can be repaid.

Over the next several months I asked the following question of four bankers (two presidents and two executive vice-presidents). "If I were borrowing for an investment that you thought might not be profitable, would you still loan the money if you knew I was capable of repaying it?"

Three said categorically and without hesitation "yes." The fourth said "Bob, I would try to talk you out of it, but in the end I would make the loan because I know that someone else would."

All gave the correct answer. The issue raises the concept of lender's liability. A banker can provide only so much advice, they cannot make up your mind for you. Judging the worthiness of an investment, and how it is managed, is the borrower's responsibility. This highlights the importance of long-term relationships. With a new customer, if the banker thought you could repay the money, they would make the loan. With a long-term relationship, the response of the fourth banker is most appropriate.

A failure to communicate can cause a dis-connect between the customer and the banker. The customer is often unrealistic about their personal financial position, and the banker often fails to adequately explain their position. Banking is complex and highly regulated. With a profit margin of less than 1%, just one bad loan out of a hundred results in a loss. Without knowing the banker's position, the customer may interpret inability to obtain what they want as intransigence or even animosity, rather than due to factors outside of the banker's control. Bankers also need to be more candid. They often relate only good things while avoiding the discussion of possible problems until they arise (as in the example above), fearing that the customer will be scared off and take their business elsewhere.

The current sub-prime/credit mess is a perfect example of the potential problems of dealing with a weak lender. Say you are turned down for a loan by two solid, conservative banks. This should be a signal that there are problems with your position. If you go to a marginal lender who is so eager for business that you receive a loan you should not have, they can get you into trouble.

THE FOUR "Cs"

When a customer applies for a loan, the bank considers the four "Cs", in decreasing order of importance.

1. Character has always been, and will always be, most important. Even the longest, most detailed, apparently air-tight

contract will not protect you when dealing with a scoundrel. If you agree to buy the Brooklyn Bridge, a million word, two-foot-high contract is worthless if the other party cannot, or will not, live up to their end of the deal. I once heard at a Boy Scout Regional Board meeting (I am unsure of the primary source of the quote) "When you have integrity, nothing else matters. When you don't have integrity, nothing else matters". In general, physicians are desirable borrowers because they are people of character.

2. Cash flow, liquidity, your income. When a bank makes a loan, the paramount financial issue is whether it can be repaid, and this requires cash. High income, i.e., cash flow, makes physicians desirable customers.

3. Financial Condition refers to your credit history and personal balance sheet, with amount of debt being most important. A bank is hesitant to loan money to someone already burdened with debt payments on a mortgage, car loan, student loans, other investments, credit cards, etc.

4. I thought Collateral was most important, but depending on the collateral, it is usually least important. At one extreme would be a $100K CD backing a $50K note (but then you really would not need the loan in the first place).

Poor collateral is an illiquid asset that can lose value. In the farmland bust of the early 1980s, farmers used land as collateral to purchase more farm land (a pyramid). When the bubble burst, the banks were left with an asset that was worth less and could not even be sold. This also applies directly to today's housing market; homes are losing value and the mortgages are under water. Collateral such as the family farm or a home that may be "precious" to the borrower may not be as precious to the lender.

Another potential problem is "impaired" collateral. If a borrower has a rental property and feels that default is inevitable, they may defer maintenance, remove fixtures, or just trash the place (another reason that character is so important).

Collateral is also of less importance because if the bank has to turn to secondary sources of repayment (i.e., the collateral), it is guaranteed they will suffer a significant loss. Bankers are appropriately fearful of "asset-based" lending.

There may be one or two times in your life you will be asked by a relative or friend to co-sign a note. Your desire to help may be noble but is terribly misguided. If they cannot pay, the bank goes after the person with the money = you. YOU SIGN A NOTE, YOU ARE LIABLE: PERIOD.

Being on a bank board of directors is prestigious, but if the bank experiences difficulties, you could have some personal liability. You should probably consider such an invitation only if you are very knowledgeable in banking or have a significant equity position in the bank.

SUMMARY OF CHAPTER TWENTY-SEVEN

- Your goal is to be able to deal with bankers on your terms, not theirs.
- Solid, long-term relationships are profitable for borrower and lender.
- Do not be seduced into an inappropriate amount of debt.
- Every word in a loan document is important, read it closely.
- Never sign a "callable" loan.
- To gain perspective, speak with someone who has suffered a foreclosure.
- Bank loans money only when they feel it can be repaid.
- Working with a weak lender can get you into trouble.
- The four "Cs" of lending are Character, Cash flow, financial Condition and Collateral.
- YOU SIGN A NOTE: YOU ARE LIABLE

VI Investing in Specific Assets

Chapter Twenty-Eight
Asset Allocation, Diversification and Beating the Market

It would appear that the three sections of this chapter provide disparate advice. The advice is different because the goals are different. The applicability relates to the sophistication and knowledge of the investor.

The less knowledgeable the investor, the more important it is to diversity and completely give up any thought of trying to "beat the market" In first section, I explain why the vast majority of physician investors, of all investors, should avoid any attempt to beat the market and will be far more successful utilizing index funds to capture market-mimicking returns and periodic asset re-allocation through regular portfolio rebalancing.

In the second section I note what I believe are the paradoxes of the advice to diversify, which I refer to as the "Myth of Diversification".

In the last section, I will show that to beat the market you must break most of the rules outlined in the first section. I must warn you (and this is not an exaggeration) that unless you are an experienced investor, passionate and willing to devote a great deal of time to your investments, trying to beat the market will make you nothing more than cannon fodder for the pros. You will be paying for their yachts.

R.M. Doroghazi, *The Physician's Guide to Investing*,
DOI 10.1007/978-1-60761-134-9_28,
© Humana Press, a part of Springer Science+Business Media, LLC 2005, 2009

THE IMPORTANCE OF DIVERSIFICATION: WHY YOU SHOULD NOT TRY TO BEAT THE MARKET

The principal goal for the average investor is to minimize risk while at the same time capture market-mimicking returns. The easiest, safest way to track the market is by disciplined income-averaging into a vehicle, either a mutual fund or ETF, with the lowest expense ratio. For stocks, this would be the S&P 500 Index and/or the Wilshire 5000 Index. The other requirements to achieve your goal are to diversify across multiple asset classes and optimize asset allocation by regular portfolio rebalancing.

If you let winners ride and minimize losses, you need to be right only 60% of the time to be a successful investor. One huge loss will negate many gains. In Table 1, the first investor hits four grand slams, but there was one investment outside of his area of expertise, such as a limited partnership in a highly leveraged piece of real estate, resulting in a complete loss. The four spectacular investments were almost negated by the one debacle.

The other investor has four positions that generate modest, attainable gains, and one position that just breaks even. But the overall gain is 10%, a full 25% more than 8%. If you talk to anyone who has accumulated wealth, they will tell you their first goal is to preserve that wealth. The first rule of investing is similar to the first rule of medicine: FIRST, SUFFER NO HUGE LOSS.

A well-diversified portfolio decreases risk and volatility and enhances return. Different asset classes can, but do not

Table 1
Difficulty in Overcoming a Complete Loss

Investor A	Investor B
$100 × 50% gain = $150	$100 × 15% gain = $115
$100 × 40% gain = $140	$100 × 15% gain = $115
$100 × 30% gain = $130	$100 × 10% gain = $110
$100 × 20% gain = $120	$100 × 10% gain = $110
$100 − 100% loss = $0	$100 × no gain = $100
$540 = 8% gain	$550 = 10% gain

necessarily, move independently, their performance shows varying degrees of correlation. Two oil stocks, such as Exxon Mobil (XOM) and ConocoPhillips (COP) will show a high degree of correlation. XOM and Apple (AAPL) are both stocks, but in different industries, so will show less correlation in price. Stocks and bonds may both go up (the 1980s), both go down (the 1970s) or bonds will go up while stocks go down (the 1930s and from 2000 through when this book goes to press). Stocks may show variable correlation to real estate. Some asset classes can even show an inverse correlation. During periods of rising interest rates and inflation, gold and commodities will shine while bonds tarnish. By being widely diversified across a range of asset classes, you can decrease volatility and preserve return because losses in one asset class may be offset by gains, or lack of losses, in other asset classes (For completeness, I must note that during a crash, such as 1987, the correlation of long positions in all asset classes approaches one, i.e., everything goes down).

Figure 1 illustrates a relatively tradition allocation of financial assets.

You will hear on the financial shows or through reading that someone has suggested a change in their recommended asset allocation, such as increasing stock exposure from 60% to 65% and decreasing fixed-income exposure from 40% to 35%. This is what they are referring to.

The most desirable asset mix changes over time, often significantly. In fact, it is asset allocation, being in the winners and out of the losers, that is the key to generating superior returns (*see* third section). It would have been very desirable to have

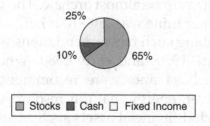

Fig. 1. Asset allocation of traditional financial investments.

been completely out of the NASDAQ from 2000 to early 2003, just as it would have been very desirable to have been in the NASDAQ from 1995 to 1999. It would have been very desirable to be in gold and silver from the early 1970s through 1980, out of the precious metals for the next two decades, and back in since 2000.

Stocks (equities) must be the core position of all portfolios. Stocks are the main asset class that generates real (after taxes and inflation) growth. A portfolio that does not have significant stock exposure will lose purchasing power over time. An investment that does not keep up with inflation is a loss. Because the US dollar has been depreciating for some time, and because some foreign economies have been growing faster than ours, and will probably grow faster than ours after the current slowdown runs its course, your stock portfolio must also have exposure to non-US markets, both via the large US multi-nationals, such as the stocks in the DJIA, and through direct exposure to the foreign markets.

Many investment advisors in the late 1990s were stating as fact there was not a need to diversify. Stocks were the only game in town, the road to riches. Just buy stocks, almost any stock, but especially those in the area of technology. The internet, computers, software, semiconductors, you can't lose. Forget price to earnings ratios, price to sales ratio, and dividend yield (dividends are important). Such traditional methods for valuing stocks were no longer applicable. These were replaced by phrases such as "the new paradigm." Cash, bonds, gold, commodities and old economy, smoke stack stocks were for old fogies. Value investors, such as Warren Buffett, and bond mavens, such as Bill Gross, were clearly so out of touch with the new paradigm as to be almost archaic. The thought of owning a gold or copper mine was antediluvian.

The people making such recommendations were probably in diapers in the late 1970s and early 1980s when the previous generation of such savants were recommending only hard assets – gold, silver, energy, natural resources and commodities. They predicted financial assets such as stocks and bonds would be dead forever.

The suggestion not to invest in other asset classes routinely comes at the wrong time, at the market top, at the exact time a prudent investor should be taking profits from the investments being hyped and rotate to other types of assets. I do not call this diversifying. To take profits in one class of assets that has had their multi-year run, that has topped out, to rotate to another class or group of assets, is a normal evolution of investing.

Fortunately, Modern Portfolio Theory provides both the intellectual basis and the practical framework to assist you with optimal asset allocation through regular portfolio rebalancing. Assume the target allocation of your $1 M portfolio is 60% stocks and 40% fixed-income. Say stocks are up 20% per year for 2 years while interest rates remain stable at 5%, giving you $864 K in stocks and $441 K in bonds. Your portfolio is now 66.3% stocks and 33.7% bonds. To return to the 60/40 allocation, you sell an appropriate amount of stocks and buy a corresponding amount of bonds. Regular portfolio rebalancing, once or twice a year, forces you to realize the goal of all investors, namely, to sell high and buy low.

I devote Chapter Fourteen to the importance of cash. The long-term return on cash is inferior to almost other asset classes. But cash has a power that nothing else has – you can buy anything and you can buy it right now. When you discover one of those real opportunities that occur approximately once a year (*see* Chapter Ten), unless there is cash available, or you can borrow money, the only options are to miss the opportunity or be forced to sell another investment (remember the commission to both buy and sell the investments will decrease your profit).

I consider a Certificate of Deposit (CD) both cash and a fixed-income investment. It is certainly the latter since you will receive a specific rate of interest for a pre-determined period of time and you will also receive the principal when the CD matures. It is also cash because it can be redeemed at anytime, although there is an interest penalty if cashed prior to the date of maturity. It is also cash because it can be used as collateral. Suppose you wish to buy a piece of real estate. You have a CD that matures in 3 months and you wish to use this money as the down payment. The bank will provide a bridge loan to cover the down payment until the CD matures.

I love CDs and feel they should represent the vast majority (or even all) of your money allocated to fixed-income investments. I have never seen a similar recommendation so I will detail why I prefer CDs to bonds:

1. Spread your money around. Try to have CDs at most of the banks in town. You have influence with the bankers where you have deposits, and you also have influence with the bankers where you do not have deposits because they see that you have money and want your business.
2. CDs really are money in the bank. You know what you have and it will only go up in value.
3. Everyone understands a CD.
4. There are no commission charges to purchase or redeem a CD. You just walk in and walk out. Contrast this to the direct ownership of a bond, where there are commissions to buy and sell, a spread between the bid and ask (you may only discover this after the sharpies clip you) or even the best managed, most efficient bond mutual fund, where there will always be some management fee. If a bond mutual fund pays an aggregate interest rate of 5% and the management fee is 0.5%, you have lost 10% of your profit.
5. CDs are not "callable." Except for Treasuries issued since 1985, most bonds have call features. If you do not understand this concept, you should not be buying an individual bond.
6. CDs at the vast majority of banks are insured by the FDIC/FSLIC for up to $100K (temporarily increased to $250 K) per account per institution (be sure to confirm this when you purchase a CD). Some bonds are insured by private companies, some are not. The current credit crisis has proven in spades that **the only guarantee you should ever accept is that of the US Government**.
7. Banks have failed and more will fail. If you are above the FDIC/FSLIC limit at any institution, you are courting disaster. Although others will probably disagree, I would suggest you bust the CDs, take your lumps on the interest rate penalty, and move your money to a safer place.

8. Even if you are below the limit, if the bank fails, your money could be tied up for some time. If the bank is publicly traded, I suggest you monitor the stock price. If it takes a nosedive, you may wish to withdraw your money. One way to monitor the health of financial institutions is via the Uniform Bank Performance Report, available at the website: http://www4.fdic.gov/UBPR/UbprReport/Search Engine/Default.asp

9. A physician does not have the ability to evaluate the credit worthiness of each individual bond issuer. The major bond rating agencies, such as Standard & Poors and Moody's, are currently taking (well-deserved) heat for their rating of debt that ended up being just junk.

10. Liquidity is not a significant problem with a CD. If you absolutely must have the money, there is generally an interest penalty for early withdrawal, but you do have your money. A good idea is to have multiple CDs and stagger the maturity so that cash is almost always available. If you have twenty CDs of varying duration and maturity, one CD will be maturing every few months.

11. You do not need to be concerned about interest rates. No one can control interest rates or predict them, so why worry about them? With a CD, you know how much money you have and the interest rate. In fact, some banks do allow you to "step-up" to a higher interest rate once during the term of the CD.

12. After the current financial crisis abates, I believe we will enter a period of inflation and rising interest rates. The longer you are locked in at an interest rate, the more "pain" you must endure until the CD matures. Thirty year bonds purchased in the 1950s and 60s were toast in the 1970s.

13. Certificates of Deposit can be purchased in your stock brokerage account, just be sure they are government insured.

Considering all of the uncertainty of bonds and all of the certainties of a CD, I suggest you avoid the purchase of any bonds besides US Treasuries (Swensen makes the same recommendation, *see* Chapter Thirty-Eight). Also be wary of investing in a bond mutual fund (Suze Orman makes the same point [1]. Utilize CDs as the vehicle of choice for your fixed-income investments.

The portfolio of the every investor should contain real estate (*see* Chapter Thirty-Two). I would not consider the equity in your home as part of your real estate investment portfolio, but I would consider any vacation or recreational property in this category. After the real estate market and economy have stabilized, I would suggest about 15%, give or take 5%, depending on your comfort level, of your entire investment portfolio be in real estate.

Despite the rhetoric, I believe it has been our government's desire to devalue the dollar. As Richard Russell of the *Dow Theory Letters* has been saying for years, to fund the national debt and the future unfunded liabilities, our government must "inflate or die". I feel "hard" assets, such as gold, commodities, natural resources and collectibles, have an important place in the portfolio of all investors (*see* Chapter Thirty-Three).

Table 2 outlines and Figure 2 represents a well-diversified portfolio that generates growth, should help you maintain purchasing power and preserve wealth during a period of inflation, and also provide safety should we experience real deflation. Please remember that these are only general numbers, they should differ depending on general market and economic

Table 2
Asset Allocation

Asset Class	Target
Stocks	
Domestic	25%
Foreign, Developed	15%
Foreign, Emerging	5%
Real Estate	15%
Hard Assets, Precious Metals, Commodities	15%
Fixed-Income (CDs and US Treasury Bonds)	15%
TIPS (Treasury Inflation Protected Securities)	10%

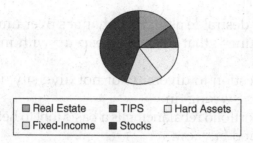

Fig. 2. Asset allocation of entire investment portfolio.

conditions, and the needs of the individual, especially your age. Choose what you are comfortable with and what seems right for you. My allocation to fixed-income is lower and my allocation to hard assets is higher than you will see elsewhere.

Let me make a point about the discipline of investing. You must always have cash for daily bills and emergencies. Cash includes your routine daily checking account and money market account. I consider everything else investments – CDs, stock market accounts, mutual funds, everything else of value. Once I get something into the "investment" category, I am loath to pull it out, except for another investment or for some other absolutely unavoidable, unexpected bill that must be paid on time, such as taxes. This self-imposed discipline helps prevent the purchase of large, often impulse-driven items such as a boat or motorcycle. It also makes you a more successful investor. In general, investments must be held for months or years to have a reasonable chance for a profit. If you are constantly buying and selling investments to have cash available for daily bills, the commissions/fees will be very significant and there will be little chance to realize a profit.

SUMMARY OF THE IMPORTANCE OF DIVER-SIFICATION

- FIRST, SUFFER NO HUGE LOSS.
- Diversification can help minimize risk and volatility and maximize return.
- When you have wealth, your first goal is to keep it.

- The most desirable asset mix changes over time.
- An investment that does not keep up with inflation is a loss.
- The suggestion to diversify, or not diversify, is routinely given at the wrong time.
- Regular portfolio rebalancing is a basic tool to help investors sell high and buy low.
- All portfolios should contain cash, stocks, fixed-income, real estate and hard assets.
- I prefer CDs (and US Treasury Bonds) as the vehicle of choice for fixed-income investments.
- Once money is in the "investment" category, leave it there.
- THE ONLY GUARANTEE TO ACCEPT IS THAT OF THE US GOVERNMENT.

THE MYTH OF DIVERSIFICATION

I always disagreed with the dogma that your home was your best investment (*see* Chapter Sixteen). Similarly all standard advice states it is mandatory to have a widely diversified portfolio. In this section I explain how the quest to diversify can cause mistakes.

The "Myth of Diversification", that you must have multiple positions in multiple asset classes, mandates investments outside your area of expertise. I submit this will increase, not decrease, your mistakes. Peter Lynch (*see* Chapter Thirty-Eight) notes than when a successful business moves out of their area of expertise, they invariably stumble, which he refers to as "diworsification".

Just as physicians specialize, I encourage you to special in a particular area of investing. You should feel comfortable, and in fact, be encouraged to direct a greater percentage of your portfolio toward your area of expertise rather than slavishly commit funds to assets you do not understand to stay "appropriately diversified". I believe it is illogical to buy positions just for the sake of diversification when you can make a larger, and almost certainly more profitable, investment in your area of expertise.

The best example of sticking to what you know is the Great One, Warren Buffett. It was suggested that he diversify from stocks, into, for example, real estate. He said essentially – "Why? I can make 30% a year in stocks, why should I even consider anything else."

Mark Twain did go a bit too far when he said "You can keep all of your eggs in one basket, but you must watch that basket closely". *Every* investor needs some degree of diversification, or you could end up suffering the same fate as the poor souls who lost their jobs and their life savings when Enron, Bear Stearns and Lehman Brothers went under. But do not let the quest for a "financially correct" amount of diversification intimidate you into making investments you do not understand. With 5 seconds to go and down by one, would you rather give the ball to your least used sub or Larry Bird? Play to your strength, not your weakness.

SUMMARY OF THE MYTH OF DIVERSIFICATION

- Over-diversification may increase your investment losses.
- Diversification is illogical. It forces you to invest outside of your area of expertise.
- BUT: All investors need some amount of diversification.
- Investing is like medicine. The greatest way to maximize returns is to specialize.

BEATING THE MARKET

The advice in the first section of this chapter sounds terribly boring. You ask yourself "Where is the glory, where is the glamour? How can I brag in the doctor's lounge or at the country club about just sending in a check every month to the S&P 500 index fund and rebalancing my portfolio twice a year"? You are a bright physician, a stud, you know you have what it takes to beat the market. What are your chances?

Not good, not good at all. Because of inflation and the increase in corporate profits, the long-term trend of the market is higher. Thus just because your portfolio is increasing in value does not necessarily mean you are out-performing, or even tracking, the market. You must also understand that trying to beat the market is like the NFL on Sunday afternoon, the number of winners equals the number of losers. Actually, because of the extra drag of commissions, fees, and the spread between the bid and ask, the number of losers is actually greater than the number of winners.

Of those who do beat the market, especially over the short-term, half are just lucky (think of the dot.com, internet "geniuses" of the late 90 s). Studies show that over a long period of time, only about 20%, one in five, of the actively-managed mutual funds out-perform the S&P 500. Considering that these funds are managed by professionals, I would put your chance of beating the market at less than 5%.

Income-averaging, sending in a check every month, re-investing all dividends, and periodic rebalancing of your portfolio. It sounds so easy – and it is! The problem is that many do not know about this concept, some don't care, and the majority are not sufficiently disciplined to stick with it.

With this disclaimer clearly in mind, I will tell you what is required to beat the market. First and foremost, you must be willing to work very, very hard. This must be your passion. If you are not willing to spend *at least* one hour a day reading and studying, you will fail. There are many very smart people out there, who are devoted, who have spent years in school and training, 10–12 hours a day, their entire adult lives, studying how to beat the market. If you do not have this passion, this commitment, and this intellectual capacity, do not even try. It is the money the pros make from you that allows them to beat the market.

Studies have examined the contribution of the factors involved in beating the market (I have rounded the numbers to simplify the discussion).

1. Superior stock selection-5%
2. Market timing-5%
3. Asset allocation-90%

Forget #1 and #2, let's go where the money is. This may seem overly simplistic to the point of being banal, but to beat the market, you must know when to follow the trend, to hang in there and ride the bull (such as stocks from 1982 to 2000). *And*, at the major turning points you must be a contrarian, taking profits in yesterday's winners (sell high) and investing them in yesterday's losers (buy low).

In my experience, the vast majority of people who think they are contrarians are just fooling themselves. Having one different stock in your portfolio does not make you a contrarian. You must stake out a position completely different than the lemmings (or penguins, depending on the pole). In late 1999, early 2000, were you buying the can't-miss, will-go-up-forever dot. com stocks, or were you cashing out, or even shorting the NASDAQ (which I did)? In 1980, were you buying gold at $800/ounce and silver at $50/ounce, or were you buying 30 year Treasuries with a coupon of 15%, a risk-free investment that beat even stocks over the next decade? In 1999, were you buying commodities when gasoline was cheaper than bottled water, and gold was $300/ounce? In 2005, were you buying or selling real estate (I sold my Lake Ozark rental condo in June, 2005)?

I believe the main reason people are not contrarians is because they cannot accept criticism. "You bought what? You sold what? Dude, you have got to be kidding. I thought you were a smart guy. That's so risky, no savvy investor would touch that with a 10 ft pole". Your consolation is knowing you were right, and having a bushel of money in the bank.

To beat the market, you must also hold concentrated positions. If you have more than about 20 positions, you are a "closet indexer", with the result that higher transaction fees, compounded by inferior stock selection, will probably cause you to under-perform the market. For any position to have an appreciable effect, it must be greater than 5% of your portfolio. I would consider a concentrated, non-diversified stock portfolio to be 8 to at most 15 positions, with none smaller than 5%, and the largest being 15% or even more (Note: At one time in the 1960s, American Express was more than 40% of Warren Buffett's portfolio).

For completeness, I must make several points. Whenever any position represents more than 5% of your portfolio, the risk of Gamblers Ruin begins to increase appreciably. I also point out that another way to augment return is to use leverage (margin). The chaos and near-destruction of our financial system in 2008 highlights the insanity and malevolence of too much debt.

SUMMARY OF BEATING THE MARKET

- There are many more losers than winners among those who try to beat the market.
- Know when to follow the trend and know when to be a contrarian.
- Asset allocation is paramount.
- Take large, concentrated positions.
- Do not even try unless you are willing to work very, very hard.

REFERENCE

1. Orman S. The Road to Wealth: A Comprehensive Guide to Your Money. New York: Riverhead Books, 2008.

Chapter Twenty-Nine
When to Buy

There are separate chapters for when to buy and when to sell because the rules and the psychology are quite different.

A local hotel owner told me that the profit on an investment is made when it is purchased, not when it is sold. The first rule of investing is that it is impossible to make money when over-paying for an asset.

But you are tempted to buy none-the-less because things just look good. Consider the stocks of Exxon Mobil (XOM) and Potash Saskatchewan (POT). I choose these as examples because they are excellent companies with great management and a sound financial base. There is no argument about the quality of the company or their products. The issue is price. To overpay for the stock of even a great company, or any asset, precludes a profit. You are investing to make money. The glamour or prestige of a stock or any asset is immaterial. In fact, these features almost always detract from the potential for profit.

Suppose the stocks of the Dow Jones Industrial Average (DJIA) were purchased in August 1929. The market was high, but times were so good it just seemed that you had to own stocks. The DJIA did not return to its 1929 peak until 1954. Twenty-five years, an investing lifetime, just to break even. The stocks of the Nikkei purchased at its peak of 39,000 in 1989 are still down 70%. They will need to go up 12% per year for the next 10 years just to break even. Three decades, or

R.M. Doroghazi, *The Physician's Guide to Investing*,
DOI 10.1007/978-1-60761-134-9_29,
© Humana Press, a part of Springer Science+Business Media, LLC 2005, 2009

possibly longer, of dead money. I will talk more about the fallacy of buy and hold forever in the next chapter.

Now for the psychology of buying low. There are several phrases worthy of mention:

1. "Buy when there is blood in the streets." (Baron Meyer Rothschild)
2. "When other people are greedy, you sell. When other people sell, you should be greedy" (Warren Buffett).
3. My favorite:
   "When other people are yellin', you should be sellin'.
   When other people are cryin', you should be buyin'."

Let me provide several examples of "cryin'." There is an ad for a condo in an over-built area of Florida: No down payment, no rent for eighteen months. That is "cryin'." The auto companies are "cryin' " to sell all of the gas-guzzlers on their lots: Zero down, zero percent interest and zero payments for six months. They may actually make less than zero since some people will drive the car for six months, return it to the dealer and just walk away.

Just because something has fallen in price, because it is less expensive than it was earlier, does not mean it is a good buy. Salesmen often use this as an inducement. A home was originally listed at $250K and the price has been reduced to $225K and again to $210K. Look at it this way; the price was lowered because it was over-priced in the first place. A collectable was $7K three years ago but is now only $5K. Even though something is less expensive than before, possibly much less, it may still be very overpriced. Cisco (CSCO) peaked at $82 in 2000. The stock may have appeared a great buy at $60, more than 25% off its peak. It bottomed in the teens and eight years later still trades in the 20 s. This represents a 65% loss after buying a stock that "looked cheap". Citigroup (C) was $56 in 2007. It then dropped to 40 with a fat dividend of more than 6%. Had you jumped in at that time, with the stock 25% of its high, you would have been wiped out as the stock collapsed to $1.

This is called a "value trap" If something that is falling in price looks cheap, with a low P/E and a fat dividend and trades at below book value, it may be because it is destined to get much cheaper. Benjamin Graham, the father of the concept of value investing, made a fortune in the 1920s, but jumped back into the market far too early and recorded cumulative losses of 70% from 1929 to the bottom in 1932 [1]. I believe (many do not) that technical analysis can help avoid this value trap.

The phrase "buy the dips" was immortalized in the bull market of the late 1990s. "Buy the dips" reached paradigm status and was the rule of the day for momentum investors. "The Bear" has clearly exposed the fallacy of this concept. "Buy the dips" could be buying the abyss. The one sure way to be wiped out is to add to losing positions. Think about it. You buy at 50, buy more at 40, buy more at 30, and if it goes to zero, you are broke. Do not "average down", do not add to losing positions.

Corporate insiders, such as officers of the company and those on the Board of Directors, may buy on weakness because their intimate knowledge of the company suggests that a stock is under-priced. The average investor should only buy on strength, not weakness. If insiders sell on weakness, you better high-tail it for the woods, because they feel prices are going lower.

Being a contrarian is the essence of buying when everyone else is selling. People will be lamenting their losses, stating empathically they have no desire to ever purchase stocks or bonds or real estate again. In general, it is fairly easy to determine when things are bad, when there is "blood in the streets."

The real issue is having the courage to buy when things look bad. The more dire the situation, the worse things look, the more money that can be made, but the more courage, and good judgment, is required. Your study suggests that something is undervalued, and it is time to buy, but at this exact moment you may begin to question your judgment. You will think, "If this is such a bargain, why aren't five other people lined up in front of me to buy? Am I missing something? Am I wrong? This seems such an obvious bargain to me, why isn't it this obvious to everyone?" I admit this is a non-egalitarian comment, but I believe it is an accurate observation: what seems obvious to a few may not be obvious to the majority of people. In the end, it just amounts to confidence in your judgment. It is not easy, it is really very difficult, but it is the essence of buying low.

I once recognized a real opportunity, but in the end lost it because I did not have enough confidence in my judgment. I collect baseball cards and sports memorabilia. Some time ago, one of the most important baseball cards in the hobby was up for auction. At that exact time there was some weakness in prices. The bidding was going very slowly. It was obvious that the card would bring much less than what I thought it was worth. Instead of making me even more eager, I admit I was scared away. I found all sorts of excuses to not buy it. Are prices collapsing? Is something wrong with the card? In the end, I did not even place a bid.

What a mistake. The card went for one-half of what I thought it was worth and would now bring many times what it sold for then. It would be the proud centerpiece of anyone's collection. I wish very much that I had bought the card but I also learned to have more faith in my judgment.

This is the essence of investing; buying something for less than it is really worth. Eventually, and eventually may be a painfully long time, the market will recognize this value and a profit will be realized.

If an investment goes down after the purchase, you should re-evaluate the position, specifically, has there been a change in fundamentals? It is mandatory to ask such questions on any large investment that turns sour. Did the stock go down because of an analyst downgrade? To me this is not a change in fundamentals and means nothing. Compare this to a biotech company that has only one product. The CEO has just been indicted for falsifying research data and the FDA does not approve the drug. Mice were being injected with prune juice rather than a new genetically engineered monoclonal antibody. Or the only mine of Acme Copper and Gold was nationalized by the local dictator. These are changes in the fundamentals.

Do not try to buy at the absolute bottom since this will result in missing many opportunities. Trying to buy at the absolute bottom and sell at the absolute top is motivated by greed and will invariably result in losses. I am quite comfortable in giving up 5% to let the trend clearly declare itself rather than buying or selling at the wrong time.

This is not to say that when negotiating a price or making a purchase you should not try for as favorable a price and terms as possible. Of course you should. The point is to not miss an otherwise good, or great, opportunity, by holding out for the last penny. It is like losing a dollar, or possibly more, to save a nickel.

Consider again Cisco (CSCO). You feel that a fair value for CSCO is $20. The stock drops to $17. Your in-depth analysis suggests that this is under-priced so you must step up and buy. In one month CSCO falls to $16. Was the purchase a mistake? Not necessarily. What matters is the value of the stock in six months or a year. If a year comes and the stock is still $16, was the purchase a mistake? No. If the purchase had been made after a thorough fundamental and technical analysis, it was just not a profitable investment. But analyze the situation so that knowledge can be gained. More likely the stock is up and has produced a nice return. (A tongue-in-cheek, and insightful, comment that applies to this situation: What is the definition of a long-term investment? Answer: A short-term investment that is losing money).

TECHNICAL ANALYSIS

I utilize both fundamental and technical analysis to guide my investments. Fundamental analysis examines the business: the product(s), the industry, the competition, the management, the finances, amount of debt, etc. For example, from my fundamental analysis I believe we are in a secular bull market in hard assets and a secular bear market in financial assets that has years to run (*see* Chapter Thirty-Three).

The weakness of using only fundamental analysis is that what a stock "should" do means nothing, let the market action confirm your thesis before investing. Say in early 1999 you came to the conclusion that the internet, dot.com stocks were over-priced, so you sell them short. Your fundamental analysis was correct; two years later the stocks were busted. But in the interim they went to the moon and you were busted. I use fundamental analysis to determine what to buy or sell, and technical analysis to help with the timing. A quote from John Maynard Keynes sums up the weakness of fundamental analysis: "The market can stay irrational longer than an investor can stay solvent".

The only solid data we have is history, what has already happened. Projections are just projections, no one can predict the future. By studying changes in price and volume (and other data), technical analysis attempts to identify patterns (just as we do in medicine) in hopes of estimating the probability that these patterns will recur in the future. The essence of technical analysis is summed up by one of the maxims of investing "Buy on strength, sell on weakness".

There is a significance, a logic, behind a new high or a new low. When something goes to a new high, the fact that investors were never willing to pay a particular price before and are then willing to pay an even higher price often indicates a fundamental change. The same when something goes to a new low; investors who were previously unwilling to part with their asset will now settle for an even lower price.

Momentum investors ignore fundamentals and just follow the trend. In fact, this is very common in the futures and other markets. It is possible to make money, sometimes a great deal of money, but your position is held with little or no conviction, so you need to be the first one out the door or risk getting trampled. I discourage pure momentum investing.

Likewise, some who rely on only fundamental analysis, will derisively, sometimes even with a haughty arrogance, dismiss technical analysis as no more than voodoo practiced by chart geeks. I prefer to use every tool at my disposal, anything that can give me an edge. I believe fundamental analysis tells you what to buy and sell and technical analysis provides valuable ancillary data on when to pull the trigger.

I have provided several references for a more detailed discussion of technical analysis [2, 3].

SUMMARY OF CHAPTER TWENTY-NINE

- The money is made when an asset is purchased.
- It is impossible to make money by overpaying for an asset.
- Buy on strength, not weakness.
- Never buy just because the price is down.
- A sure way to be wiped out is to add to losing positions.
- You must re-analyze any investment that takes a down-turn.
- Buy when there is blood in the streets, but this requires tremendous personal confidence.
- Fundamental analysis determines what to buy or sell, technical analysis helps with timing.

REFERENCES

1. Graham B. The Memoirs of the Dean of Wall Street. Edited by Chatman S. New York: McGraw-Hill, 1996.
2. Headley P. Big Trends in Trading: Strategies to Master Major Market Moves. Hoboken, NJ: John Wiley & Sons, 2002.
3. Kahn M N. Technical Analysis Plain and Simple: Charting the Markets in Your Language. Second Ed. Upper Saddle River, NJ: Financial Times Prentice Hall, 2006.

Chapter Thirty
When to Sell

Bernard Baruch made a fortune in the stock market in the 1920s and had the presence to take profits before the market dropped into the Great Depression. He subsequently served as an advisor to Presidents until his death. His quote: "I got rich by taking profits too early." This is the psychology of taking profits-sell too early, not too late. Knowing when to sell is the most difficult aspect of being a successful investor.

I will make an analogy to show how truly difficult it is to sell "too early." How many people can you name who retired "too early", when they were still on top? George Washington retired on top. Johnny Carson retired on top. Jim Brown, the greatest football (and lacrosse) player ever, retired at age 29 still on top, leading the NFL in rushing his last year (see below). Rocky Marciano retired as undefeated heavyweight champ. After this the list gets pretty short. Selling too early, like retiring too early, is not easy.

Let me provide an everyday example of when I did not sell too early. About 5 years ago, I had intended to trade in my car. But another major expense came up so I waited. Within six months, the transmission fell out of the car. Having your trade-in towed to the dealership does not put you in a particularly strong negotiating position.

You may have heard the term "locking in" your profits. A profit has not been realized until an asset is sold. The

R.M. Doroghazi, *The Physician's Guide to Investing*,
DOI 10.1007/978-1-60761-134-9_30,
© Humana Press, a part of Springer Science+Business Media, LLC 2005, 2009

investment may have appreciated ten-fold but this is just a number on paper. In general, you must sell to realize a profit.

It is not uncommon for a stock to perform well for a period of three to five years because business and market cycles often last a similar period of time. The safest period to buy and sell a stock is during the middle of this time, because there is a margin of safety on both ends.

But rather than be content with a nice gain, greed rears its ugly head and you try to hold out for every last penny of profit. Now you can lose everything. The problem is psychological. The price that you paid for an asset, or at which you hope to sell, has no meaning to anyone else in the entire universe. It has no basis whatsoever in fact. The market does not care what you paid for a stock or at what price you wish to sell or what your profit or loss may be. To believe otherwise is fantasy, like blowing mental bubbles.

The stock drops in price, but you're tough, and it has been drilled into you to buy and hold, so you try to ride it out. You are sure it will come back and even break to new highs. To sell now would be like putting your tail between your legs and running away. Now you are a goner. The stock drops further. Intransigence bordering on belligerence replaces an impartial evaluation of the situation. The price drops further and is now below the purchase price. Only now do you sell – for a loss! What was once a significant profit on paper is now a real money loss (A basic rule is to never let a good gain turn into a loss). It is human nature. It can and must be conquered. Do not try to pick the absolute top or the absolute bottom because it is impossible. The desire to milk an investment for every cent is just greed. Remember this – bulls can make money, bears can make money, but pigs get slaughtered. Take your profit out of the fat part, the easy part, the middle.

This is done by selling at the time when every fiber in your body wants to hold on for more profit. What if the price rises another ten percent after the asset is sold? You may be tempted to say, "I could have made another 10%." I would say this sounds greedy and that the sale was made at a perfect time, i.e. you did not sell too late. What if the price increases another

50% or even more? If the asset was sold for intelligent reasons, then further increases in price suggest speculation and you should be happy indeed for selling and realizing a profit before the inevitable stampede for the exits. If you did leave some real money on the table, learn from it while you console yourself with the profit you did make. Remember this financial homily:

YOU WILL NEVER GO BROKE TAKING A PROFIT

A beautiful example of selling "too early" is illustrated by Sir John Templeton. Templeton pioneered investing outside the US, and entered the Japanese market in the 60s and 70s. He made great profits for his shareholders by selling several years before the end of the Japanese stock market bubble of the late 1980s. During those last several years before the top he was criticized for getting out too early, for missing the great Japanese bull market. Critics were saying he was too old and had clearly lost his touch, after all this was a new era of investing in Japan. Traditional measure of valuation – price/earning ratio, dividend yield, etc. – no longer mattered. Twenty years after the peak, the Japanese market is still down more than 70%. Templeton's selling "too early" was clearly one of the great stock market calls of the twentieth century. Just as it takes courage to buy when things look terrible, when there is blood in the streets, it takes courage to sell and take profits too early, before it is too late.

Schiller's book *Irrational Exuberance* [1] examines manias such as the Japanese market of the late 1980s and our stock market of the late 1920s and late 1990s. How many dot.com geniuses, who for a brief period of time were multi-millionaires on paper, now wish they had read Schiller's book and sold "too early."

Making and accumulating money is not easy. It is very hard. As noted in Chapter Two, 10% a year is a reasonable return on investment. When you have made more money from an investment than you ever dreamed possible, when you are congratulating yourself for being so smart, for being such a genius, when you have dollar signs in your eyes, when you are calculating your percent per year (or per month or per week) gain, when everything is going right, when you are dreaming of retiring early – then sell!! You actually may be able to retire early!

This brings up a very important point: If you are investing to realize a specific financial goal, when you have reached that goal, you *must* sell. No matter how good things look, no matter how sure you are that the investment has further to run, you must sell. Remember, in this situation you are not investing to maximize gains, you are investing to fund your goal.

In the movie "21", it is the young man's goal to save $300,000 to attend Harvard Medical School. After several months on an MIT-centered black jack team, he has accumulated $320K, which he unwisely keeps in the roof of his dorm room. When the team starts to get some heat, his girlfriend reminds him that the only reason he joined the team was to save money for med school, and he had reached his goal. But he gets greedy. When the bad guys catch up, he not only is beaten with brass knuckles, but they also take the money. When you reach your goal, do not be greedy, you must sell.

Although not quite as dramatic, such things do occur in real life. I have friends who were saving to build their dream house. By the late 90s, their nest egg was double what was needed and more than they imagined they would ever have. Had they sold then they could have paid cash for the home and still had six-figures in the bank. They committed to the new home, but then the paper gains of the dot.com stocks evaporated as quickly as they came. Ten years later they are still paying on the mortgage. I have another friend who in 1999 had more than enough to retire. He is now in his late 60s, but because of the stock market bust, he is still working 3 days a week. When you are investing to fund a goal, and you have reached your goal – Sell!

How does the above discussion of selling too early not contradict a saying that everyone has heard, namely, cut losses but let profits ride? Buying a stock and then selling two months later for a ten percent gain is not letting profits ride (although there is nothing wrong with this if the situation dictates). Selling a stock after it has appreciated five or ten-fold over a three to five year period or thirty-fold over a ten-year period is letting profits ride.

In the years leading up to the terrible bear market of 1973–74, there was a group of stocks called the "Nifty Fifty", which included such well-known names as International Business Machines (IBM), Avon Products (AVP), and a hand full of companies no longer in business such as Digital Equipment. They were called "one decision" stocks, the only decision being to buy and hold forever. Nothing lasts forever.

There is no one decision stock. When Warren Buffett was asked his favorite holding period for a stock, he replied forever. This may be Buffett's favorite holding period but it is certainly not his only holding period. In 1969, the "go–go" stocks were being hyped and recommended regardless of price. Buffett thought the market was so over-priced that he liquidated his limited partnership and offered his investors the option of a return of their money or staying with his new investment vehicle, Berkshire Hathaway (BRK). Buffett was right. The market dragged on for several years and even rose to a new high in early 1973 before descending to the depths of the second worst bear market of the twentieth century.

Just before the October 19, 1987 crash, Buffett quietly sold all of the stocks owned by Berkshire Hathaway except his three core positions – Washington Post (WPO), Capital Cities (ABC television network) and GEICO Insurance. Buffett held these not only because of the business itself, but because he personally knew and trusted the management. On about October 12th, Buffett also cashed out the stock portfolio of Berkshire's profit-sharing plans. Although the turnover at BRK is low, it is not fixed in stone. Buffett does not hold stocks forever.

I have heard many times that for any discipline, in retrospect, it will be shown that 50% of what you were taught will eventually be proven false. Unfortunately, no one knows prospectively which half is right and which half is wrong. For people on the inside, within the system, I believe the primary concern is which half is wrong. For someone like me, who has had no formal financial training (please do not say that it shows), and is not encumbered (shackled) by pre-conceived dogma, I wonder which half is right. I can look at things from a different perspective and draw different conclusions.

I believe that the mantra of buy and hold forever is an illogical, intrinsically flawed concept. No company maintains their competitive edge forever, and only a rare few are king of the hill for even five or ten years. In the 1950s, General Motors (GM) was arguably the most powerful company in the world, the symbol of America's industrial might. In the summer of 2008, the stock is barely in double figures, its lowest level since 1955. If you had bought at that time and blindly held and reinvested all dividends, every share you purchased over the last 53 years would be under water. This book may stay in print longer than GM can avoid bankruptcy. (Note added in proofs. GM declared bankruptcy 6/1/09).

The bull market of the 1980s and 90s, the most powerful in our history, lulled investors into believing they did not have to think. If making money did not require any work or study, we would all be rich. Investment trends come and go. Vicious secular bear markets that can destroy you financially have occurred and will continue to occur. I have already provided multiple examples of investments that were dead money for a quarter century or more. At the secular bear markets lows of 1932 and late 1974, I doubt there were many believers in the buy and hold strategy. As of the fall of 2008, the market is down as compared to 9 years ago, and appears headed lower. Some investments never come back, such as tulips in 17th century Holland. Buy and hold the winners, whether that be for two months or twenty years. Get rid of the* losers, the quicker the better. Your first loss should be your biggest one. You love your family, never fall in love with an investment. Think of an investment as you would a home, sooner or later they all have to be sold. Everyone has to take profits sometime.

When the economy appears to be weakening, some who wish to remain fully invested will rotate to more "defensive" stocks, things they feel people need/want no matter how the economy fares, such as health care, food, alcohol, smokes, etc. Their reasoning is that these stocks should hold up better when the market turns down.

When I first heard of this strategy, I admit I did not understand it. As I have studied and thought more about the concept, I find it illogical.

1. The people who stay fully invested abhor the thought of "market timing", that anyone can predict which way the market will go. Changing your investment mix when you think the market will go down sounds like trying to time the market to me.
2. Where is the logic to willingly hope you will lose less? The secular bear market of 1973–74 resulted in a 50% loss in the major averages. I would not consider it particularly successful investing to lose only 40% rather than 50%.
3. I believe this is an example of "hiding" behind an academically pleasing concept rather than thinking for yourself. I remind you that the goal of investing is to make money.
4. Would you like an idea for a great defensive portfolio? How about – CASH?

Unless you are trading in a tax-free account, taking profits will generate a tax liability. There is no doubt you should try to minimize taxes (taxes destroy wealth), but likewise, do not let this desire cause you to make poor investment decisions. I know of situations where people knew it was time to sell an investment, but were so paralyzed by the specter of the tax bite that they allowed a good part of the profits to slip away. They got their wish, they minimized their taxes by minimizing their profits. Look at it this way: You are lucky you can pay "the man" because you made some money.

Do not get "shaken out" or "scared out" of a good investment. Nothing goes straight up. Your self-confidence and courage will be severely tested. It is difficult to watch paper gains evaporate (I am not good at this. I like to take profits). Almost all stocks at some time can and will go down 20 or 30%, occasionally as much as 50%. If the fundamentals (and technicals) suggest that the investment is sound, then hold. Otherwise the investment will be sold at the worst time, at its low. A panic sale is always a loser, the worst time to sell.

Likewise, when a decision has been made to sell a stock that is truly performing poorly, it is invariable that too small a portion will be sold. The stock will drop further and another small portion, rather than the entire position, will be sold. This is the financial equivalent of Chinese water torture. If the decision has been made that a stock is a loser, just sell the whole position and forget it. Your basic goal is always to preserve capital. If the sale was an error and the stock again moves upward, it can be repurchased.

There is no better way to describe how to cut losses than a conversation between Mayor Richard J. Daley (see below) of Chicago and President Lyndon Johnson. Daley was at the White House lobbying for federal aid for various Chicago projects [2]. As he began to leave, Johnson said "Listen, Dick, I've got a lot of trouble over there in Vietnam. What do you think about it?" Daley paused and said "Well, Mr. President, when you've got a losing hand in poker, you just throw in the cards." "But what about American prestige" Johnson asked. "You put your prestige in your back pocket and walk away" replied Daley. If you have a loser, forget the darn thing, sell it, and live to fight another day.

A variant of a loser is a non-performing asset. Everyone has some. They should be searched out and aggressively sold. Non-performing assets are "dead money," they are not earning any gains or dividends. People tolerate non-performing assets mostly because of inertia and emotion. The lawn mower that gave you good service for twelve or thirteen years is kaput and you have purchased a new one. Instead of letting it just sit in your garage taking up space, sell it. People and shops that repair lawn mowers will usually give $20. They repair and resell them or otherwise use them for parts. Twenty bucks is twenty bucks. Or you have clothes that have you have not worn in years. Give them to charity and take the tax deduction (my preference) or put them in a garage sale.

This advice is not to suggest that you become a regular at the pawnshop or junkyard. That would be personally, and professionally, unwise. But it could be a nice introduction to capitalism, and entrepreneurship, for your children. If you have something that fits this description, tell your children "sell it and you get to keep half." You get one half of the sale price but they may get the experience of a lifetime.

Or you collect something (*see* Chapter Thirty-Four). Items purchased when you began your collecting career may no longer fit your tastes or style, or the focus of your collection.

This is a normal evolution of collecting. You have ten items worth $100 each. They are of marginal quality, not particularly rare or desirable, and do not fit your long-term collecting plans. There is little doubt that in 5 years they will still be worth $100 each. Sell them all. Invest the money in your favorite index fund or buy a more desirable collectible worth $1,000. One one thousand dollar collectible is at least twice as valuable as 10 one hundred dollar collectibles.

Another way to evaluate if an asset should be sold would be to consider that if you did not own it but had the cash, would you buy it? This has little to do with whether the asset is up or down in price, but is a way to force you to evaluate the fundamentals. If an asset has become so over-priced that you would never pay this amount to purchase it, you feel it is clearly not worth the price, then sell. If something is down in price only because of the price fluctuations that occur from time to time, selling would be the wrong decision. But if a stock is down in price because the company is performing badly and you would never purchase the stock, then sell it. Another example would be a stock that you rode all the way down. Sell it and re-invest the money in a position that has a brighter prospect of price appreciation.

This brings up a general point: The leaders in a previous bull market, especially if prices reached the manic level, are rarely the leaders in the next bull market. It will be interesting to see how long it takes the financial stocks to recover from the current credit crunch. Cisco (CSCO) peaked at 82 in 2000 and 8 years later still trades in the low 20s. It could be years (or for the tulips, never) for these stocks to return to where you purchased them or their previous highs. You must look elsewhere for the leaders of the next bull market. In general, the stocks that hold up best during the bear market and turn up first will be the leaders of the next bull market.

An immediate sale should be considered if there is evidence of malfeasance, wrongdoing, criminal activity, cooking the books, or any sort of dishonesty. It is the Cockroach Theory: when you see one of the little buggers, there are sure to be more. Do not look back, but learn from the experience. If this is an investment with little or no liquidity, such as a limited partnership or other closely-held entity, obtain legal advice immediately to protect yourself and limit your liability.

The Cleveland Browns are not named after Jim Brown, as I thought when I growing up, but for coach Paul Brown. Brown had been tremendously successful at Ohio State, and was hired to coach the Cleveland franchise in the new All America Conference, formed just after WWII to compete with the NFL. The team was named by a vote of the fans, and Brown was held in such high regard in Ohio that the team was named for him. The Browns, with Otto Graham at quarterback, dominated the AAFC, and after merging with the NFL, that league also.

Daley's license plate was Illinois 708222, the number of votes he received when first elected mayor in 1955. His son and current Chicago mayor Richard M. Daley now has the license plate.

SUMMARY OF CHAPTER THIRTY

- Anybody can play a winner. The real winners know when to fold the losers.
- Get rich by taking profits "too early."
- A profit on paper is just that. An asset must be sold to lock in a profit.
- Your perception of the value of an investment has no basis in reality and means nothing to any other investor.
- Never let a good gain turn into a loss.

YOU WILL NEVER BO BROKE TAKING A PROFIT

- When you are congratulating yourself on your investment genius – SELL!!
- When you are investing for a particular goal – sell when you have reached your goal.
- Selling too early takes courage.

- There are no one-decision investments.
- Staying fully invested and defensive rotation are illogical.
- Do not fall in love with an investment.
- Do not let tax concerns trump sound investment decisions.
- No investment goes straight up or down. Your willpower and courage will be tested.
- Aggressively sell non-performing assets.
- The leaders of the last bull market are rarely the leaders of the next bull market.

REFERENCES

1. Shiller R J. Irrational Exuberance. Princeton, NJ: Princeton University Press, 2000.
2. Cohen A, Taylor E. American Pharaoh: Mayor Richard J Daley, His Battle for Chicago and the Nation. Boston: Little, Brown and Co, 2000.

Chapter Thirty-One
Stocks, Bonds and Mutual Funds

STOCKS AND THE STOCK MARKET

For this general discussion, stocks refer to the shares of corporations that are traded on the major exchanges, the New York Stock Exchange (NYSE), the National Association of Security Dealers Automated Quotations (NASDAQ), and the American Stock Exchange (ASE).

It is important to be able to evaluate individual securities as well as the general stock market and the economic picture as a whole. All are important since about 70% of the price of an individual stock is determined by the fundamentals of the company and 30% is influenced by general market and economic conditions.

Reading general material can provide ideas applicable to your investments. Newton's laws of gravity and motion were considered fact until the late 19th century, when it was noted they were not accurate when approaching the speed of light. Einstein's work provided rules that did not break down at the extremes. Consider the behavior of stocks at the extremes of their range. The stocks of even the best-run companies, with great management and great products (such as General Motors), were ravaged by 1932. Likewise, the stocks of even the most worthless dot.com companies, with little sales and no profits and sometimes not even any products, companies that are now just memories, were carried to preposterous highs by

R.M. Doroghazi, *The Physician's Guide to Investing*,
DOI 10.1007/978-1-60761-134-9_31,
© Humana Press, a part of Springer Science+Business Media, LLC 2005, 2009

the stock market mania of the late 1990s. But in general, good companies out-perform bad companies and over the long-term, it is a company's ability to generate profits that determines how well its stock performs.

The two general categories of factors to consider when evaluating specific stocks and the market in general are fundamental and technical factors. In the last chapter I detailed why I believe technical data can provide valuable information, especially to determine when to buy and sell.

For a discussion of fundamental analysis, such cash flow, debt, book value, etc., I refer you to Graham and Dodd's classic *Security Analysis* [1]. I believe all investors can do a better job than they think in evaluating the fundamentals of a company.

As a start, what do you personally think of the company's product? Have they opened a new frontier, such as Amgen (AMGN) or Genentech (DNA) 20 years ago, or a new way of doing business, such as Wal-Mart (WMT), or are they a leader in an industry that will revolutionize society, such as Microsoft (MSFT) or Google (GOOG), or are they a fertilizer company, such as Potash Saskatchewan (POT), in a world that wants more and better food? The company may make a quality product but be in a dying industry. It is of no consequence who manufactures the best butter churn or buggy whip.

You must also consider macro-economic factors, conditions at the level of the national and international economy. After World War II, Japan and Germany were in shambles, Great Britain and France were on the winning side but were essentially broke and had been devastated. The Soviet Union had been laid barren by fighting the Wehrmacht for five years and was ruled by the misanthrope Stalin, who killed 30–50 M of his own people in the name of revolution. China was mired in a civil war between the nationalists, led by Chiang (and Mrs.) Kai-shek, and the communist, led by Mao, a man as evil as Stalin. The United Stated was the only industrial democracy left standing. Not surprisingly, the 1950s in the United States were characterized by a spectacular bull market fueled by our productive, military, financial and technological superiority. There was almost no inflation and essentially full employment.

Contrast this to the 1970s. There were several oil/energy crises. Inflation became the norm. There were even temporary price controls. The stock market, adjusted for inflation, dropped approximately 75%.

Nothing goes straight up or straight down. In general, you want to be invested in stocks when they go up and decrease exposure (i.e. by taking profits along the way) when the market goes down. A correction is defined as a 10% drop in a major average. These have occurred on the average of every 15–18 months since World War II. They are part of the normal market process and attempting to avoid them would almost certainly be counterproductive and result in under-performing the market.

A bear market is defined as a 20% or greater drop in the major market averages. Cyclical bear markets occur on the average of every four years and last an average of about 11 months. With just a little common sense, taking profits at the appropriate time, and paying attention to both fundamental and technical factors, it is possible to minimize losses, or even profit by going short, during a bear market. But even if you do not try to avoid these cyclical bear markets, it is possible to do well in the long term because the market averages usually return to their previous highs and even make new highs within a year or two.

Three or four times a century devastating, or secular, bear markets occur, where losses may be 50% or greater. These usually occur at times of major social, political, and economic disruption, such as the Great Depression, and the first oil crisis and inflation of the mid-1970s. *Secular bear markets can and must be avoided.* Your primary goal in a secular bear market is to lose as little as possible. If a stock drops 50%, it must double just to get back to baseline. The period of time required for this to occur can represent an investing lifetime. It took the DJIA 25 years (1929–1954) to recover from the Great Depression. The Japanese market peaked at 39,000 in 1989. Twenty years later it is still around 12,000, a loss of almost seventy percent. During secular bear markets, where 85% of stocks are down, the buy and hold strategy is counterproductive.

Since 1900, there were four secular bear markets in the United States. From January 1906 to November 1907, the DJIA dropped from 103 to 53, a loss of 48%. It took ten years to recover and it was not until the mid-1920 s that the market was able to break out and stay above this level for a significant period of time. From 1929 to 1932, the DJIA dropped from 381 to 41, a loss of 89%. It took twenty-five years to recover. From January 1973 to December 1974, the DJIA dropped from 1051 to 577, a loss of 45%. However, when adjusted for inflation, the loss was almost 75%. The Dow had actually touched 1,000 in 1966, and was still below 900 in August 1982 before exploding upwards. Thus the period of nominal (non-inflation adjusted) dead money lasted sixteen years. After adjusting for inflation, the DJIA did not return to the 1966 high until 1991, again 25 years, a quarter century.

From August to October 1987, the DJIA dropped from 2,772 to 1,738, a loss of more than 36%, with a 508-point, 22% drop on October 19th, the greatest percentage-wise single day loss in our market's history. Lowry Research (www.lowrysresearch. com) and Martin Zweig, both relying on technical analysis, were able to avoid that calamity. The market, however, regained this lost ground in approximately two years and then exploded upward during the 1990s. The economy was basically sound and the market recovered.

The fourth secular bear market of the twentieth century began as we closed out the second millennium. The NASDAQ peaked on March 10, 2000 at 5,048 and bottomed in October of 2002 at 1,108, a loss of 78%, almost as severe as the DJIA suffered in the Great Depression. The NASDAQ is currently below 1,700, still down 65% from the high. Even when the NASDAQ doubles, it will still be short of its previous high. Over this same period, the DJIA was down more than 35%, and the S&P 500 was down 50%. As of September 2008, the DJIA and the S&P 500, even after adding in the skimpy dividends, are down as compared to 9 years ago (subtract another 20% after factoring in inflation).

We are currently in a secular bear market because our nation is in a time of political and economic upheaval and decline. The final unwinding of the housing bubble will not be pretty. The 20th century was the US century, the 21st century may not be.

1. The US dollar will not be the world's reserve currency much longer, it is no longer "as good as gold". A dollar buys an

amount of gold essentially invisible to the naked eye. Over the last 9 years, the DJIA has lost more than 80% of its value compared to gold.

2. We are fighting a war that costs us billions of dollars a week and the lives of thousands of our brave young men and women in a country that wants us to go home.

3. From the end of WWII until the 90s, the average American's savings rate was about 10%. Two generations have never experienced any semblance of tough times, they have no concept of what it means to sacrifice. Our savings rate is negative – we spend money we do not have, that we must borrow from the Chinese, who save 40% of what they make, which is about 10% of what we make.

4. There are obscene amounts of debt at all levels of our society. By the time this book appears in print, our national debt will be 10 trillion dollars. Add to this another $5 trillion just put on the books from the nationalization of mortgage giants Fannie Mae (FNM) and Freddie Mac (FRE) and the "bailout" of at least one-half a trillion dollars currently being debated in Washington. The government's only recourse to fund this debt will be to print more money, further debasing the dollar. Our current accounts deficit is $700B per year – every day we send $2B overseas. Foreigners are buying up our country with the money we send them for TVs and video games.

5. People were using their homes as ATMs rather than paying off a mortgage they never should have received in the first place. Home foreclosures have reached Great Depression levels.

6. When oil hit $140 per barrel, the oil reserves of the exporting countries had an estimated value of $150 trillion, approximately three times the combined value of all of the world's stock markets (*Barron's*, 7/14/08). The next 2 to 3 decades will see an unprecedented transfer of wealth to these mostly non-democratic countries, where 50% of the population (i.e., females) are often considered barely more than chattel.

7. Our private banking system is on the ropes. Bear Stearns (BSC), Lehman Brothers (LEH), American International Group (AIG), FNM, FRE, Washington Mutual (WM), Wachovia (WB) and Merrill Lynch (MER) are either history or have

been taken over. The government expects scores or even possibly hundreds of more bank failures.

I will not bore you with any more depressing, but true, facts. We are in a secular bear market because of the structural problems in our society and our financial system. In the late 1990s, people came to expect returns of 20% or more per year. Ten percent returns, the average for the 20th century, were considered chump change. In a secular bear market you should be delighted if you just get your money back. John Bogle (of the Vanguard Group) and Warren Buffett said recently that 4–7% stock market returns will be the norm for some time to come. This will be especially important when considering long-term objectives, such as saving for your children's education and for your retirement.

One of the basic ways to evaluate a stock and the market in general is to consider the price to earnings (P/E) ratio. This is exactly what it says – take the price of the stock – say $20, and divide it by the earnings of the last year – say $1 – to obtain a P/E of 20. This is what an investor is willing to pay for $1 of earnings. But people look ahead. If a well-run company with a great product in a great area has demonstrated increasing earnings (such as POT over the last several years), an investor is willing to pay a higher price for this stock and its presumably bright future.

There are several reasons to consider only the P/E ratio of the last year, the "reported" P/E. First is that this is the traditional method, allowing easy comparison to previous data. Second is that evaluating a stock by "forward-looking" price to earnings ratio is fraught with hazard. Earnings in the future, even just the next 12 months, are estimates, no more than someone's guess, and are invariably overly-optimistic. The use of the "estimated" P/E can be used to justify almost anything. You could say "the P/E on the last year's earnings is 147, but if extrapolated to 6 years from now, it is only 27." Such reasoning is often used to justify speculation. I prefer to be a little more realistic.

Another basic measure of a stock is the dividend yield. I have already emphasized the importance of dividends. Dividend yield is particularly useful in determining when the stock market as a whole is over-valued, under-valued or fairly valued. In the twentieth century, the average dividend yield of the DJIA and the S&P 500 was approximately 4.5%. The average trailing P/E of the S&P 500 was 15 to 16.

I will use various data to illustrate the degree of the stock market mania in the U.S. in the late 1990s and early 2000 and what one may find at the final bottom of this secular bear market. At the market peak in early 2000, the dividend yield of the S&P 500 was 1.2% (just one-quarter of the historical yield). The P/E of the S&P 500 was at least one-third higher than the P/E in September 1929, the high point of the market before it descended into the depths of the Great Depression. The P/E of the NASDAQ 100 was almost 100. (Due to a variety of aberrations, even these numbers are significant underestimates of the true P/E as compared to previous time periods). The end result is that the stock market of March 2000 was 50% to possibly 100% over-valued *as compared to the market of 1929*.

In *Irrational Exuberance* [2], Shiller reviews the most significant investment manias in history. He concludes that the subsequent bust after a mania mirrors the mania itself – i.e. – there is a crash. Manias never end nicely. There is pain, despair and significant economic dislocations.

Richard Russell of the *Dow Theory Letters* (www.dowtheory letters.com) points out that at true secular bear market bottoms in the U.S., the dividend yield of the DJIA and the S&P 500 is 5 to 6% or even higher, and the P/E ratio of both is between 5 and 10. At the 2002 market lows the dividend yield of the S&P 500 was 1.9% and the trailing P/E was slightly more than 30. The current (September 2008) dividend yield of the DJIA is about 2.6%. Dividends would need to double or the DJIA would need to drop 50% to generate a dividend yield of 5%. These numbers have nasty implications, but history does tend to repeat. I suggest some cash to help dull the pain.

SUMMARY OF SECTION

- The fundamentals of a company and general economic conditions influence the price of a stock.
- Technical factors are important.

- Utilize both technical and fundamental data to determine when to buy and sell.
- Stock market corrections occur on average every 15–18 months.
- Cyclical bear markets occur on average of every four years.
- Secular bear markets occur three or four times a century. They can and must be avoided.
- Your primary goal in a bear market is to lose as little as possible.
- Consider Price to Earning ratio (P/E) and dividend yield when evaluating the stock market.
- We are currently in a secular bear market that began in 2000 and will end?

BONDS

Bonds are an I.O.U. You lend money to a government entity or corporation and they agree to pay you, the lender, a predetermined rate of interest (referred to as the coupon rate because in years past coupons were on the side of the bond. They had to be clipped off and redeemed for the bond holder to be paid) for a defined period of time. The lender is then repaid the face value of the bond at maturity.

There is also a zero-coupon bond. They do not pay interest along the way, but rather are sold at a deep discount to the final redemption value. For example, using round numbers, the Treasury sells a 30-year $10,000 bond for $3,000. No interest is paid in the interim but the Treasury will redeem the bond in 30 years at the face value of $10K. If you wish to sell the bond before maturity, the value is determined by current market interest rates and time to maturity. Because of how interest is computed, these bonds are best suited for retirement accounts as compared to taxable accounts. Because no interest is paid along the way, if the bond issuer goes bankrupt before the bond matures, you have nothing. The *only* zero coupon bond I would consider are Treasuries. In fact, the *only* bond of any kind you should consider are Treasuries.

The value of a bond is determined by two main factors, credit risk and interest rate risk. The more credit-worthy the customer, the lower the interest rate they pay because the greater the likelihood they will repay the debt. Contrast this to the local loan shark, who must charge 20% interest per week because of the unreliability of his clientele. Higher risk requires higher rates, lower risk with better credit rating can obtain lower rates (This is also the case when you apply for a loan. If your personal financial statement looks like Fort Knox, you will receive the best interest rates).

The other main factor that determines a bond's value is interest rates. In general, the longer the maturity period, the higher the interest rate. The lender must receive greater compensation because their money is tied up for a longer period of time.

Bond values and interest rates move in opposite directions. When interest rates rise, the value of a bond drops. It took me some time to understand this concept, and it is very important, so I will provide a simplistic explanation. Suppose one year ago I purchased a $10,000 bond paying interest at a rate of 5%. The current rate of interest on a similar bond is 6%. No one will purchase my bond for face value paying 5% interest when they can go next door and buy a bond paying a higher rate of interest. My bond has lost value. If I wish to sell it before maturity, I must accept a lower price. The face value of the bond falls so that the buyer will receive market interest rates. A $10K bond paying an interest rate of 5% yields $500 of interest income in one year. If interest rates are now 6%, I would need to sell my bond for $8,333 (8,333 × 6% = $500 interest). A similar explanation holds if interest rates drop. My bond is now paying above market rates, so I could sell the bond for more than face value.

RISING INTEREST RATES ARE BAD FOR BONDS
FALLING INTEREST RATES ARE GOOD FOR BONDS

You may have heard that bonds are less risky than stocks. I prefer to look at risk as an overall concept, so I do disagree with the blanket statement that bonds are less risky than stocks. Over the very long term, stocks out-perform bonds, but over shorter periods of time, this may or may not be the case. There have been periods of five years or longer when bonds out-perform stocks. From 2000 to the present, Treasury bills have out-performed stocks with less volatility and a guaranteed return. Likewise, T-bills may be a "conservative, risk-free" investment over the course of a day or a week or a month (because you will get your money back) but over the course of 20 years they are "risky" because of the inferior rate of return and inflation. In the end, *all* investments have risk.

In general, bonds tend to do well when the economy is doing poorly. Interest rates are low because business activity and the demand for credit are weak. From 1929 through the 1930s, bonds, if the borrower could repay the debt, out-performed stocks. This may be when the perception that bonds were less risky than stocks arose. Contrast this to a 30-year bond purchased in the 1950s or early 60s when long-term interest rates were less then 5%. By 1980, the prime interest rate was 21% and the rate on the 30-year Treasury bond was 15%. A bond purchased in the mid-1960s was decimated by 1980 (In Latin, decem=ten. In the Roman army, if men were cowardly in battle, they suffered decimation. The cohort, men and officers, were divided into groups of ten. They chose lots, the loser was killed by the other nine men. This did not exactly inspire loyalty, and was not practiced by Julius Caeser, or his grand-nephew, and adopted son, Octavian (Augustus) or thereafter).

The principle problem with bonds is that no one can predict the direction of interest rates over the short term. However, interest rates do move in very long-term trends. Rates peaked in the 1920s and then dropped and stayed low throughout the 1930s and until after World War II. Rates at first rose slowly but then accelerated upwards until peaking in 1981. Rates fell spasmodically over the last two decades and are again at multi-decade lows.

So now for the big question: Where do interest rates, and thus bond values, go from here? I feel that after the current financial crisis abates, long-term interest rates will head higher and the multi-decade bull market in bonds will be over. For investors holding a large bond position with longer maturities, there is the possibility of real pain if interest rates rise significantly.

For these reasons and the other caveats detailed in Chapters Twenty-Eight and Thirty-Eight, I feel the average investor should not purchase individual bonds and should be hesitant to buy into even the best bond mutual fund. Instead, I feel you should utilize Certificates of Deposit (make sure you are not over the FDIC/FSLIC insurance limit) as the vehicle of choice for your fixed-income investments.

SUMMARY OF SECTION

- Bonds are not necessarily "less risky" than stocks. All investments have risk.
- The principal factors affecting a bond are credit risk and interest rate risk.
- No one can predict the direction of interest rates.
- Rising interest rates are bad for bonds, lower interest rates are good for bonds
- The only bonds you should invest in are those issued by the US Government.

MUTUAL FUNDS AND EXCHANGE TRADED FUNDS (ETFs)

In Chapter Twenty-Two (the Perniciousness of Fees) I introduced the general topic of mutual funds in the context of how mutual funds charge fees, what to look for and what to avoid. I will now discuss the various types of mutual funds, compare them to ETFs, and make suggestions.

My first recommendation is to again remind you to never buy a mutual fund with any load or commission. This includes front-end load, back-end load, surrender charge and 12b-1 fees. The following discussion concerns only no-load mutual funds.

The first general category of mutual funds is index funds. These funds track a particular index, such as the S&P 500, the

Wilshire 5000, the DJIA, etc. Index funds should be the core position in your portfolio. Because they are passive, no decision is required on what to buy or sell, the fund just stays balanced to the particular index, and fees are low. Index funds allow you to participate in the long-term growth of our economy.

There are other benefits. All dividends and gains should be re-invested so they can be magnified by compound interest. There are two small boxes on the application that ask if you wish to re-invest all dividends and gains. Check yes. Another advantage is that almost no capital gains are distributed, and thus liable to taxes. This is especially true for the S&P 500 Index Fund. It is rare for a company that has been performing well (and thus generated capital gains) to be dropped from the S&P 500. The only reasons for an index fund to realize a capital gain would be to sell stocks to rebalance the fund's portfolio so that it continues to match the index or if a company is taken over by another company. In practice, these effects are very minimal. Thus almost all the accrued capital gains of companies such as General Electric (GE) Pfizer (PFE) or Microsoft (MSFT) remain in the fund as unrealized, and untaxed, capital gains. Do not overlook this subtle, but very significant, advantage of index funds.

Exchange-Traded Funds (ETFs) are best understood when compared to no-load index mutual funds. ETFs are similar to index funds because they track a particular index, such as the SPY (S&P 500 Index), DIA (Dow Jones Industrial Average) or the QQQQ (NASDAQ 100 Index). The principle advantage of ETFs, and it is very significant, as compared to mutual funds, is their flexibility. Because ETFs are stocks, they can be traded throughout the day, as compared to mutual funds, where you only receive the price (NAV, net asset value) at the end of the day. ETFs also provide several advantages for short-selling, which I will discuss in more detail in Chapter Thirty-Five. In addition, ETFs based on the major indexes may be even more tax-efficient than comparable mutual funds, and fees are generally similar.

The major disadvantage of ETFs in comparison to mutual funds is that because they are stocks there is a commission to buy and sell. There is talk of offering "actively-managed" ETFs. They will invariably suffer from the same weaknesses of actively-managed mutual funds, i.e., Wall Street professionals will profit at your expense.

Another disadvantage of ETFs is determining the instantaneous NAV on securities that are illiquid at that particular moment. For example (*Wall Street Journal*, 3/17-18/07) there was a large drop in the Chinese market on February 27, 2007. One ETF that tracked that market closed down 9.9% although the index it tracked was down just 2.1% during Chinese trading hours. (The flip side is that you could have been on the receiving end rather than the losing end of the 7.7% discrepancy. There is nothing wrong with being lucky, except when you are unlucky).

Exchange Traded Notes (ETNs) are similar to ETFs in that they trade like a stock and typically track a market index. However, their basic financial structure is different in that they essentially represent a pledge from a bank or financial institution to pay the holder the return of a specific index. The current credit crisis has shown that the pledge of sometimes even the biggest banks or brokerages just may not be all that it is built up to be. ETNs have not garnered much market share.

In the final comparison, the ability to trade an ETF throughout the day provides a flexibility just not available with mutual funds. But because of commissions, it is also quite impractical to income-average with small sums into an ETF such as the SPY, which trades for about $90 per share. But overall, I think the advantage clearly goes to ETFs. For a more in-depth discussion of ETFs, go to my website www.thephysicianinvestor.com and see issues #16 and #17 of my newsletter. Also see Yahoo Finance! ETF Center http://finance.yahoo.com and www.indexinuverse.com for more information.

The other general category of mutual funds is those that are actively-managed. These may be general funds, which invest in any sort of security they feel will generate a profit, or sector funds, which invest in some specific area. I have already mentioned elsewhere that many studies have shown that the average actively-managed fund under-performs the index to which they are compared. There are also sector funds for every area imaginable – health care, electronics, banks, gold, natural resources, etc. Because at any one time some sectors are out-performing the general market and some are under-performing, sector funds should probably not be considered a core holding in your portfolio. Rather, they should be considered as inter-mediate-term holdings, such as one to five years, to capture the gains of a sector during its strong cycle, then take profits and move on.

There are also bond mutual funds of all types – government bonds, corporate bonds, municipal bonds, high-yield (junk) bonds, etc. For the larger states, there are municipal bond funds restricted to that state, allowing you, for example, in California or New York, to invest in a fund that is free from both federal and their state's taxes. Some bond funds focus on specific maturity periods, such as 5 years, ten years etc.

International funds invest in all areas of the world. Some invest in all major areas and countries of the world, some invest only in one area, such as Europe or Asia, and some invest in only one country, such as Russia, China, Japan, etc. As men-tioned in Chapter Twenty-Eight, I recommend 10–15% of your entire portfolio be allocated to non-US equities. If the dollar continues to depreciate over the long term, and if selected foreign economies grow faster than ours, both of which I believe will be the case, investing in foreign countries, and thus indir-ectly their currencies, would be an excellent option.

There are mutual funds and ETFs that are leveraged, i.e., they move 2 or even 3 times a particular index. They may be structured to move in correlation with, or inverse to, the index. The leverage makes them quite volatile. Because of the flexibility of being able to trade ETFs during the day, in this situation they should be used to the exclusion of such mutual funds.

Another potential disadvantage of an actively-managed fund as compared to an index fund is if the fund has had a good run and sells some positions, the gains will be distributed to the investor. This is usually done towards the end of the year, generally in late November, early December. This compares to an index fund, which often has little if any capital gains to distribute.

A very significant tax liability could arise if you buy into a fund just before it distributes a large amount of gains. Say you purchase shares on December 1st and the fund makes its yearly distribution on December 2nd. An investor could be unlucky enough to have 5% or even 10% or more of the money just invested given right back as taxable gains, as happened several years ago at Fidelity Magellan. In one day you are down 2–5%, or possibly more. I would suggest that before you make a deposit toward the end of the year, especially a large one, into a mutual fund that you check with them on what day they plan to distribute gains. This is a good example of where attention to detail can save you money.

A mutual fund will distribute gains back to the investor, but can only distribute losses when they are offset by gains. Think of it as the jump-ball arrow in basketball that alternates to indicate possession. In this situation, the arrow always points in the direction of the IRS.

There are two situations involving a genuine no-load but actively-managed mutual fund that should prompt you to re-evaluate the investment. First is when the fund manager changes. The other situation is when a poorly performing fund is merged into another fund. Violà. No more record of that fund's inferior performance (This is called survivorship bias, and when added into the statistics, further worsens the performance of actively-managed funds as compared to the passive index funds). I suggest a quick exit when this occurs. Of course, the best way to avoid this potentiality is to avoid actively-managed funds.

So what are my recommendations for the vast majority of investors?

1. There is never a reason to use any mutual fund with a load, commission or extra fee of any kind.
2. Send in a check every month, which is called income-averaging. Less shares are purchased when the market is up, but more are purchased when the market is down (buy low). With this disciplined, common-sense approach, keeping in

mind that during the secular bear markets that occur three or four times a century you want to significantly decrease your stock market exposure, you should have the greatest chance of maximizing gains.

3. Utilize passive, index-based vehicles, either ETFs or mutual funds, with the lowest expense ratio.
4. Avoid actively-managed funds.

SUMMARY OF SECTION

- Index funds, or the corresponding ETF, should be the core holdings of your stock portfolio.
- Consider a position in sector funds that are out-performing.
- ETF's offer flexibility not available with mutual funds.
- Disadvantages of ETFs include commissions to trade and difficulty in determining instantaneous Net Asset Value (NAV).
- Income averaging – disciplined consistent investing – is the best approach for the physician investor to accumulate wealth.

REFERENCES

1. Cottle S, Murray R F, Block F E. Graham and Dodd's Security Analysis. 5th Ed. New York: McGraw-Hill, 1988.
2. Shiller R F. Irrational Exuberance. Princeton, NJ. Princeton University Press, 2000.

Chapter Thirty-Two
Real Estate Other than Your Home

GENERAL POINTS

Real estate should represent a significant position in every investor's portfolio. Financially, real estate shares features with equities (stocks) and bonds. It is similar to the former in that it can appreciate and usually tracks inflation well. It is similar to the latter in that it produces a dividend (rent). Not surprisingly, its return of 7–8% is midway between the 10% return of stocks and the 5% return of bonds.

Before detailing why real estate should be a core holding, a discussion of the potential negatives is warranted. "You can't lose on real estate, it always goes up" has been exposed for the myth that it always was. *All* investments have risks. With the bursting of the real estate bubble, home prices in the US are down for the first time since the Great Depression. Comparing anything to the Great Depression should give you pause.

In the first edition, I said "I feel we may currently(early 2005) be experiencing a real estate bubble, similar to our stock market bubble of the late 1990s, similar to the Japanese stock market and real estate bubble of the late 1980s. Shiller, the author of *Irrational Exuberance* [1] has recently voiced similar concerns.... When there have been multiple years of gains and within the last year prices are up another 25–30%...you are almost

R.M. Doroghazi, *The Physician's Guide to Investing*,
DOI 10.1007/978-1-60761-134-9_32,
© Humana Press, a part of Springer Science+Business Media, LLC 2005, 2009

certain to be buying at the top.... Keep your powder dry, there will be some real bargains in several years".

As of the summer of 2008 home prices nation-wide, according to the Case-Shiller index, were down 23% from their peak. How much farther will real estate fall, and over what period of time? Will the drop be sudden, or prolonged and agonizing? I do not know, but consider this:

1. Remember the concept of regression to the mean. As it applies here, the markets that experienced the greatest run-up will probably be the ones that have the most to lose. Examples would be Las Vegas, Florida, and both coasts. However, I doubt that any market will be immune.

2. What is the mean? I suggest we start with what the pro says. Prof. Robert Shiller of Yale called the stock market bubble in *Irrational Exuberance* [1] and the real estate bubble in *Irrational Exuberance: Second Edition* [2]. Shiller showed that since 1890, when adjusted for inflation, real home prices in the US went up an average of only 0.6% per year. The only periods that deviated significantly from this were post-WWII (which was not speculative-there were two decades of pent-up demand fueled by a real increase in wealth), and 1997–2004, which was obviously speculative. Over the latter period, real home prices nation-wide were up 52%, suggesting there still may be a lot of "regressing" to go. I suggest that a reasonable mean would be to consider what the property sold for in 2000–2002, before the great speculation really heated up. Considered from another point of view, homes usually sell at about 2.8 times the average family income. At the height of the bubble, the average home was about 3.9 times average income (a 39% premium).

3. The first mistake investors make in any bear market is not to have taken profits in the preceding bull market. The second mistake is be enticed back in too early. Things look cheap because they are destined to get cheaper. Don't be a hero and try to pick the bottom. One very smart young man I know on Wall Street told me he is quite content to give up the first 5% of any bull market rather than jump in too early. Just as markets overshoot on the upside, they also tend to overshoot on the downside. Just because prices regress to the mean does not mean they will stop there.

The best way to estimate the value of real estate is to look at it as you would any other investment, i.e., what is the anticipated return? The time-honored goal for rental property is a return after expenses of 10%, referred to as the capitalization rate, the NOI (Net Operating Income) in the first year of ownership, divided by the purchase price. If the monthly rent is $1,000 and expenses are $100/month, the NOI is $900. Take that number times 120, and you would be willing to pay $108K for the property ($900 per month is a 10% return on a property costing $108K).

To highlight the extent of the speculation at the height of the recent bubble, many (supposedly) sophisticated investors were accepting capitalization rates of 6% or 5% or even lower. They were assuming (hoping) that further price appreciation would be sufficient to make up for the meager rental return. In the above example, they would pay $130 or 140K for a property that would traditionally fetch about $110K. Keep your powder dry, hang on to your cash and preserve your borrowing capacity, because before this is over you will find some real bargains.

If you find a desirable property but feel it is over-priced, either someone (not you) will over-pay, or it will just sit, and sit, and sit, until the seller is sufficiently motivated to lower the price to a realistic level. Remember, it is impossible to turn a profit if you overpay. Be patient! We may not hit bottom until 2009 or 2010.

Location, location, location. What ten or fifteen years ago was in the most fashionable area of town may now be in an area that is not as desirable or even undesirable. Even a great property in a great location may not do well if it is over-leveraged, poorly managed or the tenants do not take care of the property (always have a security deposit).

There are several reasons real estate has traditionally done well and will continue to do well in the long term. As they say, they are not making any more land, the supply is clearly limited. This fact is already quite apparent in the center of large cities, such as Manhattan, Boston, San Francisco and Washington DC. Because of the financial, educational, business, and governmental base of these areas, it is a prerequisite that people live in close proximity. These areas are also exciting because there is so much to do. As society continues to progress and the population continues to increase, there will be an even greater demand for real estate.

In general, the longer an investment is held, the greater the potential for profit. An investor buying a stock has an almost infinitely higher chance of realizing a profit if the position is held one year as compared to just one day. Stocks can be traded on-line by the touch of the button.

Compare this to real estate. Selling real estate is cumbersome. It may take weeks or months or longer in a down market, or if the property is over-priced, and the commissions are significant. You do not sell your home in a panic as occurs when the stock market drops and stocks are sold in a panic. These factors essentially force you to hold real estate longer, which in the end increases the likelihood of a profit. Think of this as a sort of system-enforced patience.

The leverage of a mortgage increases the potential profit. A piece of well-chosen real estate is often a sound investment with a 20% down payment. Compare this to purchasing a stock with only 20% down and 80% margin (the average investor cannot make such an investment since this is greater than the usual margin requirements allowed by the Federal Reserve). The purchase of a stock on 80% margin would be a terribly flimsy investment.

Consider the following as a reasonable example of the finances and profit potential of the purchase of a rental property. A $200K property is purchased with a 20% down payment of $40K. If the property was chosen appropriately, the rent should cover the expenses and mortgage payment on a 15-year note. After fifteen years, your $40K has grown to $200K, a more than 11% compounded annual rate of return.

But the gain could be even greater. There is also (1) depreciation, with its favorable short-term tax consequences, (2) the interest on the note and the expenses to maintain the property are tax-deductible, (3) hopefully there will be an increase in the value of the property and 4) it should be possible to raise the rent as time goes on, further improving the positive cash flow.

This is identical to a corporation that regularly increases dividends. This excess cash flow can be used for anything such as paying off the note early or for other investments. A properly chosen piece of rental property may produce a 15% compounded annual rate of return. The limiting factors to such profit are straightforward, namely, having the money for the down payment, choosing the right property, paying an appropriate price, the work and time of managing the property, good tenants, and patience.

I feel it is mandatory to finance investment real estate with a fixed-rate, non-recourse note with no early repayment penalty. Adjustable-rate notes are just gambling. The two decade bull market in bonds that started in the early 1980s is over (*see* the preceding chapter). Considering that interest rates are currently at multi-decade lows, and that inflation will probably worsen over the long term, interest rates will likely be higher 5–10 years from now. A non-recourse loan means that the bank's only collateral is the property. If you sign a recourse note, the bank has the "recourse" to also come after your other assets.

Real estate traditionally performs well in an inflationary environment. During inflationary periods, financial assets, such as cash and bonds, lose value. People turn to real assets to preserve wealth, with gold, commodities, collectibles and real estate the prime examples. In addition, if the property was financed with a fixed-rate note (vida supra), the debt is being paid off with dollars that are both cheaper and easier to come by.

BUT, the current situation is not traditional. We have deflation in the real estate and stock markets. This is a vicious and precarious situation. History shows that credit bubbles end in a crash, because the liquidation of debt is deflationary. Mr. Ben Bernanke, current Chairman of the Federal Reserve, is a student of the Great Depression. I believe he will do everything within his power to prevent the deflation in the housing market from spreading to Depression-like deflation in the general economy. Once prices began to spiral downward the cycle is very difficult to stop. Unfortunately, I am not sure we have yet dodged the bogey man of deflation.

Real estate is devastated by deflation. Not only is the property worth less, but because almost all real estate is purchased with some debt, the dollars used to pay off the loan are both more valuable and harder to come by. To read more on the subject, *see* Robert Prechter's book *Conquer the Crash: You Can Survive and Prosper in a Deflationary Depression* [3].

We will eventually have inflation in the general economy because we are fighting deflation by printing money. The National Debt will be ten *trillion* dollars by the time this book is in print and is increasing at a rate of two billion dollars every day. We have added trillions to the books via the government takeover of mortgage giants Fannie Mae (FNM) and Freddie Mac (FRE) and other companies. Our leaders have chosen to sacrifice the dollar to prevent Depression-like deflation. This is not just my opinion. About four years ago, Paul Volcker, one of the most capable Chairman ever of the Federal Reserve, whose actions in the late 70s and early 80s saved the dollar, predicted a 75% chance of a third-world style debt crisis in the United States within the next 5 years. When recently asked about this prediction, he said "what do you think we are having now?" Few people in the world have more credibility in financial circles than Volcker. Vigyáz, in Hungarian means "look out for danger."

My suggestion to best protect yourself against possible deflation is to be out of debt and have plenty of cash. You do not want your home being sold on the courthouse steps with all of the other foreclosures. To hedge against inflation, own some gold (*see* the next chapter).

SUMMARY OF SECTION

- Every investment portfolio should contain real estate.
- Real estate shares features with both stocks and bonds.
- Use the capitalization rate to value rental property.
- I fear the real estate market has not yet reached bottom.

- Finance rental property with a fixed-rate, non-recourse loan.
- Real estate traditionally does well in an inflationary environment but is devastated by deflation.
- We may not yet have dodged the bogey man of deflation.

OWNING A PROPERTY OUTRIGHT

There are several situations, in addition to your home, that you should consider the direct purchase of real estate as an investment.

The first is vacation or recreational property. A typical example is a home or condo in areas you like to go on vacation or just relax. Examples include anywhere on the water, whether that be a seacoast, riverbank or lake, such as Lake of the Ozarks in this area. I must make one recommendation. The most desirable properties are the ones right on the water. Do not purchase a "second tier" property, one not directly on the water. These will never be as desirable and it is quite unlikely they will appreciate as rapidly. You do not want to be forced to look around someone else's trees or shrubs or home to see the water. You want that unobstructed view, those gorgeous sunrises or sunsets, the sounds of the waves, to be right outside your window or balcony. Real estate is like collectibles. People want the best and there will always be someone willing to pay for it. Buy the best property you can afford (note I emphasize you can afford. Don't get carried away!). These will be the most fun and have the greatest appreciation potential.

Other examples of desirable areas include snow skiing areas, resorts, land for hunting or hiking, historical areas, islands, and properties in general in areas that are warm during the winter, such as the southeast, south, gulf coast and southwest. Because of the lifestyle they offer, properties on a golf course are becoming increasingly popular, both as a home and as a vacation destination. Just as you should always buy on the water, always buy on the golf course, do not buy a second tier property.

Remember there is a practical aspect to vacation property. Not only is cost important, but how long it takes to get there is much more important for the vast majority of people looking for a second home, or any piece of recreational property. A 75-mile drive can be easily accomplished two weekends a month as compared to a full day's travel with multiple airplane connections to get from the upper Midwest or Northeast to a beachfront home in the Florida Keys.

As society becomes wealthier more money will be spent on recreational property. Only so much can be spent on a home (albeit sometimes very much), car, electronics and other basic needs. This leaves more discretionary income to be funneled into recreational property. I also believe this will apply to collectibles (see Chapter Thirty-Four).

Although I strongly recommend you own recreational/vacation property, remember this is a discretionary purchase. Unless you are presented a very compelling opportunity, let the dust settle on the current real estate mess before making a commitment.

One question that always arises with vacation and recreational property is if you should purchase a stand-alone home or a condo. The majority of people probably find stand-alone homes more desirable. The appreciation potential is almost always greater than a condo because you own the land. With a condo you must also deal with the other owners, which can sometimes be a royal pain. Another potential problem with condos relates to the financial health of the complex. For established, going concerns, this is usually not an issue. For condos that have not yet been completed and turned over to the owners association, if the developer goes belly up, you could be in a very ugly situation. This is a real possibility in the current real estate market.

The principle features that make condos desirable are the lower price and lack of maintenance. Unless you are willing to pay others to perform the maintenance on a stand-alone home, a good part of your precious vacation time will be spent on maintenance and upkeep such as mowing the lawn, raking the leaves, painting, etc. Whatever you choose should suit your preference and needs but do not forget this very important and practical issue.

You can own a property for personal use only or for both personal use and as a rental. The great part of the later option is that you can cover some portion of the mortgage payments with the rental income. There are real estate firms that will rent/ manage the property. As with everything there is a down side. If you rent the property the IRS limits personal use to no more than the greater of fourteen days or 10% of the days that the property is rented. Some people do not like the thought of other people sleeping in their beds. To some people this is not an issue. It is completely up to you.

There are other ways recreational property can produce income. If you want a property for outdoor activities such as fishing, hunting or camping, look for something that also has agricultural potential (If you are "land-locked," i.e., you do not have direct access to a road, make sure that you have your right-of-way in writing). Agricultural land has, so far, resisted the general downturn in real estate. If you purchased a property because of the nice lake that can also be row cropped or planted in trees, all the better.

Another upside of owning recreational property is that its use by family and close friends will generate considerable goodwill. I assure you when someone can save $250 or more a day, and stay in a nicer place, and fix their own meals rather than be forced to eat out, and do their wash, they will remember your generosity for a long time. Don't be stingy; allow your good fortune to bring enjoyment to others. I do have one rule when I let others use my condo: the place must be left cleaner than they found it.

There are other factors to consider with vacation property. It is not uncommon for people, after they retire, to sell their home and move into what was previously their recreational/vacation property. This is especially common if the property is in a warmer area. This is also an excellent example of how patience and good planning can pay long-term dividends.

Or, you may not move to the area, but know the area so well from years of vacations that you purchase a second unit as a full-time rental investment. I did this in 2002 when I purchased a second condo unit at the Lake of the Ozarks as a full-time rental property (and sold it in June, 2005 at the top of the market).

At least at the Lake of the Ozarks, the first-time buyer holds their property an average of only three years. Some people are moving up, but most have found this just was not for them and sell (real estate agents love this because the high turn-over generates commissions). My first point is to make sure the property is what you want before you buy. Promise yourself you will use it every-so-often. My other point is that if you find you do not like it, get out and cut your losses. I know several people who used their property sparingly or not at all for years before they finally faced reality and decided to sell. It is a terrible waste of resources to let a six-figure investment just sit. Use it or sell it.

The time-share concept waxes and wanes in popularity. The upside is that these cost only a fraction of buying a similar property, and you have considerable flexibility. You do not feel as "locked in" as when you own a property, and time share credits can often be traded to visit other destinations. Look on a time-share as a convenience, it is *not* an investment, you will not make money on a time-share.

The second situation where you should consider buying a property outright and then renting is when you can rent to a relative or close friend, essentially an "inside" deal.

The best place to start is with your parents. There are several possibilities. If your parents are middle class, lower middle class or of more humble origins, it is probable that a good deal of their wealth is the equity in their home. Your parents may have a net worth of $250K, but $200K is the value of their home and $50K are CDs in the bank. They could afford a better life style if they could tap the equity in their home.

There are two options. One is a "reverse mortgage" from the bank. Rather than discuss the pros and cons in detail, let me just make the same general comment I made about borrowing from your own retirement account: I just do not like the concept and feel they should be avoided. A much better option, presuming your parents' home is a reasonable investment in and of itself and they wish to continue to live there, is to purchase the home and rent it back to them. Your family has already saved 6% because there was no real estate commission, you have a perfect tenant, and it should be possible to structure things such that, with an appropriate down payment, the rent covers your mortgage payments and other expenses. Or if your parents wish to move into a smaller or different home or a condo, you should purchase this and rent it to them. There is almost no reason for your parents to rent from anyone but you.

By doing this you have a great investment and a nice piece of rental property that will hopefully be paid for free and clear in ten to fifteen years. And your parents have $200K (or whatever the equity in their home) to do anything they have always dreamed of, but never pursued because they did not have the money. I have one physician friend who is such an astute investor that he was able to help his parents invest the money they received when he bought their home that the income generated from their investments not only covered their rental payments but allowed them extra spending money without having to touch the principle.

One suggestion: Be sure your siblings are fully aware of how everything is structured so there are no hard feelings down the line, because when they see what a nice investment you made at the "expense of their inheritance", they will be jealous.

There was an article in *Barron's* (4/5/04) with the catchy title of "Kiddie Condos". Rather than paying for room in a dorm or apartment, with nothing to show after four years of college, it suggested the possibility of buying a condo in the area of the school and renting it to your child. The children have a nicer place to live, and if it is a two bedroom, the other bedroom can be rented to a roommate, further helping to defray the costs or even showing a profit. The parents can accumulate equity and also gain from depreciation and hopefully appreciation of the unit. The key to any rental is to keep it rented to a tenant who pays their bills on time and takes good care of the property. To rent to a relative or close friend, someone you can trust, is money in the bank.

Remember that this property, as with any piece of real estate, must be purchased with the realization that it will at sometime be resold. The property must not only fit your needs but also have features potential buyers find desirable. Because you would probably be holding such a property for only 3 or 4 years (unless you have multiple children that plan to attend the same school), the current real estate market has just about killed this idea. But keep it in your memory banks for future reference.

Granted, such opportunities do not occur often, but you do not need many opportunities to accumulate real wealth. Say you identify one such opportunity every five years – twice a decade. You purchase your first rental property (as a reminder, not selling a previous home is a real possibility) at age 40 with a 10 to 15 year note. You buy a property every 5 years at a cost of $150K. When the first property is paid off the income can be applied to help pay off notes on the later purchases. By age 65 you own five properties free and clear worth at least $5 \times \$150K = \$750K$ (plus potential appreciation) with a net rental income of 40–50 thousand dollars per year. One half of your retirement. It can be this easy. To be Warren Buffett or Bill Gates requires genius. But mere discipline and patience can be enough to allow you to retire with comfort and financial security.

I have one other suggestion for a near "no-brainer" real estate investment. This involves buying into the real estate of your practice. There are two important reasons to consider this: (1) If you think it is nice when someone else pays you rent, wait until you pay yourself rent. It is financial ecstasy. (2) Because this involves your practice, you maintain a degree of input and control, both financially and as it relates to the politics of your practice vis-à-vis your partners.

But there can be two significant negatives. The first concerns the size of the group. These are typically set up as partnerships where everyone has an equal vote. When there are two to four partners it is usually, but not always, easy to reach a consensus. But if there are 25 or 30 partners, you will quickly realize why our forefathers established our great country as a republic rather than a democracy. The more people, the more difficult it is to get anything accomplished.

It is also essential that the criteria for the buyout when you leave or retire be clearly stipulated (I believe a mandatory buyout is in the best interests of the partner and the partnership). If they are not, you may be dealing with retired partners who now live in Arizona or Florida and do not have the same interests as you. Or worse, if a partner has died, you could be dealing with an estate lawyer or bank trust department or family member whom you have never met. These situations can be terribly messy. This also illustrates a general point: it is always easier to get into something than it is to get out. Be careful.

Of course, you may purchase any other piece of rental property such as a home, condo, duplex, small apartment building or office building. Either a relative, such as your spouse, a grown child or a sibling or a retired parent could manage the property for you, or there are professional rental management firms whose job it is to manage such properties. Although I incessantly preach self-reliance, I do not recommend you personally attempt to manage rental property while actively practicing medicine. Your time, worth $100–$200 an hour, is much better spent taking care of patients. In addition, I am sure you already receive enough phone calls about patients with headaches, constipation and nausea without receiving calls that a sewer has backed up.

I suggest the physician investor avoid the direct purchase of undeveloped land as an investment. I am not discussing recreational land, but undeveloped land. There are at least three reasons. The first is financial. Undeveloped land produces no income, so because of insurance and taxes and other expenses and payments on the note (if the land was not purchased with cash), there is a negative cash flow. Second, land cannot be depreciated, as compared to the favorable tax consequence of depreciating a structure such as a home. Third, the profit potential in developing land is not in the land but in the developing. One of the basic ways to profit from any investment is to be able to unlock value not apparent to others. Being a successful developer is quite difficult. The successful developers I have met are really solid business people. I also know several solid business people who tried their hand at development and failed. It would be very difficult if not impossible for even an astute physician investor to be a successful land developer.

You may also invest in any other type of real estate in any way that a company or partnership may be structured. These must be evaluated on their own merit, but remember my comments elsewhere regarding the frequent problems with physicians and limited partnerships, especially those sold through a broker.

SUMMARY OF SECTION

- Strongly consider the purchase of recreational/vacation property.
- Always buy on the water or the golf course. Avoid second tier properties.
- Use your recreational property or sell it.
- Be generous and let others use your recreational property.
- People want the best and there will always be someone willing to pay for it.
- Look for opportunities to rent to family or close friends.
- Do not attempt to manage or develop real estate yourself.
- Buy into the real estate of your practice, but be sure the buyout is defined.

REAL ESTATE INVESTMENT TRUSTS (REITs)

REITs are companies that own and manage real estate. Their structure mandates that 90% of the profits be paid out as dividends, so the yield is high, typically in the range of 5–10% per year.

The two general types of REITs are equity REITs, which invest in properties, manage them for rental income, and then sell them, and mortgage REITs, which invest in and realize income from mortgages. In general, equity REITs more closely follow the real estate market and should be the ones in which a physician invests because they have shown greater long-term returns than mortgage REITs (In the long run it is always more profitable to own a company than lend it money).

There are REITs for every type of real estate; Apartments in large cities, small cities, office buildings nationwide or in Boston or Chicago or San Francisco, industrial complexes, malls, warehouse, even medical office buildings. See the website www.Reit.com for more information on REITs.

REITs have several desirable features. First is the dividend yield. Second is that the shares trade on the major stock exchanges, just as the shares of Potash Saskatchewan (POT) or Peabody Energy (BTU). This provides instant liquidity as compared to owning a property outright, which may take considerable time to sell. REITs are professionally managed, but just as with any management team, there are above average and below average performers. If you prefer capital gains rather than dividends, REOCs (Real Estate Operating Companies) are structured to favor capital gains.

You may purchase the stock of a specific REIT, or buy shares in a mutual fund or ETF that specializes in REITs (see the Specialty-Real Estate screener at Yahoo Finance! ETF Center http://finance.yahoo.com). These vehicles allow you to invest in real estate at only a tiny fraction of the money that would be required to purchase even a small condo.

The stocks of REITs trade every day, and thus the prices change daily, although usually not very much. Compare this to your home or a rental property. It is very unlikely that when you drive up to your home in the evening you say "my home has gone down $237 in value today or my rental property is up exactly $8 today."

Historically, REITs provide diversification because they show less than a 50% correlation with the general stock market, and tend to out-perform or under-perform the market for periods lasting years. Thus if REITs have gone through a period of underperformance, it may be a time to buy. Likewise, if you are ahead 40% in three years (20% total dividends and 20% capital appreciation) it may be time to take profits and re-allocate the assets.

SUMMARY OF SECTION

- REITs offer the possibility to invest smaller amounts of money and liquidity not possible when owning a property outright.
- The long-term performance of equity REITs is superior to that of mortgage REITs.

REFERENCES

1. Shiller R J. Irrational Exuberance. Princeton, NJ: Princeton University Press, 2000.
2. Shiller R J. Irrational Exuberance: Second Edition. Princeton, NJ: Princeton University Press, 2005.
3. Prechter R R. Conquer the Crash: You Can Survive and Prosper in a Deflationary Recession. Hoboken, NJ: John Wiley & Sons, 2002.

Chapter Thirty-Three
The Precious Metals and Commodities

GOLD AND THE PRECIOUS METALS

Accept the fact: The once-mighty U.S. dollar is no longer "as good as gold". You can no longer go to the Treasury and exchange your paper money for specie (coined gold and silver) on demand. People the world-over are losing confidence in fiat currencies and trading their intrinsically worthless paper money for real assets, such as the precious metals, diamonds, collectibles and commodities. But you must understand: gold is not going up, the value (purchasing power) of paper money is going down. I have been bullish on the precious metals since gold was $380/ounce in the fall of 2003. Although there will be corrections along the way, I believe the bull market in the precious metals and commodities has many years to run.

Gold has been money since the beginning of civilization. It is malleable, it does not rust, it does not tarnish, its' financial and visual luster are eternal. Gold salvaged from the floor of the deepest ocean or buried for thousands of years retains its value. Gold is the only commodity produced not to be consumed. It is estimated that 85% of the gold ever mined is still above ground. If you are holding a one ounce gold coin in your hand, it probably contains several molecules once held in the hand of Alexander, Caesar or Napoleon.

R.M. Doroghazi, *The Physician's Guide to Investing*,
DOI 10.1007/978-1-60761-134-9_33,
© Humana Press, a part of Springer Science+Business Media, LLC 2005, 2009

The painful, and shameful, reality is that the dollar has fallen so far that it is worth only 1/1000 an ounce of gold, an amount essentially invisible to the naked eye. Gold is wealth because it can only be produced by the sweat of a man's brow. Paper money can, and is, created and manipulated by the wish of politicians. History has shown that all paper money eventually becomes worthless. Gold has no counter-party risk, it stands alone.

An investment, such as a CD at the bank, the stock of a corporation such as Proctor and Gamble (PG), or a piece of rental property or farmland, produces a return. Gold is not an investment, it is a storehouse of wealth. Because it can be difficult to appreciate or determine something's value when viewed in isolation, let me provide some perspective by comparison. In Old Testament times (about 500 BCE), in the Great Depression, and in 2008, one ounce of gold purchased 300 loaves of bread. In Roman times, an ounce of gold purchased a fine toga. Today an ounce of gold still purchases a fine suit. The year I was born gasoline was 19 cents a gallon. One dollar purchased enough gas to get you from Columbia to St. Louis (about 120 miles). One ounce of gold bought enough gas to get you from NYC to St. Louis and back. Today, one ounce of gold still buys enough gas to get you from NYC to St. Louis and back, while a dollar won't even get you across town.

A good way to evaluate the precious metals is to compare the ratio of the DJIA/gold, that is, how many ounces of gold are required to purchase the Dow Jones Industrial Average. When the ratio is high, financial assets are expensive and gold is cheap. When the ratio is low, gold is dear and it is time to buy financial assets. The average over the last century was about 10.

After the bull market of the Roaring 20 s, the DJIA peaked at 381 in 1929. Gold was $20.67 per ounce (as it had been since our currency was established in 1792), a ratio of almost 20/1. As the market sank into the Great Depression, the DJIA bottomed at 41 in 1932. In 1933, after Roosevelt called-in (confiscated is a more accurate word) and shortly thereafter re-valued gold to $35/ounce, the ratio had fallen to almost 1/ 1. Financial assets were cheap, it was the buy of the century in the stock market.

In 1966, the DJIA briefly touched 1,000, while gold was fixed by the Bretton-Woods agreement at $35/ounce. The ratio was almost 30 to1, indicating financial assets were expensive and gold was cheap. With President Johnson's deficit spending of the mid-to-late 60 s, inflation began to accelerate. In 1971, when the French demanded gold for their depreciating dollars, Nixon was forced to close the gold window. The last link to the gold standard, and the discipline it imposed, was broken. Inflation and gold skyrocketed. The stock market tanked, the second worst bear market of the twentieth century. By 1980, the DJIA and gold were both at 800. The 30:1 ratio was again back to 1:1. Gold was expensive and stocks were again cheap.

In 1999, the DJIA was above 10,000, and gold reached its 19-year low of $255, coincident with the Bank of England's sale of one-half of its gold. The ratio was more than 40:1, the highest ever, and marked the beginning of the current bull market in the precious metals and the bear market in financial assets. Since then the DJIA has lost more than 80% of its value compared to gold.

Of course I have no idea where gold goes from here, but history suggests that before this bull market in the precious metals is over, the ratio will continue to drop and may again approach parity. In 2003, James Turk, who writes the *Freemarket Gold & Money Report*(www.fgmr.com), predicted gold would reach $8,000 per ounce. The number sounds like pure fantasy, but if history repeats and the ratio falls to 3:1 or 2:1 or even 1:1, gold will be far into 4 figures.

Because of incremental monetary demand, silver rises faster than gold in precious metals bull markets. It usually requires about 50 ounces of silver to buy one ounce of gold. In early 1980, when the Hunt brothers tried to corner the silver market, gold was $800/ounce, and silver was $50/ounce, a ratio of 16:1. At silver's low in 1991, during the precious metal bear market, it took more than 90 ounces of silver to purchase one ounce of gold. If gold goes to $3,000 per ounce and the ratio drops to 20:1, silver would be $150/ounce.

Again, these numbers seem terribly unrealistic, but it has happened before. Be reminded also that a good deal of the gains in a bull market are at the very end, when things get hysterical and frothy, at the blow-off top. As a comparison, in 1995, when the NASDAQ crossed 1,000, did you believe that in March, 2000, it would be 5,000?

Your core position in the precious metals should be US-minted bullion coins in your personal possession. Take delivery and keep the gold in your safe deposit box at the bank. Because one of the reasons you are buying gold is as an insurance policy, it would be desirable to have some outside the United States. Remember that in 1933 it was made illegal for US citizens to hold gold, and considering the recent intervention of the government in the markets, including banning the short sale of many financial stocks, it is not inconceivable that if things got really rough, the government could again call in the gold. Unfortunately, since September 11th, it has become extremely difficult to open a bank account outside the US.

Until recently, I recommended the purchase of only 1 oz Gold Eagles, because on smaller denomination gold coins and silver, the mark-up was proportionally higher. However, if gold goes anywhere near where Turk suggests, a single 1 oz gold coin will be thousands of dollars, and a pound of gold will approach six-figures, thus limiting liquidity. I now also recommend the purchase of gold coins smaller than one ounce, and 1 oz US Silver Eagles. Not only will their liquidity be greater, but it will allow people with smaller amounts to invest to enter the market. Gifting will also be more practical. I love my nieces and nephews, but not enough to give them a 1 oz gold coin, whereas a 1 oz Silver Eagle would make a nice birthday or Christmas present.

(Note: As this book goes to press, the US-minted gold and silver bullion coins have almost disappeared from the market.

One ounce gold Buffalos are no longer available. We are seeing an example of Thomas Gresham's observation during the reign of Queen Elizabeth I that "Bad money drives out the good").

There are many ways to invest in the precious metals in your brokerage account. Probably best for the average investor is through a gold/precious metals mutual fund, as offered by almost all of the major mutual fund companies. There are Exchange Traded Funds (ETFs) for gold-GLD and IAU-which each represent 1/10 ounce of gold, and silver (SLV), which represents 1 ounce of silver. An ETF for platinum may also be available by the time this book appears in print. Note that profits from these precious metals ETFs are taxed at the collectibles rate of 28%, as compared to the 15% rate on long-term capital gains. This is not an issue in a retirement account.

The mining stocks are leveraged, that is, they tend to go up, and down, faster than the price of the underlying metal. In addition, in a stock bear market, they can behave more like stocks, i.e., they go down. You can buy the stocks of individual miners, but I would discourage this unless you have considerable time to spend researching the individual issues. A much better option is the ETF with the ticker GDX, which represents a basket of mining stocks.

How much should you invest in the precious metals? I recommend a position representing *at least* 5% of your investible net worth. If you believe we are in for a period of significant inflation, and that the government's officially published figures under-estimate the true rate of inflation, I submit that you should hold a position in the precious metals.

My recommendation on gold and the precious metals makes most mainstream investment advisors apoplectic (a semi-archaic term which means to have a stroke). I could be wrong. If you purchased gold in 1971 and sold in early 1980, you were an absolute genius. If you purchased gold in early 1980 because you thought it would go up forever and that financial assets were dead, you endured a quarter-century of pain. If you began purchasing gold in 2003, your investment has far out-per-formed the DJIA and the S&P 500.

People say gold is risky. It was not as risky as Fannie Mae, Freddie Mac, Bear Stearns, Lehman Brothers, AIG, or general motors Washington Mutual. Or you go into the forest, chop down a tree and grind it into pulp. You make half the paper into napkins that say Happy Birthday. You slap Ben Franklin's kisser on the rest and say it's worth a hundred bucks. I think that is pretty risky. Buy some gold.

To read more about gold, the precious metals and the depre-ciation of the US dollar, see the first four references at the end of this chapter [1—4].

COMMODITIES

You can live without many things, from the latest, most glamorous high-tech gadgets to even an auto or a television, but you cannot live without commodities. They are the food, fuel, metals and fabrics you consume every day of your life. Yet any mention of investing in this diverse and essential asset class is often dismissed with curt and corre-spondingly un-insightful comments such as "I've heard they are very risky".

I strongly recommend you read *Hot Commodities* [5] by Jim Rogers, from which some of this discussion is taken. Rogers was one of the first to appreciate the current bull market in commodities, and his book provides many details and insights.

Rogers quotes the work of Barry Bannister [6, 7] which shows that "stocks and commodities have alternated leader-ship in regular cycles averaging 18 years". The current bull market in commodities began in 1998/99 when, adjusted for inflation, commodities were as low as during the Great Depression. Of more importance to this discussion, it sug-gests we are only about half way through this bull market in commodities.

Warren Buffett and John Bogle (founder of the Vanguard Group) recently suggested we are in for a prolonged period of under-performance in the stock market, with 4—7% annual returns more likely than the !0% compounded returns of the twentieth century. This fits nicely with this data, and suggests that the relative under-performance in equities (i.e., the current bear market that began in 2000) will continue until the mid-to-late teens, when the commodity bull market will end and it will be time to rotate back into financial assets.

The best way to maximize gains, to make real money in this commodity bull market, in any bull market, is to literally "ride the bull". Stake out your position early and just hang on. There are corrections in all bull markets, and they can be fast and brutal. But being confident in your position, knowing you are in a long-term bull market, allows you to hold on when things get scary. Trading in and out, trying to be slick and beat the market, rarely works, and when it does, it is usually just luck. You invariably get whipsawed, buying high and selling low, missing out on much of the gain, or even suffering a loss.

Before discussing how you can profit from this bull market, let me tell you what you must avoid. Many have the impression that commodities are risky because of the stories of investors, from (supposedly) sophisticated professionals at large institutions and hedge funds to amateurs like your uncle Jimmy, who lost their shirt in the commodity market. The problem was not investing in commodities per se, but the inappropriate use of leverage (margin).

For example, a gold futures contract represents 100 oz of gold. If you deposit the entire value of the contract with the broker ($100 K if gold is $1,000/ounce), you are un-leveraged. Although there are differences, for this discussion it is similar to owning 100 oz of gold outright. If gold drops $60, a 6% loss, you are down $6,000. But if you purchased the contract with a minimum margin deposit ($5K in this example), a $60 move against you not only wipes you out, but you owe the broker another $1,000. As highlighted by the credit crisis of 2008, over-leveraged investments court disaster.

In some respects, commodities are even less risky than financial assets. Your capital on deposit with the broker can be invested in short-term T-Bills to generate interest income. A commodity cannot go bankrupt. The bonds of a corporation, the sovereign bonds of a country, and stocks, can all become worthless, but an ounce of gold, a pound of copper, a bale of cotton, and a gallon of gasoline, will always have some value.

Rogers makes two suggestions for the average investor. The first is to buy a broad index, or basket of commodities, analogous to the S&P 500 Index for stocks. The best known indices include the Reuters-CRB Futures Price Index, the Dow Jones-AIG Commodity Index, and the Goldman Sachs Commodity Index.

Buying an index rather than attempting to beat the market by buying individual positions is a broad theme in investing. Index investing allows you to minimize fees and avoid underperformance because of poor selection, while capturing the broad move in the market. In some circumstances, index investing is even more tax efficient.

Rogers also recommends investing in the commodities themselves, rather than surrogates, such as the companies or countries that produce commodities.

The tradition way to invest directly in commodities is through the futures market (*see* Chapter Thirty-Five). I would recommend this only for sophisticated investors. A much better option for the average investor is via a mutual fund or ETF. Because there are many options, and new products are being offered all the time, you will need to research this yourself. All of the large mutual fund companies offer commodity/natural resource-related funds. Also see the website www. etfconnect.com.

SUMMARY OF CHAPTER THIRTY-THREE

- The US dollar is no longer "as good as gold".
- Gold is not going up, the purchasing power of paper money is going down.
- Gold has been money since the beginning of civilization.

- Gold is not an investment, it is a storehouse of wealth.
- To gain perspective, compare gold to the Dow Jones Industrial Average.
- Silver outperforms gold in precious metals bull markets.
- Your core position should be US-minted bullion coins in your personal possession.
- I suggest at least a 5% position in the precious metals.
- It would be desirable to have some gold outside the US. The government called in the gold in 1933, it could happen again.
- Stocks and commodities alternate leadership in regular cycles averaging 18 years. This suggests we are only half way through the commodity bull market and the stock bear market.
- Stake out your position early and "ride the bull".
- Commodities cannot go broke as can financial assets.

REFERENCES

1. Turk J, Rubino J. The Coming Collapse of the Dollar and How to Profit From It. New York: Currency-Doubleday, 2004.
2. Lewis N. Gold: The Once and Future Money. Hoboken, NJ: John Wiley & Sons, 2007.
3. Bonner B, Wiggin A. Empire of Debt: The Rise of an Epic Financial Crisis. Hoboken, NJ: John Wiley & Sons, 2006.
4. Schiff P D, Downes J. Crash Proof: How to Profit From the Coming Economic Collapse. Hoboken, NJ: John Wiley & Sons, 2007.
5. Rogers J. Hot Commodities: How Anyone Can Invest Profitably in the World's Best Market. New York: Random House, 2004.
6. Bannister B, Forward P. The Inflation Cycle of 2002 to 2015. Equity Research Industrial Portfolio Strategy. Legg Mason, April 19, 2002.
7. Bannister B. War, Legacy Debt, and Social Costs As Catalysts for US Inflation Cycle. Legg Mason, May 16, 2003.

Chapter Thirty-Four
Art and Collectibles

COLLECTIBLES

I have always been fascinated by detail, what makes one thing different than something else. Whenever I find a subject that interests me, I read as much about it as I can. I have also always been fascinated and held a respect for antiquity. The look, the touch, the feel, and the story behind something: who made it, why they made it, why was someone careful enough to preserve it or how was it lucky enough to survive to the present day.

With these sorts of tastes and interests, it is not surprising I am a collector. Collecting is fun and enjoyable, and a great way to spend quality time with the family, from going to an antique mall to watching "Antique Road Show" together on TV. Collecting can also be used as just one more way to teach your children how to invest their money and introduce them to a potential life-long interest.

Bright, inquisitive people almost always have interests outside their primary vocation, and this often includes hobbies and collecting. I believe that my deep interest and knowledge of baseball at least helped me gain acceptance to the Massachusetts General Hospital for my medical internship and residency.

Dr Mark Siegler, currently the Lindy Bergman Professor of Medicine at the University of Chicago, and one of the world's foremost authorities on medical ethics, was a very junior faculty

R.M. Doroghazi, *The Physician's Guide to Investing*,
DOI 10.1007/978-1-60761-134-9_34,
© Humana Press, a part of Springer Science+Business Media, LLC 2005, 2009

member when I was a 3rd year medical student. In my letter of recommendation, Mark noted my photographic memory and encyclopedic knowledge of baseball. He said that such a passion and ability to acquire so much knowledge indicated the mental acuity and desire to do the same in medicine.

My interview at the MGH was before a panel of senior physicians including Dr. Arnold Weinberg, Asst Chief of Medicine, Dr Kurt Isselbacher and Dr. Peter Yurchak. I was nervous to the point of being petrified. The interview began with Dr. Weinberg saying "Bob, in the 1941 World Series, Tommy Henrich reached first base on a missed 3rd strike. Who was the catcher?"

I instantly replied "Mickey Owen", and without thinking said "OK, who was the pitcher"? He did not know, nor did any of the other esteemed physicians who held my professional future in their hands. I shook my finger in Dr. Weinberg's face and said proudly "It was Hugh Casey".

I then said to myself "Bob, you just embarrassed the Assistant Chief of Medicine of the Massachusetts General Hospital and all of his big-shot Harvard friends. This is not good".

I was not only accepted, but over the years I have received phone calls from people I didn't know asking me to repeat the story. At a University of Chicago event in 2008, a classmate that I had not seen in the 31 years since graduation had heard the story and asked me to clarify a few details. Having hobbies and interests outside of medicine can pay both intellectual and professional dividends.

I have come up with what I call Doroghazi's Rule of Collectibles. Until the Industrial Revolution, almost everything a worker produced was consumed immediately in their daily lives. However, as society becomes wealthier, with more discretionary income, I believe more and more money will be directed into collectibles (and recreational land (*see* Chapter Thirty-Two), personal experiences, and charity (*see* Chapter Forty). Only so much can be spent, although admittedly quite a lot by some folks, on clothes, electrical gadgets, a car and a home. People always want things that cannot just be mass-produced in a factory, something others don't have, things with a restricted, finite supply, such as things that were made yesterday. There are only so many 19th century tables and chairs, so many ante-bellum mansions, and so many sci-fi movie posters from the 1950s.

However, there is no other area of investing where knowledge of the subject is more critical to success. Although I strongly encourage you to consider collecting as a pleasurable way to spend your free time, I must point out that few people realize a reasonable return from the money spent on collectibles. Be sure what you spend either generates sufficient enjoyment or an adequate profit.

Remember, there are only two differences between adult's toys and children's toys: adult's toys are more expensive and children don't finance their tinker toys or video games with a loan from the bank.

Three factors determine the value of all collectibles:

1. Desirability. The baseball cards of Charles "Whammy" Douglas, Clarence "Choo-Choo" Coleman, Bob "Ach" Duliba, and Stan "The Man" Musial were produced in similar quantity. Whose card do you think is more valuable?
2. Condition. A 1959 Topps Bob Gibson rookie card graded Gem Mint 10 by PSA (Professional Sports Authenticator) would realize $15,000 or more at auction. The same card affixed to your bicycle fender with a clothespin to generate a "putt-putt" noise when you rode around the neighborhood behind the DDT sprayer might not even be sellable.
3. I had a friend who was a Yankee fan. In 1961, he took his Mickey Mantle and Roger Maris cards, put the backs of the cards to each other, and stapled them together so he could keep them in his back pocket. These cards in mint condition would be worth thousands. Even if he still has the cards today, their only value is in his memories.

There are many other issues to consider when collecting:

1. A collection *must* be focused. The terms superior, profitable collection and eclectic are almost mutually exclusive. A collection of cars will probably just be a bunch of cars. But a collection of Chevrolet Chevelles from the late 60s and early 70s, with a 396cc or 454cc engine, will be a world-class collection. The best, most focused collections are always the most profitable collections.

2. Knowledge. The importance of information has already been mentioned many times elsewhere. Knowledge is power. If you recognize value not apparent to others, you can profit. The premier dealers and auction house personnel know as much about their area as physicians know about medicine. The knowledge base of some dealers and collectors is astounding and never ceases to amaze me.

3. Quality. Everyone wants the best, and there will always be someone willing to pay for it. The most beautiful diamond in 2008 will be a beautiful diamond in 2108. Stuff that was junk in 1908 will be junk forever.

4. You must start small. Your knowledge base and experience are less, you are more likely to make a mistake. It is also almost invariable your tastes will change and mature as you gain more knowledge. It is not uncommon for items purchased early in your collecting career not to be part of your final collection.

5. Patience, patience, patience. The premier pieces may be unavailable for years or even decades. The most spectacular collections, with the best items, often become available only when the collection is liquidated after the collector's death. Purchasing something just to fill a slot is a terrible waste of resources. Wait for what you want then go for it.

6. Collectibles and art are the "canary in the gold mine", the ultimate discretionary purchase. When times are good and people are flush, prices go bonkers. At the first hint of bad times, prices can go into the dumpster. Not surprisingly, except when a collection is being liquidated because of the death of the collector, most premium pieces only appear on the market when prices are strong, at the top. The sophisticated insiders know when to sell.

7. Prices of the most desirable pieces increase geometrically, not arithmetically. Coins are graded on a scale of 4—70. Say there are 20 coins graded MS-64 that sell for $1,000 each. There are 7 coins graded MS-65, and they sell for $5,000 each. But there is only one coin graded MS-66. It could easily bring $20,000—$25,000 or even more. Everyone wants the best, and someone will always pay for it.

8. Buy only from reputable dealers. This is one of the most difficult aspects of collecting. Who are the reputable dealers? Re-read Chapter Twenty "Who Can You Trust?" In the end, the only thing every collector can rely on is their own judgment and knowledge base. You and you alone can best determine the reputable dealers.

9. Forgeries abound. On almost every episode of "Antique Road Show" they have a forgery. Some years ago the Boston Museum of Fine Arts had a display on forgeries.

   No one is too wealthy to avoid be taken. In 1985, a member of the Forbes family paid $156,000 for a 1787 Chateau Lafite Bordeaux, engraved with "Th.J", thought to once be part of Thomas Jefferson's cellar. It, and many other "rare" wines that subsequently appeared, turned out to be fakes [1]. It really was vinegar (vin = wine, aigre = sour).

10. One good item is better than many cheaper ones. One $10K collectible is worth far more than ten $1K collectibles. On the better work, you only have to find one buyer, on the others you have to find 10 buyers (unless they are a set of something). The higher price is saying the item is more desirable.

11. Third-party grading services. "Hands-off" (i.e., they do not trade in the product), third-party grading services have had a significant impact in coins, baseball cards, comic books, and other areas.

   Using baseball cards as an example, a card can be sent to Professional Sports Authenticator (PSA) and for a fee graded according to a pre-defined scale (I am not recommending PSA over any of the other services, I just use them as an example). If they feel the card is authentic and unaltered, it will be assigned a grade from 1 to 10 (the highest), and encapsulated in a hermetically-sealed plastic holder that is quite light and helps preserve the card.

   Such services have had a tremendously positive impact. Grading has become more standardized, the vast majority of forged and altered material has been weeded out, and significant credibility has been created where little existed before.

   The services also generate a Population report, essentially a census, noting how many cards have been graded and how many have been assigned to each grade. Using the 1933 Goudey Babe Ruth #181 as an example, hundreds of cards have been authenticated but only one has received the grade of PSA Gem Mint 10. This card is arguably the best 1933 Goudey Ruth #181 in existence. Such grading and publication of a census report has unlocked the value of these items, especially the premium material. Everyone wants the best.

12. What will be valuable in the future? As far as I can tell, no one knows. This is why it is so important to buy what you like. If you do have a good eye and good judgment (and did not over-pay), then you will have a collection you like and may make a few bucks. If the investment angle does not materialize (which is usually the case), you still have a collection you like.

13. Larger works are generally more desirable than smaller works. A $20 gold piece is much more valuable than a nickel or dime of the similar quality and rarity.

14. Control ego. If it is your desire to have the best, most prominent, most important collection, you *will* be disappointed. Someone will have always more money to spend. It is like trying to be the richest person, you are just setting yourself up to fail. Dealers know how to play to this ego, they know when they have you hooked and can just reel you in.

15. Have a good relationship with the quality dealers. Physicians have favorite referral sources. Businesses have favorite customers (remember the 80/20 rule, 80% of your business comes from 20% of your customers). Dealers offer the premium material to their preferred customers first. Many of the best items never see the open market. Many pieces are "sold" before the dealer buys them. A client offers a piece to a dealer. Before purchasing the item, the dealer will call a customer they know collects in this area to determine their level of interest. Many times the sale is consummated even before the dealer makes the purchase.

16. Bid for yourself. Either attend the auction personally, or bid over the phone or on the internet. Never submit a written bid

that allows the auction house to bid for you. Your bid may not be fairly executed, and there is an excellent chance you will purchase the item for your limit bid and not a penny less. This has happened to me, so I say again, never let the auction house execute your written bid at a live auction, no matter how (apparently) sterling their reputation.

Likewise, if you do attend an auction, especially a smaller, local auction, such as an estate sale, beware of a "shill", a plant who pushes up the bids. If you cannot see the person in the audience bidding against you, ask they be pointed out. It could be the auctioneer's brother-in-law.

17. Dealer's opinions of other dealer's material. Most dealers will "talk down" other dealers' material, and until I figured this out, it caused me to miss some good items. The dealer who gives you their true opinion (good or bad) of another dealer's material is worth their weight in gold.

18. Hype. The more hype, the more I am turned off. When you buy a piece, the description will be glowing. A year later when you wish to sell it back to the same dealer, you will be stunned to learn what an undesirable item you have. "Doc, I have one of those in inventory right now that I have been trying to sell for 4 months". This is a game, and you must learn how to play it.

19. The more original, the more desirable. You must resist the urge to have your collectible changed, refinished or altered in any way. It is actually the built up gunk and grime, formally called the "patina", that is important to insure the piece's originality.

20. Liquidity is usually poor. It can take time, sometimes months, to sell a collectible, and there are always commissions that are usually in the range of (at least) 15—25%.

SUMMARY OF SECTION

- Collecting is fun but is usually not profitable.
- The value of all collectibles is determined by desirability, condition, and rarity.

- There is no area of investing where knowledge is more important.
- Always buy the best.
- Buy what you like. It has the best chance to be profitable.

ART

The human mind is the most amazing creation of the natural world, and its most defining quality is the ability for abstract thought. Only a few animals besides humans can look into a mirror and comprehend they are looking at themselves. The earliest examples of writing, using symbols to transfer and preserve a thought on papyrus or parchment or a clay tablet, appeared in the 4th millennium BCE.

About 50,000 years ago, there was an acceleration in the development of human intelligence. Archaic *Homo sapiens*, and ultimately *Homo sapiens sapiens*, won out in their 500,000 year struggle with *Homo erectus* in Asia and *Homo Neanderthals* [2] in Europe and the Middle East (thal, pronounced "taal", without the "h", means valley in German. The first skeleton was discovered in Joachim Neander's valley, thus Neanderthal). It was also at this time that the drawings of mammoths, horses, elk, and other animals began to appear on the walls of caves in Lascaux, Chauvet-Pont-D'Arc, and elsewhere.

Art is one of the defining characteristics of a culture. What better way to adorn public buildings, temples and homes than with art. Art *is* one of the finer things in life.

This advice is not directed to those who can afford to spend $1—2M on a George Caleb Bingham genre painting, such as "The Jolly Flatboatmen" (Bingham was from mid-Missouri, and I live on Bingham Road). Such people either have a great deal of money and are sophisticated connoisseurs of art, or just have a great deal of money with little knowledge of art, but wish to display the expensive works of famous artists on their walls to try to impress others (this is the case much more often than you think). This advice is for those who have attained a solid financial base and are starting to generate some discretionary income, and can afford to spend several thousand dollars or more on art.

After writing the first edition of this book, it was my desire to speak with an art dealer or gallery owner to get the inside scoop on what you need to know when buying art. Only after 5 tries did I get someone to speak to me, and only then with the promise that I would not "out" them, because it *would* hurt their business. With markups of 100% or more, it is easy to see why they are such a secretive bunch.

The first point when buying art is whether the artist is dead or alive. With "expensive, dead-guy art", such as Rembrandt, Monet or Frederick Church (you would never believe the painting of an iceberg could be so spectacular), all of the facts are out, everyone knows the story. Without information others do not have, it is impossible to gain an advantage and generate a reasonable return.

Forgeries abound in "dead-guy" art. I have read articles about world famous dealers who turned out to be crooks. Forgeries can fool even legitimate dealers and auction houses. You must do your own homework, and even seek out independent opinions. A healthy sense of skepticism is essential.

You must also be on the lookout for authentic, but stolen, art. You may wonder how it would be possible to sell the stolen work of a famous artist, but it happens all the time. Think of it this way: For $1M, you could have a $50M painting hanging on your wall. You must know the provenance. Julian Radcliffe operates Art Loss Register, which maintains the world's largest database on stolen art (*Forbes*, 12/24/07). If you are considering such a purchase, contact them.

The best chance for a collector to make money in art is to have a good eye and buy from a living artist. This is everyone's dream, to find the "next" Picasso, while the works are still affordable. But it will be your children or grandchildren who reap the financial rewards, because it is only over this period of time that the artist has died (no more supply), and others have come to appreciate what you recognized decades before.

How do you develop an "eye" for art?

1. You have an advantage. Not only are physicians bright, but they are trained observers, and often possess innate abilities that lend themselves to developing an eye for art.

2. Develop an eye for art just as you develop your abilities as a physician, i.e., study and work hard. Read all you can, go to museums, attend lectures, shows, and gallery openings, talk with others, and see all of the works you can.

When purchasing art, you must rely on your own judgment. Do not buy on the recommendation of others, because you will buy what they like rather than what you like. Never, ever ask the gallery owner or artist what you should buy because you will be the owner of the dog they have been trying to unload for years. Never take an interior decorator with you to buy art. You will buy what they want to buy, and pay a commission to boot, a lose-lose situation. Do not send your spouse to buy art; they will buy what they want, which by definition, is not exactly what you want. A much better suggestion is to say to your spouse "you decorate that wall, I'll do this wall". You both get exactly what you want. Never buy art on sale, *never*. A sale is the terminal event in an artist's career, an indication their work is a disaster.

If you purchase the art of a living artist at a gallery, the markup is 100%. You pay $10K for a painting, the artist gets $5K and the gallery keeps $5K (when is the last time you made that kind of money on call?).The markup in NYC, and other high-end, glitzy vacation destinations such as Maui, Nantucket, Key West, etc., is even greater. If you buy a $10K painting in NYC, the artist gets $3K and the gallery keeps the rest. My advice: If you see something you like at a gallery by a living artist, don't buy it, walk out, and contact the artist directly.

There can be other benefits of building a relationship with the artist. If you are a return customer, you have a better chance of getting their better works. Many artists at some time in their life will have a rough spot (try being a successful investor when you get a paycheck only 3 or 4 times a year, and have no idea when it is coming or how much it will be). Because of the relationship, you may be able to quietly pick up quality work at below the artist's usual price.

Prints usually sell for only a fraction of the cost of an original. The smaller the print run, the better, but except for print #1, the number is of no significance. Giclées are expensive to produce and of high quality, whereas offset prints are barely more expensive to produce than high quality wall paper. The cost of framing is usually more than the cost of the print.

Beware of what I call susceptible situations, where you can be seduced into buying something you never intended (I have done this, but it will not happen again). Examples include when you are on vacation, especially the high-end destinations mentioned above, or on a cruise ship. Do not buy art at a charity auction. I guarantee you this will happen at least once during your life so I will repeat it. This will save you many times the cost of this book.

DO NOT BUY ART AT A CHARITY AUCTION

The free drinks have an astounding ability to loosen your checkbook (they also accept credit cards), and you want to look like a generous big-shot in front of the rest of the crowd.

Also note that when you present the receipt to your accountant to claim a charitable deduction, you will be reminded that you can only claim the amount paid above the fair market value. You paid $2K, but the fair market value is $3K: sorry Charlie, not one penny of deduction on a painting you never really wanted in the first place. Just give the charity the money, because the whole amount is deductible.

About 15 years ago, we were at a premier showing in one of the glitzy places mentioned above. The paintings were all in the $50—150K range. There were at least two very aggressive sales people for every patron in the gallery. To have a little fun, I said to my wife, in a loud voice "Dear, I really like these paintings, what should we buy"? That was a big-time mistake. We were hounded for the rest of the evening, and I could not wait to get out of there. It never pays to be a smart aleck.

Table 1
Important Issues in Collecting

A collection must be focused
Knowledge
Buy quality
Start small
Patience, patience, patience
Collectibles are a discretionary purchase
Prices increase geometrically
Buy from reputable dealers
Forgeries abound
One good item is better than many cheaper ones
Third-party grading services
Buy what you like
Larger works are more desirable than smaller works
Control ego
Have a good relationship with quality dealers
Bid for yourself
Beware of dealer's opinions of other dealer's material
Beware of hype
The more original, the more desirable
Liquidity is poor

SUMMARY OF SECTION

- Art is one of the finer things in life.
- Is the artist dead or alive?
- Forgeries abound with "dead-guy" art.
- Even authentic pieces may be stolen.
- Rely on your own judgment. Never buy on other's recommendation.
- Never buy art on sale.
- The markup at galleries is 100% or more.
- DO NOT BUY ART AT A CHARITY AUCTION.

REFERENCE

1. Wallace B. The Billionaire's Vinegar: The Mystery of the World's Most Expensive Bottle of Wine. New York: Crown, 2008.
2. Johanson DC, Wong K. Lucy's Legacy: The Quest for Human Origins. New York: Harmony Books, 2009.

Chapter Thirty-Five
Other Types of Investments

SELLING SHORT

Everyone knows how to profit on a "long" position. Buy low, hope the price goes up, and then sell high. You pocket the difference. Selling short is doing the exact same thing but in reverse order. Sell high, hope the price goes down, then buy it back at a lower price. You pocket the difference. Selling short is not complicated and allows you to make money when something goes down. It is a basic technique of investing worth your time and effort to understand.

There are many misconceptions about short selling. When things go down, people often look for a scapegoat. In the bear market of 2000–2002, the short sellers took a great deal of (inappropriate) heat and criticism. They were referred to as vultures, profiting from other people's losses, they were at least partially blamed for the market decline itself (a great example of blaming others for your own errors) and some even went so far as to call selling short un-American. In 2008, short sellers were blamed for driving down the financial stocks, and the government took the unprecedented step of even banning the short sale of almost one thousand financially-related stocks.

To the contrary. Short sellers provide an important function to help prevent unwarranted speculation. Selling short helps cap speculative price rises and because a short seller must buy

R.M. Doroghazi, *The Physician's Guide to Investing*,
DOI 10.1007/978-1-60761-134-9_35,
© Humana Press, a part of Springer Science+Business Media, LLC 2005, 2009

back stock to cover their position, they provide support in a down market. Short selling helps contain volatility on both the high and low ends of the price spectrum.

Selling short is not complicated, it is not wicked, and it is not un-American. If you own a stock and think it will go down, you sell. That is not wicked or un-American. If you do not own a stock and think it will go down, you can sell it short. What is the difference?

Do not underestimate the importance of short selling as a tool to preserve capital, or even make money, during a bear market, when other investor's portfolios are being ravaged. If the market drops 20%, and by selling short, you can break even, you have protected 2 years of standard return. In a secular bear market, when the averages can drop as much as 50% or even more, if you can just break even it is possible to protect an entire decade of gains. Ten years or more of gains. Being able to preserve capital, or even profit, when others suffer significant losses could be the seminal event in a lifetime of successful investing.

Consider this perspective: If the market is up 20% and you are up 25%, and you can continue to beat the market by 5% every year, you could make a 7 or 8 figure salary on Wall Street. If the market is down 25% in one year, and by holding some cash and short selling you were able to break even, you beat the market by 25%. All you need to do is track the market for the next 4 years, and you have generated the same world-class returns with less volatility.

Throughout this book I stress the importance of patience as one of the cornerstones of the accumulation of wealth. It often requires months or longer to realize a ten to twenty percent gain on a long position. Because things always go down more quickly, often much more quickly, than they go up, it is possible, in fact often the case, that you may realize a ten to twenty percent gain in several days, weeks or months on a short position.

This is how selling short works. You "borrow" the shares of a particular stock and sell them on the market. The cash proceeds are placed in your account (While a short position is active, you are paid interest on what you are ahead, but you pay interest, because you are on margin, if you are behind). This is where the first misconception arises – how do you "borrow" stock? The brokerage firm does this. Suppose I place an order with my broker to sell short 100 shares of Acme Computer and Software (I use "Acme" because it is the name of everything on the Road Runner cartoons and on the Three Stooges, yet I am not sure I have seen an Acme anything in real life. Acme means "the highest point: peak syn see summit (Webster's)". The brokers have thousands of accounts. Many individuals and institutions that have accounts with the broker sign as part of their account agreement that the shares in their account may be "borrowed" for exactly this purpose. Sometimes the broker borrows the shares from their own account or occasionally must borrow the shares from another broker. The broker does the paper work (it is actually all done electronically), borrows the shares for you and then executes the trade. ("Naked" shorting, without first borrowing the shares, is illegal although apparently not uncommon).

Suppose you short Acme Computer at 150. One week later it has dropped to 120, a 20% gain. You are satisfied with this profit and "cover" your short position with an order to buy back the shares. The broker executes the trade as they do any other. The money left in your account after paying for the shares is the profit.

Things that are essentially "unique" cannot be sold short because at some time in the future they must be repurchased. You cannot short a collectible, such as a painting or piece of antique furniture or baseball card, or a specific piece of real estate. If you think the price of such an asset will drop significantly, you would just sell it.

As with everything, there are negatives. What are the negatives of selling short?

1. The possibility of loss is infinite! Many discussions on selling short state this so definitively at the outset as to almost preclude any further discussion of the subject. To provide a medical analogy, I would note the typical discussion in the lay press of the group of cholesterol-lowering medicines know collectively as the "statins." Great emphasis is placed on the approximate one in one thousand occurrence of rhabdomyolysis and the 1–1½% incidence of significant (but reversible) abnormalities in liver function tests. Yet barely a word is written that statins decrease the risk of stroke, heart attack and death by up to 30–50%.

With a "long" position (if not leveraged) all that can be lost is the amount invested. If you purchase a stock at 10 and it goes to 0, you have suffered a 100% loss. If a stock is shorted at 10 and it goes to 50, you have lost 400%. You would have either covered or been forced to cover by the brokerage house long before such a loss occurs, but it is possible.

2. Margin requirements for short selling tend to be higher than on long positions.

3. It may be difficult, or even impossible, to short a stock that is thinly traded. Stocks that trade millions of shares a day – such as Apple Computer (AAPL) – may be shorted instantaneously, whereas thinly-traded stocks, stocks with poor liquidity, may be difficult or impossible to borrow and sell short.

4. In years past, and sometimes today, there may be a "short squeeze." This can occur with a stock that is thinly-traded and heavily shorted. Say a stock appears so over-valued to so many investors that a very significant percentage of the float (total number of shares available to be traded) are sold short. The stock goes up, and the short sellers, to prevent further losses, must buy shares back. But because there are so few shares available, the price is forced higher. Now more shorts need to cover, and the price is forced ever higher. This was a routine maneuver during the 1920s when speculators formed "pools" to manipulate prices up or down. It is instructive on how the market works, and it does occasionally occur.

5. Do not short a stock just because it is over-valued, you could get clobbered. You feel a stock is fairly valued at $10 per share. It goes to $20 a share and you short it. But the stock continues to go up and up – and up, such as the dot.com stocks of 1999 and early 2000, or the Japanese market of the late 1980s. Do not short a stock just because it is over-valued. It could go up further to become tremendously, ridiculously over-valued. A stock *must* break in price before selling it short. For example, the stock sold short at 20 one year later has fallen to two. But in the interim it went to 70, and you were forced to cover at 40 for a 100% loss. You were completely correct in your appraisal of the stock but were killed by poor timing and not paying attention to the technicals.

6. The Securities and Exchange Commission (SEC) was formed in 1934. One of its initial regulations was that stocks could only be shorted on an "up" tick, that is, sold short at a price higher than the previous trade. The fear was that short sales without any intervening increase in price would act as a self-reinforcing positive feedback loop causing prices to cascade downwards. In 2006, I believe quite unwisely, the SEC repealed the uptick rule.

7. Short selling requires exceedingly close, essentially day-to-day, monitoring of the position. To make big money on a standard long position, patience, usually measured in months or years, is required. With short selling, just the opposite is mandatory. The typical duration of a short position is days, weeks or months. Take your ten, twenty or thirty percent profit and get out.

8. Short selling requires a different personality and mindset than the traditional buy and hold investor.

9. I believe that as soon as you execute a short sale, you must put in a good-till-cancel (GTC) limit order to cover the short at whatever your target price. Because stocks can collapse and bounce back so quickly, sometimes measured in minutes, you could easily miss receiving the best price by 5 or 10% or more. Another reason for a GTC limit order to cover is that occasionally when markets are down big-time, brokers can get swamped, both over the phone and on-line, and you cannot reach them with an order.

10. If a stock goes ex-dividend while you are short, you must pay the dividend. Say that among all of its thousands of accounts, your broker holds in "the street's name" (their name) 100K shares of Acme Computer. The company pays the broker the appropriate amount of dividend, and the broker distributes the money to the stockholders' accounts. If you short 1,000 shares of Acme, there are now only 99K shares in the street's name, so the company sends the broker only enough to cover the dividend on 99K shares. Because there is no reason for anyone to loan their shares and lose a dividend, you must make up the difference. For good or

bad, this makes it more expensive to short a high dividend stock, and much, much easier to short one that pays no dividend.

11. This point concerns ETFs. Say you wish to short the S&P 500. If you short the SPY, you must pay any dividends while you are short. But there are now short, double-short, and even triple-short, ETFs, that is, they are structured to move the inverse, or double or triple, the inverse of an index. These short ETFs pay a dividend. If you short the S&P 500 by shorting the SPY, you owe the 2% dividend. If you short the S&P 500 by going long an inverse fund, you receive a dividend, which is currently about 2%, a difference of 4%. My newsletter, Interim Bulletin #20A, 7/27/07, "An Advantageous Way to Sell Short", was the first time I saw this point in print. (You can read this and other issues of my newsletter at my website www.thephysicianinvestor.com).

I feel that a great utility of these inverse "bear" ETFs is in a retirement account. The standard retirement account does not allow short selling (because margin is not allowed in a retirement account, a wise rule). The only way you may avoid losses in your retirement account, if you feel a significant decline is in the offing, is to sell your long positions and stay in cash (there is nothing wrong with this. It certainly beats a loss). But these inverse ETFs are just a stock position so they are allowed in such accounts. They may help you protect gains that have taken years to realize.

Although it may sound counter-intuitive, it is both easier and safer to make money shorting a stock when it is closer to the bottom than to the top. A stock tops at 55 and is sold short at 50. But such a drop may only represent a period of correction, as occurs with all stocks. The stock breaks to new highs and you are forced to cover for a loss. But say you are correct and the stock drops 15 points, and you cover at 35 for a 30% gain. Great job. But consider this; the stock gets the absolute tar beat out of it and keeps going down and down and down. You short it at 20, it drops 10 points and you cover at 10 for a 50% gain. It is the same story with going long. Getting in too early is risky. Wait until the story is clear and then jump. Take the easy money.

I believe going short should be a standard tool in the portfolio of all investors. If you think prices will go up, you buy long. If you think prices will go down, you sell short. Overall, the average investor should only consider the possibility of going short for 5–10% of their investing lifetime. But during bear markets, especially the secular bear markets that occur three or four times a century (such as now), selling short may allow you to prevent the loss of years of savings. For more information on how you may profit when stocks, or the market in general, drops, see the reference by Caes at the end of this chapter [1].

THE CONCEPT OF HEDGING AND HEDGE FUNDS

Hedge funds have certainly been in the news, most often in a negative light. They are a very important investment vehicle, so you must understand the concepts on which they are built [2–5].

Webster's provides two definitions of hedge. The first: "To protect oneself financially: specif: to buy or sell commodity futures as a protection against loss due to price fluctuation".

You manufacture copper tubing, and to conduct business you must be able to guarantee your supply and your price. You set your prices once a year, so your customers, such as plumbing supply wholesalers, can make their business plans [6].

Say the current price of copper is $3.00 per pound. In the futures market you go long (buy) a sufficient number of contracts (each representing 25K pounds of copper) to meet your needs for the next year. In the interim, copper goes to $3.20. Your futures contracts now show a profit, but they are just pieces of paper, you need the metal itself. You go into the current (spot) market with the $3.00 you planned to spend, add the 20 cent profit from the futures contracts, and you have your copper at what you had planned to pay for it. If copper falls to $2.80, your futures contracts show a paper loss, but this is offset because you must pay only $2.80 for the copper. Hedging with futures allows you to conduct your business as planned.

Webster's other definition of hedge is "to minimize the risk of a bet".

Alfred Jones established the first hedge fund in 1949 using the equity long/short strategy, still the most common strategy used by about 50% of funds. Jones reasoned the risk of holding long positions could be "hedged" by simultaneously holding short positions.

The most important factors were to determine how much to allocate to the long and short positions and superior security selection. If the longs did well and the shorts did poorly, in an up market, the longs would go up more than the shorts, and in a down market, the longs would lose less while the shorts lost more. The obvious key is a superior fund manager (referred to as alpha, the extra return generated above the broad market's performance by the manager's skill).

An interesting historical note. MIT mathematician Ed Thorp, who introduced the concept of card counting in blackjack in his 1962 best seller *Beat the Dealer* [7] made a fortune in the hedge fund business with the concept of convertible bond arbitrage, as outlined is his subsequent book *Beat the Market* [8].

The usual hedge fund fees are "2 and 20", two percent of assets under management *plus* 20% of the profits. Compare this to a well-run S&P 500 index fund, where the management fee is only 15 basis points (a basis point is one one-hundredth of a percent). To merely match the average 10% return on the S&P 500, a hedge fund manager must generate a 15% return, i.e., a 50% greater profit. There are also "fund of funds" which do not manage money directly, but allocate it to what they feel are the best performing funds, adding another one-half to one percent management fee. Are such fees justifiable, or is this just a glamorous, high-class financial shakedown? (*See* Chapter Thirty-Eight on a bet between Warren Buffett and a hedge fund manager to see if this is possible).

Long-term data shows that not only can some hedge fund managers, net of fees, outperform their benchmark, but they can do it with less volatility. All rational investors would like to make more money with less volatility and to preserve capital in bear markets. What are your options?

1. You need $50–100 million dollars or even more to gain access to the best fund managers. If you have that kind of money, you already have the connections.

2. Newer funds tend to outperform more established funds, presumably because the new guys on the block are "hungrier". If you have $1–10 M to invest, you may be able to gain access to these potential opportunities. If this applies, *see* reference [2] to help you with the due diligence of how to evaluate and choose a fund manager.

VENTURE CAPITAL

Some businesses, even after initial capital contributions and borrowing from banks, do not have the funds required to expand. People may have a truly great idea, but need financing to buy the machinery and equipment, to hire other people, to perform more research and to help market their ideas before they earn a penny of profit. Venture capitalists will provide this financing in exchange for some amount of the equity (ownership) of the company.

The allures of venture capital are the exclusivity of investing in something unavailable to others and that you may be getting in on the ground floor of the next Google (GOOG). The principle downsides of investing in start-up businesses is that most businesses are never profitable and end in failure. Even if they are profitable, your money will be tied up for years.

The Columbia (MO) Chamber of Commerce recently started a group called Centennial Investors, and I was asked to join. We are "angel investors", an incubator, venture capital group, to help local entrepreneurs determine if their idea has merit and to obtain investment capital.

This has been a tremendous learning experience for me. I have seen how astute businessmen from all fields evaluate the merits of a business. For the few proposals that make the first cut, a group is formed to perform due diligence, where we look at everything, the good or service, the competition, the business model, the management, including business and personal/legal background, the financing, patents, etc. Only a few of these show sufficient potential to warrant a positive recommendation to the group.

In Chapter Ten, I say that real opportunities arise only about once a year. I can now attach a numerical figure to that advice. You are presented with 100 opportunities. Only 10 are even worth the time and effort of the due diligence process, and only one of these is worthy of an investment. Remember that number – one in one hundred.

If you make $250K a year and save 20%, it takes an entire year to generate $50K of investment capital. I propose what I call "Bob's Rule Number One"

Spend One Hour of Due Diligence for

Every One Thousand Dollars Invested

Remember the concept of due diligence whenever you are presented with any potential investment, especially a limited partnership, stock in a closely-held company, or venture capital situation such as this. Having 30 or 40 pairs of eyes look at something will give you a much better chance to identify the one in one hundred real opportunities.

DERIVATIVES

Warren Buffett said he does not understand derivatives. He even went so far as to refer to them as financial weapons of mass destruction. He was right. It appears that many of the guys on Wall Street did not understand them either. The final bill for these artificially-contrived products, created ostensibly to help spread and manage risk, but in actuality mostly to generate fees, will be in the trillions.

FUTURES

With futures, you buy or sell a contract that fixes the ability to buy or sell something at a specific price at a specific time in the future [6]. Futures can offer various degrees of leverage. For example, if gold is trading at $1,000/ounce, one contract of 100 oz represents $100,000 worth of gold. If this one contract is backed by $100 K in your account, it is un-leveraged and is little different financially than owning that amount of gold outright. If you own 7 contracts, you are leveraged at 7 to 1.

As previously mentioned, leverage works both ways. When things are good, it can be great. When things go bad, it can be unimaginably ugly.

In his book *Starting Out in Futures Trading* [9], Mark Powers begins with a discussion of one's suitability for trading. This is an insightful and masterful discussion and beautifully sums up many of the general aspects of investing made elsewhere in this book. Powers says:

- Commodity futures trading is not for everybody.
- You should not trade unless you are psychologically suited to taking large risks.
- You should not trade unless you are sure that you can control your ego and your greed.
- If you cannot discipline yourself well enough to admit a mistake on a trade and close it out at a small loss or to be satisfied with a moderate gain on a winning trade, do not trade.
- If you tend to live on hopes and dreams instead of the realities of hard facts, do not trade.
- If you think you can make money trading futures without doing some hard work, do not trade.

When opening a futures account, the multi-page document you must sign states that 80% of people who trade in futures lose money. There is nothing intrinsically evil about futures, they are just a type of investment vehicle. Rather, it is the lack of appreciation of the malevolent potential of the leverage afforded by futures that have given them, and indirectly commodities (because this is how commodities are traded) a bad name.

The options for trading in futures include managing the account yourself, hire a Commodity Trading Advisor (CTA) to provide you with advice (similar to a full-service stock broker), or have a Discretionary Individual Account, where you allow someone else to manage the account at their discretion. Although I feel we are in a multi-year bull market in commodities (*see* Chapter Thirty-Three), I would suggest futures only if you are a sophisticated investor willing to expend significant time and effort on the subject.

The two groups that trade futures are called collectively hedgers and speculators. In my discussion of hedge funds (above), I explained how hedgers, the producers and users of the commodity, use the futures markets to help conduct their business.

Now consider the speculator, such as a physician. Webster's provides several definitions for speculate, including "to review something idly or casually and often inconclusively, to assume a business risk in hope of gain or to buy or sell in expectation of profiting from market fluctuations." Mark Powers' definition of a successful speculator is "one who picks the right time to die."

Before you consider trading futures with leverage, watch the movie "War Games." As pointed out in the movie, the only way to win "is not to play the game!"

OPTIONS

There are two kinds of options contracts. A "call" gives you the right, but not the obligation, to purchase the underlying security at the exercise, or strike, price. Calls are purchased if you think the security will rise in price. A "put" gives you the right, but not the obligation, to sell the underlying stock at the exercise price. There is an inverse correlation between the price of the stock and the value of the put. As the price of the underlying stock drops, the value of the put increases. Puts are used for protection, as insurance, if things go down [10].

Not only is there a commission to buy and sell the option, but the bid-ask spread is often very wide, in the range of 5% or more. The value of the option is dependent upon the intrinsic value and the time premium. If you do not understand these concepts, do not trade options.

An option has a term, or life span, and thus a predefined expiration date. One option represents one hundred shares of stock. Because of this multiplier effect, options are leveraged, a small change in the price of the underlying security results in a large change in the value of the option. For example, say that Acme Computers is trading at 60. You pay $2 for a call (you hope the price goes up) with a strike price of 65 that expires on the 17th of next month. If the security goes to 75, your call is worth at least $10 (75–65), a 400% profit. If the stock closes below 65 on the 17th, it expires worthless and you lose your entire investment.

The advantage of options as compared to futures is that your loss is limited to what you paid for the option, whereas with futures there is no limit to your potential loss. The disadvantage is that the desired result must occur before the option expires. Say again Acme Computers is trading at 60, but you think it is a dog and is going to 45, so you buy a put with a strike price of 55. On the 17th of the month the stock price is 58 and your put expires worthless. Three days later, the company pre-announces horrendous results, and the stock drops to 38. If these results had been reported a week earlier, the put, for which you had paid $1, would be worth at least $17 (55–38). It is tough enough to make money without having to pick the day of the month that the train will come in.

In fact, seventy-five to eighty percent of options expire worthless. This alone should convince you not to trade in options. Do not consider this a challenge to see if you will be among the anointed few. Professional options traders, in fact, professional investors of all types, are often referred to as the "smart" money. The non-professional, the amateur, such as a physician trading in options, is referred to as "dumb" money. I wonder how people got that idea?

STOPS

A stop is an order that can be placed instructing that a position be sold if the price drops to a certain point. Its function is supposed to be, as the name implies, to stop further losses. It sounds like an absolutely logical technique that a prudent investor would use to prevent serious losses. But in actuality, it guarantees that you will sell at a low price.

Nothing ever goes straight up. Even the strongest, best-performing investments experience corrections, where the price may drop 20–30% or even more. Say a stock purchased at 30 has risen to 50, although you think it may have a little more upside potential. You wish to lock in profits (actually, if that is the case, sell now, "too early" and keep the entire profit) so a stop loss order is placed at 37.5, 25% below the high. The stock enters a period of correction and it goes to a low of 37.4 for a nanosecond, thus triggering your stop loss order, and then goes right back up. You are "stopped" out at the low price. Remember the saying "quit when you are ahead." Stop and stop loss orders force you to "quit when you are behind."

This does not mean you should not sell losers. To the contrary, you should have mental stops, predetermined criteria to know when a position should be sold. Suppose the above stock clearly breaks down and you sell at 32, rather than at 37.5. The few extra points you lose on the real dogs will not make up for the many times that you are stopped out of the winners.

I suggest you use only the closing prices to trigger your mental stops. Prices can sometimes be down a really scary amount during the day, only to close with a minimal loss, or even a gain. The logic behind relying on closing rather than intra-day prices is that the closing price is one that a professional investor is willing to walk away from for a day or weekend or longer. In addition, it is generally noted that amateurs trade at the beginning of the day, pros trade at the end. The trend of the market in the last half hour is the most important trend of the day.

I recommend you do not use stop or stop-loss orders.

LIMIT ORDER

These can be considered in specific situations. There may be limit orders to buy or limit orders to sell. With the former, you have researched a company and determined they have a superior product, superior management and are in a growing industry. However, you feel that the current stock price of 50 with a P/E of 20 is too high, essentially precluding the chance to realize a reasonable profit. The dividend yield is 2.5%. But if the stock could be purchased at 35, the P/E would be 14 and the dividend yield would be 3.8%, providing an excellent opportunity. Or you may already own the stock, really like it, and wish to add to your position. An order is placed to purchase the stock at a limit of 35 (or lower). Considering price fluctuations, this may allow the purchase of a good stock with a good dividend yield and good profit potential at an appropriate price.

With a limit order to sell, an order is placed to sell a position, but only if it reaches a particular price. Just as a stop-loss order forces you to sell "when you are behind," a limit order forces you to sell "when you are ahead." Limit orders may be considered in specific situations when you wish to cash out and take profits "too early."

As mentioned above, a good-until-cancel limit order is mandatory to cover a short position.

VARIANTS OF COMMON STOCK

1. Preferred Stock. A preferred stock is similar to a common stock in that it represents partial ownership of a company, but there are many differences. With a preferred stock, the dividend is fixed, so they perform more like bonds than stocks. The upside of a preferred stock is that the dividend on preferred shares must be paid before dividends are paid on the common shares. Should there be a bankruptcy, preferred shares also have a claim on the company's assets superior to that of common stock. The downside of preferred shares is that since they behave more like a fixed-income investment, they benefit little from the growth of the company.
2. Convertible Shares. I do not understand the nuances of convertible shares. I invest only in what I know. If you understand them, have at it. If not, avoid them.
3. Super-voting Shares. This typically occurs when the founding person/family/insiders still wishes to retain control of the company yet "cash out" by selling a portion of their stock. For example, the Class "A" shares may have 10 votes per

share controlled by the original owners, and the Class "B" shareholders put up an equal amount of money but have only one-tenth vote per share.

Studies have shown that the stock of companies structured in this way tend to under-perform the market. Each situation should be evaluated on its own merits, but you are being asked to invest your hard-earned money yet not have an equal say. If things get tough who do you think will come out on top?

SUMMARY OF CHAPTER THIRTY-FIVE

- Selling short is not complicated and allows you to preserve capital, or even profit, in a bear market.
- You must wait for a stock to break in price before selling it short.
- Always have good-till-cancelled (GTC) limit orders in place to cover your short position.
- You must pay the dividend while you are short a stock.
- Inverse ETFs pay rather than cost you a dividend and allow you to short in a retirement account.
- Hedging is a standard business technique for the producers and users of commodities.
- Hedge funds employ many strategies, the most common being equity long/short.
- Only one in one hundred opportunities are worthy of an investment.

Bob's Rule Number One:
Spend One Hour of Due Diligence for
Every One Thousand Dollars Invested.

- Avoid trading futures on leverage.
- Avoid options.
- Avoid anything you do not understand but that promises instant wealth.
- Do not be "dumb money".
- Avoid stop-loss orders. They force you to quit "when you are behind".

- Use mental stops based on closing prices because amateurs trade at the open, pros trade at the close.
- Consider limit orders in certain situations.
- There are many variants of common stock. They should be avoided unless well understood.

REFERENCES

1. Caes C J. Tools of the Bear: How Any Investor Can Make Money When Stocks Go Down. Chicago: Probus Publishing, 1993.
2. Biggs B. HedgeHogging. Hoboken, NJ: John Wiley & Sons, 2006.
3. Kirschner S, Mayer E, Kessler L. The Investor's Guide to Hedge Funds. Hoboken, NJ: John Wiley & Sons, 2006.
4. Bookstaber R. A Demon of Our Own Designs: Markets, Hedge Funds, and the Perils of Financial Innovation. Hoboken, NJ: John Wiley & Sons, 2007.
5. Burton K. Hedge Hunters: Hedge Fund Masters on the Rewards, the Risk, and the Reckoning. New York: Bloomberg Press, 2007.
6. Kleinman G. Trading Commodities and Financial Futures: A Step-by-Step Guide to Mastering the Markets. 3rd Ed. Boston: Financial Times Prentice Hall, 2005.
7. Thorp EO. Beat the Dealer: A Winning Strategy for the Game of Twenty One. New York: Vintage Books, 1962.
8. Thorp EO, Kassouf S. Beat the Market: A Scientific Stock Market System. New York: Random House, 1967.
9. Powers M J. Starting Out in Futures Trading. 5th Ed. Chicago: Probus Publishing, 1993.
10. Thomsell M C. Getting Started in Options. 7th Ed. Hoboken, NJ: John Wiley & Sons, 2007.

VII More Tips for Realizing Your Financial Goals

Chapter Thirty-Six
Obtaining Investment Information

In medicine, the more you read, the more you study, the harder you work, the more you know and the better your performance. It is the same with just about everything, including investing. The more you read, study and the harder you work, the better your chance of attaining your primary goal – financial security. Spending ten or fifteen minutes a month on your investments is not sufficient time to expect to realize an adequate return on your money.

Many investors note that a good number of their most profitable ideas come from reading non-financial material, from newspapers and magazines to science, history, and social and political thought, or even the classics. Throughout this work I provide analogies, insights and examples to support my opinions and advice from just such sources. Just think; *Beowulf, The Divine Comedy, The Prince, Candide, Gulliver's Travels* or the *Bible* may not only provide you with enjoyment and inspiration, but will make you smarter and could generate profitable investment ideas.

For the young investor just starting out who may have no investment knowledge at all, an excellent and inexpensive place to begin would be to read the business section of your daily newspaper. This will provide general information on the economy, the markets, and financial news of significance. In the evening there are many shows on the television that summarize the day's financial events. Choose one that seems right for you and watch it.

R.M. Doroghazi, *The Physician's Guide to Investing*,
DOI 10.1007/978-1-60761-134-9_36,
© Humana Press, a part of Springer Science+Business Media, LLC 2005, 2009

My absolute personal favorite for investment ideas and critical analysis is *Barron's* (www.Barrons.com). Alan Abelson, who pens the weekly column "Up and Down Wall Street," is the Mark Twain of our time. He is a real riot; witty, sublime and at the same time perceptive. The column on the back page of *Barron's* is written by Thomas Donlan (tg.donlan@barrons. com). I consider him one of the great social commentators of our time. I give *Barron's* my strongest recommendation as a source of both information and analysis. Each fall *Barron's* has a one day "Art of Successful Investing Conference" in Manhattan. Most of the presenters are members of the *Barron's* Roundtable, such as Felix Zulauf and Marc Faber. I have attended for the last 3 years and recommend it to you.

I have subscribed to *Forbes* (www.forbes.com) for two decades. *Forbes* has a significant social and political slant but contains very important financial information, stories, analysis and opinions. The articles in the money and investing section by Kenneth Fisher, Gary Shilling, David Dreman and others that appear towards the back pages are especially informative (I think it is a shame they dropped the column by James Grant of the *Interest Rate Observer*, www.grantspub.com). Almost every issue contains at least one story about a scam or some sort of nefarious activity perpetrated against investors. These are instructive, and frightening, and will help you develop your own sense of healthy skepticism to identify potential investment scams.

I subscribe to the *Wall Street Journal* (www.wsj.com) and it is the first thing I read every morning. It contains so much information and is so influential you should consider it. The problem for a physician in a busy practice is finding sufficient time to read it and thus justify the expense (a copy is often in the doctor's lounge or your hospital library).

I have subscribed to *The Economist* (www.EconomistSubscriptions.com) for 4 years. Along with *Smithsonian Magazine* (www. smithsonianmag.com), I consider it the best general "intellectual" journal in print. It is fascinating to see how others view us from "across the pond". *The Economist* is a great source of information on non-US economic issues, and the book reviews, medical, science and other general articles are second to none.

The *Value Line* (www.valuelineinc.com) has a stock market analysis that has been published for decades. They analyze the fundamentals of approximately 1,700 stocks on a weekly basis. It is not only a tremendous source of information and data, but will help you understand the process of how stocks, and the market, are critically evaluated. They have a 13-week introductory offer that you should consider.

The money you pay for financial and investing information *may* be tax deductible. Discuss this with your accountant.

As a physician, you will receive, free of charge, periodicals that are directed towards economic and financial issues facing physicians. I am neutral to negative on these. They do provide some information but I think your valuable time can be better spent elsewhere.

During the weekday, I use the website CNNMoney (www.cnnmoney.com) to obtain quotes and monitor the market. It is really excellent. This site also features many of the articles from its parents, CNN, *Fortune* and *Money* magazine.

StockCharts.com (www.stockcharts.com) provides excellent stock charting with accompanying technical data.

For many years I have subscribed to *Daily Graphs* (www.dailygraphs.com) which includes information on sales and earnings, daily volume and all sorts of other statistics and technical data. The same company publishes *Investor's Business Daily* (www.Investors.com). Both publications highlight technical data, emphasizing especially the Earnings Per Share (EPS) and Relative Strength (RS) ratings. As noted elsewhere, I utilize fundamental analysis to help determine which industries and stocks to buy, and technical data to help determine when to buy and sell.

There are literally thousands of other financially-related publications, surveys, newsletters, and forecasting services. I feel four are worthy of mention.

I subscribe to *Lowry Research* (www.Lowryresearch.com) The fact they have been in business since 1938 (seven decades is a long time) should suggest their analysis and recommendations are insightful. They have proven to me that technical analysis can help predict the general trend of the market. More importantly, their advice has helped me make money. Their principle thesis is that by looking at the buying power (accumulation) and selling pressure (distribution) and a variety of other indicators that one can quantify the basic driving forces of capitalistic financial markets, namely, supply and demand. In the May 20, 2002, pages MW 15–19, issue of *Barron's* there was an article written by Paul Desmond of *Lowry's* entitled "Identifying Bear Market Bottoms and New Bull Markets." I recommend you read this article, available through their website. It is the single most useful, informative article on the stock market I have ever read! Desmond stated that the stock market low of September 2001 was not the final market bottom. He was correct. I give *Lowry Research* my strongest recommendation.

Richard Russell has written the *Dow Theory Letters* since 1958 (www.dowtheoryletters.com). I have already mentioned him elsewhere several times. Russell is a genius and has tremendous credibility with me. He has been bullish on gold since about 2000 and his general market insights have been right-on. He is also amazingly prolific, livening up his daily posts with stories from WWII and comments on politics and world affairs. He has an introductory offer you should consider.

James Turk has written the *Freemarket Gold & Money Report* since 1987 (www.fgmr.com). I first heard of Turk when he was interviewed in *Barron's* six years ago. I believe he is the best gold market analyst around. He also has a website www.gold money.com.

I have written *The Physician Investor Newsletter* since 2006. I continually review and update all the issues that you will confront in your financial life. I give my view of the major market themes, and discuss subjects as diverse as embezzlement, how to spot a con man, and investing in for-profit facilities. I also try to teach you about your investments in general by reviewing things such as ETFs, the concept of hedging, and the malevolence of debt. I feel confident you will find at least one idea per year that will save you or make you much more than the cost of the letter. Go to my website:

www.thephysicianinvestor.com

to sign up for your free four month trial subscription.

SOURCES OF INFORMATION THAT ARE NOT HELPFUL

On Tuesday morning, at the market open, Acme Computers and Software announces their quarterly earnings. They are terrible, far below analysts' expectations. Because Acme is such a bell-weather the market drops 150 points. After the announcement, four analysts downgrade the stock. After the market closes, one of these analysts is interviewed and states "The market dropped 150 points today because Acme Computers and Software reported disappointing earnings." When I hear such things I must admit I am not impressed.

I would be very impressed if at 7:00 a.m. that morning, before the announcement, and before the market opened, an analyst would say, "Acme Computers and Software will report disappointing earnings", provide in detail the reasons for his or her concerns and predicts that the market will drop 150 points. "I am downgrading the stock." This would be very impressive indeed and I would pay attention to what this person said in the future.

Of course the whole subject is one of credibility. Anyone can talk, and many do. Who do you believe? What is useful information and what is worthless psychobabble? The people whose' opinion carries weight with me are the people who have been right in the past. Good examples of credible people are those who have a track record of making money. When Richard Russell, Paul Desmond or James Turk make a statement or prediction, I listen. Several times a year *Barron's* has a roundtable where people with long, credible and successful financial careers, such as Felix Zulauf, Marc Faber of the *Gloom Boom & Doom Report* (www.GloomBoomDoom.com), Fred Hickey of the *High-Tech Strategist*, and Bill Gross (of bond giant Pimco), provide their opinions. I read this intently for ideas. Or you may read a financial publication which has a particular columnist (such as those sited above in *Forbes*) who have given sage advice over the years. These people have credibility with me.

The people I do not listen to are the analysts who work at brokerage firms. Sometimes they are right, there are certainly a few who are good, but much more often they are wrong. There were several high-profile analysts from the late 1990s market mania who were indicted for giving contradictory self-serving not-impartial opinions. So and so upgrades or downgrades a particular stock or a particular sector of the market. I just yawn, try to completely filter these things out and not let them influence me one way or the other. In fact, about a year ago I was able to buy more of a stock I already owned when it dropped following an analysts downgrade. The best example of this sort of worthless advice from a brokerage firm analyst is provided by Peter Lynch in his book *One Up on Wall Street* (*see* Chapter Thirty-Eight). Lynch has framed on his wall a report from a brokerage firm that says "Due to the recent bankruptcy, we are removing this stock from our buy list." To quote Homer Simpson "D'OH!"

Another source of information that I do not allow to influence me is an interview with the CEO or officer of a company commenting on their company. Do your really believe this person will say something bad about their company? In fact, when they go out of their way to say everything is going well, you can be sure it is not. In 2008, the executives of the major financial companies that eventually went under were issuing reassuring statements right up to the day they went bust.

My ears would perk up a little bit, though, if they have praise for a competitor.

SUMMARY OF CHAPTER THIRTY-SIX

- General, non-financial reading will make you smarter and generate profitable ideas.
- Just as in medicine, the more you read and study, the more you know.
- There are many excellent financial publications. Choose the one(s) that is right for you.
- What is the credibility of the person giving the advice?
- Be wary of the opinion of brokerage firm analysts and officers speaking about their own company.

SUGGESTED READING

Following is a short list of books covering many general aspects of finance, investing and economics of general interest not referenced elsewhere.

1. Schwed F Jr. Where are the Customer's Yachts? or A Good Hard Look at Wall Street. New York: John Wiley & Sons, 1940. At the end of the day, the brokers throw all the money into the air. Whatever sticks to the ceiling is the client's, they keep the rest. I try to emulate Schwed's whimsical, satirical and insightful style.
2. Shiller, RJ. The Subprime Solution. Princeton, NJ: Princeton University Press, 2008. My book is going to press as his book will appear in print. Shiller nailed the stock market bubble and the housing bubble.
3. El-Erian M. When Markets Collide: Investment Strategies for the Age of Global Economic Change. New York: McGraw-Hill, 2008. A very smart man's impression of the changes taking place.
4. Schwager JD. The New Market Wizards: Conversations with America's Top Traders. New York: Harper Business, 1992.
5. Kazanjian K: Wizards of Wall Street, Market Beating Insights and Strategies From the World's Top-Performing Mutual Fund Managers. New York: New York Institute of Finance, 2000.
6. Train J. The New Money Masters: Winning Investment Strategies of: Soros, Lynch, Steinhardt, Rogers, Neff, Wanger, Michaels, Carret. New York: Harper and Row, 1989. These 3 books are a little dated, but good advice never goes out of style.
7. Cassidy DL. It's Not What Stocks You Buy, It's When You Sell: Understanding and Overcoming Your Self-Imposed Barriers to Investment Success. Chicago: Probus Publishing, 1991.
8. Rogers J. Investment Biker: On the Road with Jim Rogers. New York: Random House, 1994. The same Jim Rogers who wrote *Hot Commodities*.
9. Levy L, Linden E. The Mind of Wall Street: A Legendary Financier on the Perils of Greed and the Mysteries of the Market. New York: Public Affairs, 2002.
10. Sloan A P. My Years with General Motors. McDonald J, Stevens C eds. New York: Anchor Press, 1972. A history of the early automobile industry by possibly the greatest corporate executive of the twentieth century.
11. McLean B, Elkind P. The Smartest Guys in the Room: The Amazing Rise and Scandalous Fall of Enron. New York: Penguin, 2003. Rates with John Dean's *Blind Ambition* (Simon and Schuster, 1976) as a study in the corrupting power of arrogance.

Chapter Thirty-Seven
On-Line Brokers and the Internet

The first decision when choosing a broker is between a full-service or a discount broker. To quote David Swensen (*see* next chapter), chief of the Yale endowment "Investors who employ full-service brokers pay a very real something for an extremely costly nothing. The incremental fees for broker-assisted transactions purchase only a human voice (I really love this guy). Investors foolish enough to trade with full-service brokers get what they deserve. Prudent investors....execute their trades through low-cost, execution-only brokers" [1].

Now that you have decided to go with a discount broker, the next step is to determine if you wish to place a trade by talking to an agent (remember, they do not provide advice, they only execute your trade) or placing the trade on-line yourself. In the late 1980s, I transferred my account from a full-service broker to Charles Schwab (SCHW), one of the pioneer discount brokers, so I will use them as an example. The commission for an on-line trade is $8.95. A $25 surcharge is added if I speak to an agent to execute the trade. If you place just one trade a week, this is an extra $1,300 per year. If you have a one-half million dollar portfolio, you are giving away 26 basis points (a basis point is one one-hundredth of a percent) and receiving nothing in return. Although my overall computer skills are relatively rudimentary, I am quite facile in trading on-line. Considering the difference in cost, and the general

R.M. Doroghazi, *The Physician's Guide to Investing*,
DOI 10.1007/978-1-60761-134-9_37,
© Humana Press, a part of Springer Science+Business Media, LLC 2005, 2009

direction of our increasingly computer-based society, it is mandatory that you be able to execute your own trades on-line.

I have found two sources to be especially useful to obtain information regarding on-line brokers. First is to go directly to their website (*see* Table 1) and evaluate the offerings yourself. Second is "The Electronic Investor" column each week in *Barron's*, penned by Theresa Carey and Mike Hogan, and from which many of the following points are taken (electronicinvestor@ yahoo.com).

In the March 17, 2008 issue, *Barron's* published their 13th annual ranking of the on-line brokers, a composite based upon their evaluation of trade experience, trading technology, usability, range of offerings, research amenities, portfolio analysis and reports, customer service and access, and cost.

The salient points in choosing an on-line broker are the same as when purchasing any other good or service. Determine your

Table 1
Major On-Line Brokers

Broker (with ticker)	Website
AB Watley (ABWG)	www.abwatley.com
Charles Schwab (SCHW)	www.schwab.com
Choice Trade	www.choicetrade.com
E*Trade Securities (ETFC)	www.etrade.com
Fidelity Investments	www.fidelity.com
Firstrade Securities	www.firstrade.com
Interactive Brokers (IBKR)	www.interactive.brokers.com
Just2Trade	www.just2trade.com
Lightspeed Pro Trading	www.lightspeedtrading.com
MB Trading (MBTF)	www.mbtrading.com
Muriel Siebert & Co (SIEB)	www.siebertnet.com
OptionsHouse	www.optionshouse.com
OptionsXpress (OXPS)	www.optionsxpress.com
Scottrade	www.scottrade.com
TD Ameritrade (AMTD)	www.tdameritrade.com
Terra Nova Financial (TNFG)	www.tnfg.com
thinkorswim	www.thinkorswim.com
TradeKing	www.tradeking.com
TradeStation Securities (TRAD)	www.tradestation.com
Zecco	www.zecco.com

needs, how these needs can be best served, and how much it costs. No matter how enticing a good or service, do not buy or subscribe unless what you receive justifies the cost.

The investment tools offered by the on-line brokers are powerful, sophisticated and are being continually changed and updated. Almost everything can be customized. Many are down-loaded to your computer. It is beyond the scope of this work to review and compare all of the offerings and it would be out-dated anyway by the time this book appears in print. Instead, I will discuss the issues you should consider when choosing an on-line broker.

The first issue is cost. In general, the more you trade, the lower the fee per trade. Some people trade rarely, maybe several times a month or less. Some people trade 5 or 10 or more times a day. Fees at most brokers are negotiable, so if you are a frequent trader, or have a large account balance, make sure you receive the lowest possible commissions and fees.

The next issue is access to data. In general, the more you trade, the more products available to you. Brokers either perform their own research or provide access to the research of others, including links to various blogs and commentary of all kinds. There are screeners and tools which allow you to search for specific fundamental or technical indicators upon which to base a trade. Educational material and on-line seminars are available through the brokers and independent sites.

Software to "back-test" your trading strategy against a database can be down-loaded to your PC. It may also be possible to do "virtual trading", to practice trading without using real money. This may be useful to understanding the mechanics of placing trades and the capabilities of the product, however, almost any system can be tweaked and manipulated to fit the past. This does not mean it will work prospectively. Virtual trading is like playing with monopoly money. You take a risk and lose and say so what. Losing real money meant for retirement or the children's education is more painful.

Because news of any kind, from a terrorist attack to things less dramatic such as a corporate announcement or a government statistical report, can influence the market, brokers offer various degrees of "streaming", i.e., as instantaneous as possible, news. You can be alerted by email of events that fall within your parameters. The news stories can even contain imbedded quotes and charts allowing you to trade directly from the alert.

There are literally tens of thousands of websites not associated with or accessible through the on-line brokers that provide financial data, opinions, information and news. I mention some of these throughout this book when discussing the topics to which they apply.

Your trades may be simple or very complex. Trades can be initiated by data via a buy or sell alert. Orders may have multiple legs, or be multi-contingent or conditional. For example, you will buy 100 shares of the ETF GDX (Market Vectors Gold Miners, a basket of precious metals mining stocks) only if the spot gold price closes above $1,000 per ounce.

A wide range of financial products, such CDs, bonds, options, futures and forex (foreign currencies) can be traded on-line. You can trade directly in select foreign markets in local currencies, and I expect this will continue to expand. One of the basic themes I discuss throughout this book is that I believe over the long term the United States dollar will lose purchasing power and that selected foreign economies and markets will out-perform ours. I would place the ability to trade directly in foreign markets high on the list of factors to consider when choosing an on-line broker.

The competition between on-line brokers has improved the cost and transparency of order execution. Traders have more options to insure that their order is executed at the best price for them, not what is most profitable for the broker or market maker (The SEC has a rule referred to as NBBO stating that a broker must guarantee the National Best Bid and Offer prices available). Powerful tools and data that were previously available only to those on the floor of the exchanges or at the offices of the large brokers are now available to the average retail investor.

In their analysis, *Barron's* also evaluated the on-line services offered by 3 banks. If you do not trade frequently, a bank-based broker does offer convenience. *Barron's* overall rankings though were quite low, mainly because the offerings in trading technology and product range were limited.

Considering the turmoil in the financial markets in 2008, with the failure of multiple financial institutions, the issue of the safety of your money in a brokerage account is more than just idle speculation. After confirming your money market accounts are all in US Treasury paper, and you are not over the FDIC/ FSLIC limit at your bank, call your broker to determine the insurance protection on your account.

Securities, such as stocks, options and bonds, including up to $100K in cash, in brokerage accounts are insured up to $500K per customer per broker by the Securities Investor Protection Corp (SIPC), a federally-mandated, non-profit entity funded by the financial services industry. Note that money market funds and ETFs (regardless of the underlying asset) are also considered securities. Futures contracts, commodities and currencies are not covered by the SIPC. As with the FDIC/FSLIC, the SIPC does not insure a loss due to a poor investment decision or the drop in value of a security.

Rather, you are protected against nefarious activity by your broker, i.e., stealing from your account, or more pertinent now, the bankruptcy of your broker. Should the latter occur, the SIPC will return to you all securities registered in your name (Note: Securities are in "your name" only if a stock certificate in your name has been generated, which few investors do. Otherwise, all positions in your account are in the "street's name", not yours). Any losses over this are insured up to $500K. Many brokers have further coverage through Lloyd's of London. The Customer Assets Protection Company (Capco) is a consortium of brokers that also provides additional coverage in excess of the $500K provided by the SPIC.

The SIPC publishes *The Investor's Guide to Brokerage Firm Liquidations: What You Need to Know...And Do*. See http:// www.sipc.org/pdf/SIPC_brochure_Investors_Guide_To_BD_ Liquidations.pdf

Some cautious investors split their assets between brokers, and even between clearing agents for the brokers, to remain below the limit. If your broker is publicly traded, I suggest you monitor their stock price, although admittedly this may not even be sufficient, as things could conceivably go down the drain so quickly that you might not have time to act. Since the start of 2008, I have checked the price of Schwab at least once a week. To make an analogy to my discussion of Long-term Care Insurance (*see* Chapter Eighteen), it is probably wise to choose a broker with financial muscle and demonstrated long-term staying power rather than try to save a few bucks with a start-up. There is nothing wrong with being a little extra careful.

Another very real issue with on-line brokers is security and identity theft. Check with your broker on what safeguards are in place. Remember that when you call your broker and are asked your date of birth, mother's maiden name, telephone number, street address, etc., or you are required to phone in a particular type of order rather than place the trade electronically, it may be a hassle but it is to protect you.

Phishing, pronounced like and a word play on fishing, "is the criminally fraudulent process of attempting to acquire sensitive information . . . by masquerading as a trustworthy entity in an electronic communication" (Wikipedia). Pharming involves hijacking legitimate information from a server. The operant issue is that someone contacts you, either by email or instant messaging (or phone), looking for sensitive information such as account number, password, Social Security number, etc. Call the broker (or bank or credit card company) directly – NOT the number they tell you to call – to confirm the request before giving out anything. Both phishing and pharming are most commonly launched on evenings or weekends, when just such customer service is minimal. Now that I know what this is, I recognize I receive such phone calls and emails at least several times a week.

The most important piece of personal information is your Social Security number, with the last 4 digits being especially critical. For many on-line brokers, the customer identification number is usually your Social Security number, a practice that should be changed. OnGuard Online (www.onguardonline. gov) is a government-sponsored site to help with consumer security. For a fee, LifeLock (www.likelock.com) "locks" your identity to prevent unauthorized access and will help reinstate your identity if it is stolen.

Security becomes even more of an issue if you access and trade in your account by any sort of wireless device. There are wireless trading platforms for Blackberry and other mobile devices, and they are becoming more powerful, with more tools available.

Because it is unlikely that a physician-in-training or in a busy practice can spend multiple hours a day monitoring the markets or require the high-powered trading tools or instantaneous information, I suggest that the safety of your money, reasonably low cost and high marks for customer service and access be your main parameters in choosing a discount on-line broker. Their other services should meet the needs of almost every physician investor.

SUMMARY OF CHAPTER THIRTY-SEVEN

- Avoid full-service brokers.
- Place your own trades on-line.
- Choose your on-line broker based upon cost and your needs.
- Back-testing and virtual trading are not the same as putting real money on the line.
- Look for the ability to trade directly in foreign markets.
- Confirm the insurance coverage on your brokerage account.
- Account security is important. Beware of identity theft, phishing and pharming.
- Having your Social Security number as your customer identification number is not a good idea.

REFERENCE

1. Swensen DF. Unconventional Success: A Fundamental Approach to Personal Investment. New York: Free Press, 2005.

Chapter Thirty-Eight
Investment Strategies of the Pros

I love to read history. I especially love to read about great people from all walks of life, political leaders, scientists, intellectuals and military leaders. Since there are really not many truly new and original ideas, you can learn a great deal from studying people who have been successful and what made them successful. To quote Niccolo Machiavelli in *The Prince*, "For exercising the mind, the prince (the leader) must read histories and in them consider the actions of the imminent men, see how they conduct themselves, examine the reason for their victories and defeats, in order to avoid the latter and imitate the former".

I have chosen to profile four individuals. Warren Buffett is one of the most successful and probably best known investor of the post-World War II era. David Swensen's work has had a profound effect on how universities and foundations manage their endowments, and how individual investors can maximize returns and minimize risk. Peter Lynch was the tremendously successful manager of Fidelity Magellan, whose career recently hit a bump in the road. Burton Malkiel is one of the most important investment/economic theoreticians of our time.

WARREN BUFFETT

I consider Mozart to be not only the greatest musical mind ever, but possibly the greatest genius ever. There have obviously been many great composers over the years. Hadyn (who said when

R.M. Doroghazi, *The Physician's Guide to Investing*,
DOI 10.1007/978-1-60761-134-9_38,
© Humana Press, a part of Springer Science+Business Media, LLC 2005, 2009

Mozart died "there will not be another talent like him in a hundred years"), von Weber, Verdi, John Philip Sousa, George M. Cohan, Irving Berlin, Richard Rogers and John Lennon to name just a few.

But Mozart towered even over these people. He had a mind that was simply the most amazing musical computer ever. He never rewrote or changed a piece to obtain the final product. The piece was just in his head, he wrote it down once and that was it. No changes, just an instantaneous finished product. Imagine Ernest Hemmingway writing all of the works of his life just once, never, ever changing even a single word.

By age six, Mozart's father Leopold took him on tours of Europe. He would hear a piece and then, sitting at the clavier, begin to play, improvising and playing constantly with variations, changing the passages, even mimicking the local style, for hours at a time [1]. Consider what you were doing at age six. It is unlikely you were reading (much less writing) the *New England Journal of Medicine*. Or the time, apparently after hearing the piece just once at the Vatican, Mozart was able to write from memory the entire choral score of Allegri's Miserere (Miserere refers to Psalm 51, a Prayer of Repentance)

I consider Buffett to be the financial and investing equivalent of Mozart. I think he understands the science of money as no one else. Even though Buffett operates on a different plain than the rest of us mortals, there are many things that can be learned by studying his career. Much of the following information is from the book *Buffett: The Making of an American Capitalist* by Roger Lowenstein [2]. I have also added things that have occurred since the publication of Lowenstein's book.

I would compare Buffett to Einstein. Many of the ideas and concepts that ultimately resulted in the theories of special and general relativity were the results of Einstein's thought experiments. A man is in an elevator being pulled toward earth by gravity. A beam of light enters through a hole on one side of the elevator and exits a hole on the other side. How does the man in the elevator describe the path of the light? How does the path of light appear to an observer outside the elevator on the ground?

Buffett conducts thought experiments with money. He constructs scenarios, such as if there were two islands. He will then interject a variable such as a tax, a dividend, a change in productivity, a change in the business model, a change in the savings rate or whatever and play out in his mind the result and draw conclusions from this.

He will also use simple, everyday situations to illustrate his points. In one of his annual letters to Berkshire shareholders he noted that people were happy when stock prices were high and unhappy when prices were low, when he felt it should be the opposite. To explain his viewpoint, he asked "If you ate only hamburgers your entire life, would you want the price to be high or low?" Clearly, you would want a low price so you could purchase more hamburgers (stocks) for your money.

It was obvious from the beginning that Buffett (and most of the greatest investors) was interested in making and investing money. I make this point to contrast what I have seen and heard about flim-flam men, who routinely have a checkered and spotty past (*see* Chapter Twenty, Who Can You Trust?). People who are the greatest successes in any field do not do this or that and then suddenly at age 30 or 40 decide they are going to be the greatest investor in the world. Their genome directs them to their area of genius, just as Tiger Wood's genome directed him to golf and the Big O's (Oscar Robertson) genome directed him to play basketball. If someone should come to you and promise 25 or 30% returns, similar to Warren Buffett, but their past shows that they sold insurance, then shoes, then were a cattle rancher, then a missionary or preacher (watch out here) and now at age 45 they are a financial advisor, it would be wise to be skeptical.

Most people feel that one of the defining points in Buffett's career occurred in 1969 when he liquidated his partnership and returned all the money to the investors. In May of 1956, Buffett started his partnership in Omaha, Nebraska with seven investors who put up a total of $105,000. Buffett invested $100 and directed the investments. By the end of 1968, the assets of Buffett Associates, Ltd. was $104 million dollars. The 1960s were characterized by the "go-go" stocks and by ill-advised conglomeration, an example of what Peter Lynch calls "diworseification." Buffett felt the market was so over-priced and could find no good bargains that he sold all of the partnership's positions and returned everyone's money. Can you imagine any other investment advisor giving people their money back, closing up shop, and thus not generating fees, because they could not find any good investments? From 1957 to 1967, the DJIA was up at a 7.4% compounded annual rate. Buffett's partnership was up at a 29.5% compounded annual rate.

Not only was Buffett's act of returning his investor's money unique, but it also dramatizes that even the Great One feels there are times that it is not wise or prudent to be fully invested, that stocks (or any asset) may be so over-valued that the only direction is down. Buffett was not only correct in his assessment of the market but was "too early." The market peaked almost four years later in January 1973 and then over the next 22 months lost almost 50% of its value (actually much more after factoring in inflation).

Buffett said that two of his largest positions, Coca-Cola (KO) and Gillette (G), in retrospect, were so over-valued at the market top in 1999–2000 that they should have been sold. However, he felt constrained because he was on their boards, and was personally in such a prominent position, that he could not sell. It appears that occasionally success can be counterproductive.

Buffett was the premier student of the father of value investing, Benjamin Graham. Graham looked for companies selling below book value or below the amount of cash on their books, for fifty cents on the dollar. Buffett took this concept a step further. He looked for something that could not be duplicated, that was unique, essentially a monopoly. An example would be where there is only one, or a very dominant newspaper, in town. They can command what they want for advertising (although newspaper stocks have not done well recently because of the Internet, i.e., competition). Or there is a brand name. There is only one Coca-Cola. And, of course, not forgetting value investing, Buffett never overpays and almost never gets into a bidding contest.

Buffett continually emphasizes that he invests only in what he understands. No software, no computers, and no disk drives. Just railroads, newspapers, soda pop, chocolate candy, ice cream sundaes (BRK owns Dairy Queen), and money. Invest in what you know.

Buffett understands how to put money to best use. This is apparent in the structure of Berkshire Hathaway. When Buffett invests, he either buys very large positions, or more recently; buys the entire company. But he always leaves management in place. Buffett lets people who know how to make candy make candy, who know how to sell carpets sell carpets, who know how to run gas pipelines run the pipelines. Buffett uses his genius to control the allocation of capital.

Buffett's grasp of the science of money gives him insight into evaluating general trends in investing and finance. And because of his track record, and his reputation of integrity, his opinion carries great weight. He is especially adept at identifying fads and other deviations from standard investment principles that so often appear to block the logical thinking process of others. He commented early and strongly upon the importance of expensing stock options. He commented on the excesses that afflicted many corporations, and their executives, in the last 5 to 10 years. Obscene salaries and bonuses, parties, and lavish offices, all at the expense of the person who should be profiting, i.e. the shareholder. Contrast this to Buffett, who still receives a $100,000 annual salary from Berkshire and who has never sold a single share of his BRK stock (although he is in the process of donating it to the Gates foundation).

Buffett invests in insurance companies because he was the first to truly recognize the potential of the "float." (a great example of the more basic the process you can understand, the better the chance for profit). You pay the insurance company a premium on your homeowners insurance. Your home may never burn. You pay the premium on your life insurance policy. Hopefully it will be decades before you die. In the interim, the insurance company has the money to invest, which is usually put into Treasury bills or similar low-risk, fixed-income assets. Buffett puts his money to work to generate a 20% return.

Buffett emphasize you must have the appropriate temperament to invest in the stock market. An investment can and will
be down twenty or thirty percent, or even more, from time to
time. If the investor cannot cope with this volatility they will sell
at the wrong time. Selling out of fear, panic and disgust is
always the wrong time to sell.

Would you want to be on the other end of a business deal with
Warren Buffett? By definition you will be selling too cheap or
paying too dear. I applied this logic in a local business situation.
A friend and I looked at a piece of land in town, prime development land, but the price seemed pretty stiff. The seller was
one of the most solid, well-regarded businessmen around who
had built up and sold several large companies. I said, "Look at
his record, do we want to be on the other end of a business deal
with Bill?" We passed.

At the May, 2006 Berkshire annual meeting Buffett offered to
bet $1 M that over 10 years, and *after fees*, the performance of an
S&P 500 index fund would beat 10 hedge funds any opponent
might choose. Buffett has long claimed that the fees charged by
"helpers" are onerous and to be avoided.

Fortune magazine reported in June, 2008 that Protégé Partners
has taken a variation of the bet. Specifically, that 5 fund of funds
chosen by Protégé, net of all fees, over a time period of ten years
can beat the Vanguard S&P 500 Index fund, which charges a fee
of 15 basis points (0.15%).The proceeds of the bet will go to a
charity of the winner's choice.

There are handful of truly gifted investors, such as Buffett,
who can beat the S&P 500 by more than 5% over the course of
many years (The people at Protégé note they are fortunate they
are not betting against Buffett). But as a practical note, access to
such super stars requires $50 M or $100 M or even more. The
point Buffett is trying to make is that the overwhelming majority of investors are best served by the S&P 500 index fund with
the lowest expense ratio.

One final point about Buffett. He admits his mistakes. This
is often terribly lacking in the corporate executive of today.
This is the main reason I suggest elsewhere (*see* Chapter
Twenty-Six) that you should put little or no emphasis on

what a corporate executive says about their own company. In his book *How to Win Friends and Influence People*. Dale Carnegie devotes an entire chapter to the importance of admitting mistakes [3].

SUMMARY OF WARREN BUFFETT'S INVESTMENT STYLE

- Patience, patience – and more patience.
- Invest in what you know.
- Never, ever overpay for an asset.
- Occasionally things become truly over-priced – then sell.
- Admit your mistakes.

DAVID SWENSEN

Under Swensen's direction, the Yale endowment has returned a compound rate of approximately 16% per year since 1985.

In *Pioneering Portfolio Management* [4], Swensen initiated and defined the move of endowments away from the heavy reliance on domestic marketable securities (especially bonds) to emphasize a collection of asset classes expected to provide equity-like returns driven by fundamentally different underlying factors. Swensen's work has had a profound and positive effect on how universities and charities manage their investments.

This discussion will focus on *Unconventional Success* [5], which I consider the financial/investing equivalent of *Harrison's Principles of Internal Medicine* (McGraw-Hill). *Unconventional Success* should be one of your core financial books, read thoroughly, and reviewed once or twice a year. I purchased two copies, one of which I extensively underlined and notated. I sent the other copy to Swensen for his autograph (with a self-addressed, stamped return envelope) along with a copy of Issue #6 of my newsletter, which reviewed the book. He was gracious enough to flatter me with the inscription "with respect, David Swensen".

Sometimes works sound impressive academically, yet fail in the real world. *Unconventional Success* serves as a practical and intellectual template on how to manage sums from the size of your portfolio to an 11-figure endowment.

Swensen has no ax to grind, no turf to protect, he is not trying to sell anything. He gives his honest opinion, both positive, and, more importantly, negative, on scenarios or situations that confront all investors. (Note: Swensen apparently makes about $3–5 M per year. With the results he has generated for more than 2 decades managing the sums of money he has, he could *easily* make *twenty or more times* as much in private industry. I respect this).

Swensen has two basic messages:

1. You should construct a portfolio that is

   A. Well-diversified
   B. Equity oriented
   C. Passively managed
   D. Using not-for-profit managers

2. *The mutual fund industry fails America's individual investors.*

Over reasonably long periods of time, stocks out-perform bonds and cash.

Diversification provides a "free lunch" of enhanced returns and reduced risks.

Because investors often chase yesterday's winners, there is excessive allocation to recent strong performers, offset by inadequate allocation to recent weak performers (poor investors buy high and sell low). Mean reversion dictates conviction and disciplined portfolio rebalancing, which forces you to act against the crowd, to buy low and sell high. Market collapses require substantial purchases in an environment pervaded by bearish sentiment and market bubbles require substantial sales in an environment suffused with bullish sentiment. Rebalancers must demonstrate unusual determination and fortitude = guts. Excess volatility allows systematic rebalancers more chances to profit, creating portfolios with lower risk and higher return.

Rational investors (Swensen loves this term) avoid trying to select specific securities in an attempt to beat the market. Investors cannot win the active-management game. Pre-tax returns fall short of market-mimicking passively-managed funds and taxes generated by sales produce even more dismal results. Of those who do beat the market, especially over the short term, randomness (also called luck) plays a significant role in separating the winners from the loser (the Internet bubble made everyone a genius). Over a twenty year span, only 22%, i.e., only one in five, actively-managed mutual funds beat the Vanguard Index 500 fund.

Investors must be tax sensitive. Taxes destroy wealth. Laws favor capital gains over dividends and interest income by (1) lower tax rates and (2) taxes incurred only when realized. Deferring capital gains creates enormous economic value. Swensen suggests tax-deferred accounts be used for trading and interest and dividends, and long-term capital appreciation investments be directed to taxable accounts. Swensen also reminds you to be wary of tax shelters (*see* Chapter Twenty-Five).

A well-diversified portfolio holds positions in six "core" asset classes, with at least 5%, but no more than 30%, in each class. Positions less than 5% are too small to have a significant effect, and positions above 30% decrease diversification. A portfolio with 30% domestic, 15% foreign developed and 5% emerging market equities, 20% real estate, 15% US Treasury bonds and 15% US Treasury Inflation Protected Securities (TIPS) is well-diversified, generates market returns not requiring active management, trades in markets that are broad and deep and does not rely on "concoctions promoted by Wall Street financial engineers".

Domestic equities are the class of choice for long-term investors, with dividends providing the greatest portion of returns (Emphasized in Chapter Two). Over the long term, but not the short term, domestic equities correlate well with inflation.

Returns on foreign developed equity are similar to domestic equity, but the lack of correlation provides diversification.

However, foreign equity should not exceed 25% of assets because currency exposure causes unwarranted risks. Real estate has characteristics of both stocks and bonds and provides returns midway between them. It also tracks inflation well.

The debt issued by government-sponsored-enterprises (GSEs) such as Fannie Mae (FNM) and Freddie Mac (FRE) are not the same as the full-faith-and-credit of the Treasury (these two entities were taken over by the government as this book goes to press).

With few exceptions, privately offered retail real estate (limited) partnerships provide exposure to the real estate market at such obscenely high costs that the individual investor stands no chance of a fair return (*see* Chapter Twenty-Five).

Portfolio construction is both science and art, the latter including common sense, personal preference, and your level of risk tolerance. You must have a conviction to your methods, because positions lightly-held will invariably be sold at the wrong time. Likewise, unrealistic investors do not realize their limitations and are routinely over-confident.

Swensen laments that so few accept responsibility for their retirement savings. According to a 2001 Federal Reserve survey, more than one of four eligible do not participate in a 401(k), and of those that do, less than 10% made the maximum contribution. A distressingly high percentage also cash out when they change jobs.

Investors must know their time horizon. The sooner they need the money, the greater the allocation to cash, because they cannot tolerate volatility. A time horizon of less than 2 years dictates a 100% cash position (A good example would be if you are saving for the down payment on a home).

Non-core Asset Classes to Avoid

Corporate Bonds. Swensen feels all of your fixed-income investments should be in non-callable, full-faith-and-credit obligations of the US Treasury (the only guarantee you should accept is that of the US Government). Unattractive characteristics of corporate bonds include (A) Credit risk. A Triple A bond can only decline in quality. Why invest in anything where there is no upside? (B) Illiquidity. (C) Callability. This is the option of the issuer to redeem the bond before maturity, on terms always favorable to them. If interest rates rise, the investor has lost value, while the issuer is paying below market rates. If rates fall, the bond has gained value, but may be "called" (redeemed) by the issuer at a pre-set price. "Heads they win, tails you lose".

High-Yield Bonds. Suffer from a concentrated version of unattractive features.

Tax-Exempt Bonds. Markets are very illiquid and longer maturities face the uncertainty of future tax rates. Trading costs are high and "Market-makers prey on the small investor . . . avoid dealing with Wall Street sharks" (where else will you hear such a candid, and accurate, comment from someone so respected).

Asset-Backed Securities. The financial complexity makes them hard to understand (One of the most successful, sophisticated investors in the world is saying there are things he does not understand).

Foreign Bonds. Problems too numerous to detail.

Hedge Funds. (*See* Chapter Thirty-Five) "Belong in the domain of sophisticated investors who commit significant resources to the manager selection process".

Leveraged Buyout/Private Equity Funds. In the absence of truly superior fund selection (or extraordinary luck), investors should stay far, far away.

In summary "Non-core assets provide investors with a broad range of superficially-appealing but ultimately performance-damaging investment alternatives. . .Investors require unusual self-confidence to ignore the widely hyped non-core investments and to embrace the quietly effective core investments".

How the Mutual Fund Industry Fails America's Investors

I suggest you read Chapter Five of *Unconventional Success* for yourself. Swensen provides well-documented examples of how almost every major broker, money manager, and mutual fund company, almost certainly one that handles your money, has operated to maximize their profits at your expense. "When fiduciary responsibility to investors compete with corporate desire for profits, profits win".

Swensen's opinion of Morningstar is especially noteworthy. "Unfortunately, investors find no useful assistance from Morningstar, as the firm's rating system proves hopelessly naïve. Their backward-looking performance measurement metrics prove useless to forward-looking investors".

Load funds under-perform their no-load cousins by roughly the amount of the additional fees. 12b-1 fees are charged every year, and essentially represent a net transfer from fund shareholders to fund management. The transaction cost advantage enjoyed by index funds joins the long list of reasons to prefer the rock-solid certainty of market-mimicking return. Sensible investors avoid the brokerage community, opting for the lower cost, self-service alterative. Avoid broker-marketed mutual funds.

A few managers do win the active management game. Limiting assets under management represents one of the most powerful statements regarding primacy of investors interests over personal profits (more assets generate more fees, regardless of performance). Market-beating managers have concentrated positions (*see* Chapter Twenty-Eight), and must be willing to accept long periods of under-performance to produce superior long-term returns. Such managers look for a stable client base with a time horizon of longer than 3 years. The most powerful incentive for an agent to serve clients interests stems from side-by-side investments (alignment of interests).

ETF's exhibit greater tax efficiency than otherwise comparable open-ended mutual funds. The necessity of dealing with the brokerage community constitutes the most serious drawback of investing in ETFs. As time passes, the ETF market will increasingly take on the unattractive characteristics of the traditional mutual fund universe.

FINAL RECOMMENDATION

Swensen feels that "ultimately, a passive index fund managed by a not-for profit investment management organization (Vanguard or TIAA-CREF) represents the combination most likely to satisfy investor's aspirations".

SUMMARY OF DAVID SWENSEN'S INVESTMENT STYLE

- Construct a portfolio that is well-diversified, equity oriented, and passively managed using not-for-profit managers.
- *The mutual fund industry fails America's individual investors.*
- Disciplined portfolio rebalancing forces you to buy low and sell high.
- Taxes destroy wealth.
- Avoid non-core investments.
- All of your fixed-income investments should be non-callable, full-faith-and-credit obligations of the US Treasury.
- Morningstar's rating system is "hopelessly naïve".
- Investors cannot win the actively-managed mutual fund game.
- Avoid broker-marketed funds.
- As time passes, ETFs will take on the unattractive characteristics of traditional mutual funds.

PETER LYNCH

Lynch has written three books, *One Up on Wall Street* [6], *Beating the Street* [7], and *Learn to Earn* [8]. I have used these as the source for most of the following discussion and for the other references to Lynch throughout this work.

Lynch was the manager of the Fidelity Magellan Fund from 1977 through 1990. One thousand dollars invested in 1977 had grown to $28,000 by 1990, a compounded annual return of approximately 27%.

I have chosen to examine Lynch's investing style, philosophy and career for four reasons. In 2008 Lynch had a run-in with the SEC, and as Machiavelli said, we must examine defeats to be able to avoid them. The third reason is because he was so successful and the second reason is by writing these books he has outlined in detail his decision-making process. But the most important reason I have chosen to profile Lynch is that every investor can profit from many of the points he makes. Lynch is clearly a genius, but the way he evaluates investments and provides explanations that are so clear and logical, and disarmingly simple, that it merits a full discussion. For example, Lynch defines a leveraged buyout as "a company purchased with borrowed money by people who really can't afford it."

I devote Chapter Nine to investing in what you know. Lynch devotes a quarter to a third of his books to this point. To illustrate Lynch notes that physicians rarely look to medicine for their investments. A doctor, who should be investing in a drug company or medical instrument maker or a company that in some way can control health care costs, is more likely investing in an oil company. The example he uses relates to the release of the first true medication to block stomach acid secretion, the histamine 2 (H2) receptor blocker Tagamat (cimetidine) by SmithKline Beckman in 1977. Lynch also points out that the managers of the oil company are more likely investing in the stock of a drug company than in the oil business (I question this. I suspect they were investing in the oil business).Invest in what you know.

I suggest you take the following comment, which Lynch refers to as Peter's Principle #3, as one of the ten most important points of this book and commit it to memory.

Never Invest in any Idea You Can't Illustrate with a Crayon

There are several other general themes that permeate Lynch's message. Lynch proclaims, with no hesitation, that amateurs have an edge. Many professional money managers' performance is determined by how they compare to their peers, such as funds with a similar focus or some standard bench-mark, such as the S&P 500 or the DJIA. Lynch feels this often results in not being as concerned with not winning but to be more concerned with not losing. For example, if a money man-ager buys the stock of a small unknown company and the investment fails, he or she is open to criticism. Compare this to taking a position in a large, established, quality company such as Exxon Mobil (XOM), a stock that almost every large fund holds. If it goes up, it goes up. But if it goes down, you cannot be criticized because everyone else purchased the stock. Lynch feels this mindset guarantees mediocrity. (I am on the boards of a small foundation and several organizations with small endowments. If you remember this insight, you will understand the mind of every bank trust officer in the world).

Lynch feels the more Wall Street analyst that follow a stock, the less likely it is to be profitable. In essence, when everyone knows all of the information, it is difficult to have an advantage. When you have information that few others possess, you have an edge. Lynch's eyes light up and his mouth begins to water when he discovers a company that no analyst, or at most a few, follow. Obviously, just because a company is not followed by the analysts does not mean it should be purchased, but he feels it is a great starting point to investigate and learn more about the business and their product.

Another of Lynch's recurrent themes is that the amateur who keeps their eyes open will learn about companies, typically local or regional ones, six months to a year before the Wall Street pros. Lynch feels the average person comes across real invest-ment opportunities in their daily lives two or three times a year (*see* Chapter Ten on Recognizing Opportunities). He uses as an example the auto parts retailer Pep Boys, Manny, Moe and Jack (PBY). He notes that anyone familiar with the company, such as lawyers, executives, accountants, clerks, or even the carpenters and plumbers who were building the new buildings for the company's expansion, should have seen how well the business was going and purchased the stock.

Lynch provides other examples of investment opportunities from his daily life. His wife brings home L'eggs panty hose so he buys Hanes. He eats at Dunkin' Donut, stays at LaQuinta Inns. He also emphasizes these are just ideas and one must do more research, but these examples typify to him the advantage that amateurs have over professionals.

Several years ago, I noted that Gamestop (GME) had solid earnings and strong technicals. I called my personal video game analysts (sons John and Michael) who traded there often, liked the business model, and noted high traffic in the stores. I mentioned this in my newsletter, purchased the stock, and made a few bucks. I thought of Lynch the whole time.

Several other general points that Lynch makes reinforces those made earlier regarding Buffett. Look for companies with little or no competition. Competition is great for the consumer, resulting in good products, great selection, and great price. It is one of the basic strengths of our capitalistic system. Competition is not that good for a company. Rockefeller and Carnegie despised competition.

Lynch also emphasizes the importance of patience. With many stocks, often his famous "ten-baggers", a stock that appreciated tenfold, he did not make the big money until holding the stock for three, four or more years. Patience pay$$.

Lynch makes several other points worthy of mention. The more glamorous a stock, the hotter the industry, the more discussion he hears, the more he avoids it. The more mundane, the more he loves it. Lynch, of course, looks at many, many factors when evaluating a company, but in the end, it is a company's profitability, how much money they make, that eventually determines their value. He emphasizes many times that the earlier you invest in a company, the greater the risk. Let the company demonstrate that their business model works, and can be effectively duplicated outside their original geographic area, before investing. This time period is often one or two years. There is usually plenty of time, do not jump in too early (*see* Chapter Twenty-Five).

Lynch stresses, and is correct, that in the long term, stocks outperform bonds. As he notes, it is better to own the company than to lend it money. But Lynch also notes that over periods lasting up to five to ten years bonds can outperform stocks. From 1982 to 1990, despite the amazing bull market in stocks, because of the drop in interest rates from historic highs, bonds actually performed slightly better than stocks.

There is one point on which I differ with Lynch. He feels that you should always be fully invested in stocks. I have already explained in detail why there are times I feel that a fully invested position is not warranted.

In the *Wall Street Journal* (3/6/08), it was reported that Lynch settled a civil case with the Securities and Exchange Commission (SEC), alleging he "obtained numerous free tickets to concerts, theater and sporting events paid for by outside brokers". Lynch paid a fine of $15,948 without admitting or denying guilt. Fidelity paid an $8M fine to settle, also without admitting or denying guilt. Jeffries Group paid $10M in 2006 as one of the firms that supplied the gifts.

Because commissions are paid with shareholder's money, mutual funds are supposed to send trades to whichever firm offers the best price and service. Investment advisors are prohibited from accepting compensation from firms with which they do business, and have a legal duty to seek the best price for trades.

I do not personally know, or have ever met, Mr. Lynch, but his self-deprecating humor and general story strongly suggest a humble, basically good man. In a written statement, Lynch said "In asking the Fidelity equity trading desk for occasional help locating tickets, I never intended to do anything inappropriate and I regret having made such requests".

The point: The mere appearance of a conflict of interest can be as damaging to your reputation as the real thing. I am lucky that along the way I had several mentors who cautioned me on this exact point, before I was ensnared in an otherwise completely innocent but damning situation.

SUMMARY OF PETER LYNCH'S INVESTMENT STYLE

- Invest in what you know.
- **Be able to explain your investment using only a crayon.**
- Amateurs have an edge.
- In the end, profits determine the value of a company.

- You can discover investment opportunities in your daily life, so keep your eyes open.
- The mere appearance of a conflict of interest can be as damaging as the real thing.

BURTON MALKIEL

In *The Random Walk Guide to Investing: Ten Rules for Financial Success* [9], Malkiel's discussion, always direct, sometimes irreverent, supports and further details many of the points I make elsewhere. I will also make several comments on his most recent work *From Wall Street to the Great Wall: How Investors Can Profit from China's Booming Economy* [10].

Malkiel spent several decades employed as a market professional with one of Wall Street's leading investment firms. As he says, it takes one to know one. Following this he was Dean of the School of Organization and Management at Yale and is currently the Chemical Bank Chairman's Professor of Economics at Princeton. Malkiel notes that he has been a lifelong investor and successful market participant. He is thus able to back up his impressive academic credentials with an ability to make money in the real world.

In 1974, Malkiel published *A Random Walk Down Wall Street* [11]. The book is now in its ninth edition and is clearly one of the most influential works on investing in the post-WW II era. Malkiel's principal thesis is that the vast majority of professional money managers (not individuals, but professional money managers) cannot consistently, over the long term, beat the general market averages as represented by index funds administered by non-profit managers. That point has been made almost innumerable times elsewhere in this book.

The best way to review *The Random Walk to Investing* is point by point.

Basic Point #1: Fire Your Investment Advisor. Swensen agrees (see above). I remind the reader of the full-service broker who thrice dissuades me from buying stock in the baseball card company Topps (TOPP). Malkiel emphasizes that *the investment advisor's primary interest is to make money for themselves and their company, not for you* (I suggest you never forget this). He notes that the advisors always push the products on which they make the greatest commissions. He states that financial "experts" know little more than you and that "A blindfolded chimpanzee (or bare assed ape as he refers to them in *Random Walk*) throwing darts at the stock pages can select individual stocks as well as the experts." Many people comment on Jim Cramer's "Mad Money" show. Malkiel says "tune out the TV investment gurus who dispense worthless advice."

Basic Point #2: Focus on Four Investment Categories – Cash, Bonds, Common Stocks and Real Estate. Aside from my comments regarding hard assets (*see* Chapter Thirty-Three and Chapter Thirty-Four), Malkiel's recommendations are very similar to mine. He notes that over the long term, the return from common stocks (8–10%) is superior to the return from high quality bonds (5–6%). Malkiel emphasizes that investing in stocks requires a temperament that can endure significant pain because from time to time the investment will (not can, will) be down significantly.

Malkiel states that "For the most part, the stock market does a remarkably good job of pricing stocks efficiently so that they reflect the degree to which future growth is anticipated." I disagree somewhat with Malkiel on this point, although not as much as I did before. What has tempered my opinion is reading *The Wisdom of Crowds* by James Surowiecki [12] and *Wealth, War & Wisdom* (*see* the next chapter) by Barton Biggs [13], where the authors show to my satisfaction that the stock market, essentially the collective wisdom of all investors, is a fairly efficient discounting mechanism.

But in the next paragraph, Malkiel partially contradicts his own statement with a discussion of investment bubbles of the past. "Investors do need to know, however, that the stock market takes occasional trips to the loony bin." (Almost everything I have read suggests it is easier to identify the bottom than the top, to "buy when there is blood in the streets" than to "sell too early").

A collectibles dealer once told me that at any show 90% of the items for sale are over-priced or fairly priced, but 10% are under-priced. This is how I would view the markets. Most of the time, most stocks are reasonably priced. Sometimes, most or all stocks are over-priced or terribly over-priced (our market in 1929, Japan in the late 1980s, our market in the late 1990s), and sometimes they are significantly under-priced (1932, late 1974, 1982). The efficient investors can determine when the market is not efficient. This is the secret to investing, when you can realize significant profits.

The remainder of Malkiel's points are:

Basic Point #3: Understand the Risk/Return Relationship (*see* Chapter Six).

Rule 1: Start Saving Now, Not Later. Time is money. *See* Chapter Three on the magnificence of compound interest and my comments noting that the younger the person, the more valuable their money and the fact that lost money will never be recouped.

Rule 2: Keep a Steady Course. The Only Sure Road to Wealth is Regular Savings. I have already pointed out the importance of discipline and that the best investors are the best savers.

Rule 3: Don't be Caught Empty-Handed. Insurance and Cash Reserves.

Rule 4: Stiff the Tax Collector. I doubt Malkiel wants you to take this literally, but he does recommend you make full use of all tax-advantage options to save for your retirement and for your children's education. And he recommends that the "Best Tax Strategy of All" is to own your home rather than rent. One of your basic goals is to buy a home as early as financially feasible with the goal of having the mortgage paid off by your mid-40s.

Rule 5: Match Your Asset Mix to Your Investment Personality: How to Allocate Your Assets.

Rule 6: Never Forget that Diversity Reduces Adversity. Please *see* Chapter Twenty-Four for my impression of the strengths and weaknesses of diversification.

Rule 7: Pay yourself, not the Piper. Fees are either money in your pocket or in someone else's. Malkiel emphasizes the importance of fees, especially as they relate to mutual funds. He quotes John Bogle "a low expense ratio is the major reason why a (mutual) fund does well – the surest route to top quartile returns is bottom quartile expenses."

Rule 8: Bow to the Wisdom of the Market.

Rule 9: Back Proven Winners: Index funds. Malkiel and Bogle and Buffett and Swensen agree. The best way for the average investor to participate in the stock market is to income-average into the index fund with the lowest expense ratio operated by non-profit money managers.

Rule 10: Don't be Your Own Worst Enemy: Avoid Stupid Investor Tricks. This is one of the principal goals of this book.

Three months ago I started *From Wall Street to the Great Wall.* Even having to write this chapter could not compel me to finish this book. Your time and money will be better spent elsewhere. Sorry Professor, but even Bob Pettit didn't hit all of his jump shots and Cliff Hagan didn't hit all of his hooks.

SUMMARY OF BURTON MALKIEL'S INVESTMENT STYLE

- Don't listen to "experts".
- *The investment advisor's primary interest is to make money for themselves and their company, not for you.*
- Focus on cash, stocks, bonds and real estate.
- You can profit from efficiencies, and inefficiencies, of the market.
- Time is money.
- Discipline: The best saver is the best investor.
- Use all tax-advantaged options to save for retirement and your children's education.
- Index funds are the preferred vehicle to invest in the stock market.

REFERENCES

1. Solomon M. Mozart: A Life. New York: Harper-Collins, 1995.
2. Lowenstein R. Buffett: The Making of an American Capitalist. New York: Broadway Books, 1995.

3. Carnegie D. How to Win Friends and Influence People. Carnegie D, Pell AR, eds. New York: Pocket Books, 1981.

4. Swensen D F. Pioneering Portfolio Management: An Unconventional Approach to Institutional Investment. New York: Free Press, 2000.

5. Swensen D F. Unconventional Success: A Fundamental Approach to Personal Investment. New York: Free Press, 2005.

6. Lynch P, Rothchild J. One Up on Wall Street: How to Use What You Already Know to Make Money in the Market. New York: Simon & Schuster, 1989.

7. Lynch P, Rothchild J. Beating the Street. New York: Simon & Schuster. 1993.

8. Lynch P, Rothchild J. Learn to Earn: A Beginner's Guide to the Basics of Investing and Business. New York: Fireside Books, 1995.

9. Malkiel B G. The Random Walk Guide to Investing: Ten Rules for Financial Success. New York: WW Norton, 2003.

10. Malkiel B G, Taylor P A, with Mei J, Yang R. From Wall Street to the Great Wall: How Investors Can Profit from China's Booming Economy. New York: WW Norton, 2008.

11. Malkiel B G. A Random Walk Down Wall Street. New York: WW Norton, 1974.

12. Surowiecki J. The Wisdom of Crowds. New York: Doubleday, 2004.

13. Biggs B. Wealth, War, & Wisdom. New York: John Wiley & Sons, 2008.

Chapter Thirty-Nine
Some Miscellaneous Bits of Advice

A PHYSICIAN IS AN EXECUTIVE

Physicians make dozens of significant decisions every day. Few physicians realize they are executives, even fewer try to think and act like one, and none are given any training on how to be an effective executive.

First, an executive must protect, must stick up for, their employees. If someone reproaches your employee, and you do not immediately defend them, you will lose their respect, probably forever. Even if your employee was wrong, you must be the one to discipline them, not someone else (but do this later, in private). If someone has a problem with your employee, they must go through you, not to the employee directly. Likewise, you must show the same courtesy if you experience a problem with the employee of another physician.

Push all decisions as far down the line as possible. Employees who do not have input into controlling their work environment feel powerless and frustrated. One of the best ways to promote job satisfaction is to let people make decisions.

Presuming you have chosen and trained your employees well, you should be able to trust their judgment. Allow them as much responsibility as they are comfortable in handling. Sometimes I found myself saying "I don't want to hear about this anymore, you take care of it". The result was invariably to my satisfaction.

R.M. Doroghazi, *The Physician's Guide to Investing*,
DOI 10.1007/978-1-60761-134-9_39,
© Humana Press, a part of Springer Science+Business Media, LLC 2005, 2009

If you employ a nurse, a college graduate, a trained professional, and allow them to do no more than carry your bag and answer the phone, you should be embarrassed. If they are competent and worth having as an employee, you will not have them for long.

Push all tasks down the line as far as possible, and be *very aggressive* about it. All you have to sell is your time, it must be jealously guarded. Five to ten minutes of your time is worth an hour of your nurse's time. Your secretary's time is worth only half of your nurse's time. It is a big hit to your pocketbook if you do anything a nurse can do, or your nurse does something a secretary can do.

This is not Social Darwinism, you are not "dumping" on anyone, you are not taking advantage of them. You are trained to do a job, and your employees are trained to do their job. Stick to your job, and let them perform the job for which they were hired. You will be more efficient, provide better patient care, and your employees will be happier.

An executive must stay focused. Details are important, but do not allow them to distract you from the primary strategic objective. A patient comes in with an anterior myocardial infarction and a blood pressure barely palpable at 74 mmHg. You can either ask for an ophthalmoscope to look in their ears, eyes, nose and mouth, or you can stand them on their head, run in fluid and appropriate medications, and tell the cardiac cath team to also prepare for the insertion of an intra-aortic balloon pump.

At the end of the first Star Wars movie ("Episode IV, A New Hope"), the rebel fighters are making their run at the Death Star. They are no match for the evil lord Darth Vader, who is picking off the brave freedom fighters one by one. Vader hits one of the rebels, and they are forced to peel off. Vader's escort wants to follow to finish them off, but Vader says "Let him go, stay on the leader".

Let someone else drive whenever possible. Several people told me along the way I was the most efficient person they ever saw, so I think about these sorts of things a lot. In the course of a work day, the greatest waste of an executive's time is to drive. It is completely dead time, non-productive and worthless (Discussed in more detail in Chapter Sixteen, Your Home). If you see patients at out-lying hospitals or clinics, have your nurse, or some other employee of the practice, drive, or even consider a chauffer. Sounds extravagant? Your time is worth $150/hour, while you can hire a driver for less than $10/hour. And if you were on call the night before, you can get in a quick nap and hopefully not fall asleep behind the wheel and have a wreck.

CHANGING PRACTICES

Choosing the best practice is obviously one of the most important decisions of your life. Everything – tangible and intangible- goes into making this decision.

Before commenting on the financial consequences of changing practices, allow me to give some advice, which I believe applies to private practice and academia. There are no perfect practices. They do not exist. This realization usually occurs about six months to a year after starting and is like hitting a brick wall. Things are not what you imagined, something was supposedly promised, the older guys are taking advantage of you (possible, but actually fairly unlikely). One uniform refrain from young associates is that they are working hard, seeing many patients and the older guys are making money from their toil and labor. The young physician lacks the perspective of time and does not realize that the older guys (a generic term for male or female) have been working for ten, twenty or thirty years to allow the young physician to enter a ready-made practice where they are busy from the outset. The older guys were fighting battles and doing things twenty years ago to start the practice that the new associates would now probably consider below them. The bottom line is that you must think very long and hard before changing practices. There is no perfect practice.

If things truly are not working out, you must be brutally honest with yourself. Is the problem them or me? If the difficulty is the latter, then changing practices is not the answer and will not solve the problem.

The financial consequences of changing practices are devastating. If changing practices necessitates moving, there are all of the financial losses involved with selling a home and buying a new one, uprooting the family, and other related expenses.

Changing practices will also delay by at least several years when the big salaries will be made. You do not lose the first year's salary, but rather it is the last year's salary, the big salaries, that are lost. This seems counter-intuitive but is true.

Suppose an associate starts at $125,000 a year with partnership in two years.

2009 – $125,000
2010 – $125,000
2011 – $250,000}
  ↓   } 20 years at $250,000 per year
2030 – $250,000 Total 22 years of practice

Now suppose you work for one year, feel you are being taken advantage of, and change practices. You start all over again.

      2009 – $125,000
Start over 2010 – $125,000
      2011 – $125,000
      2012 – $250,000}
        ↓   } 20 years at $250,000
      2031 – $250,000 Total 23 years of practice

The person who changes practices actually loses three times. Up front there is the loss of the difference between $125,000 and $250,000. There is also the loss of the compounding of this difference for all subsequent years ($125,000 compounded at 10% annually for 20 years is more than $840,000). In addition, you must work an extra year to make the last $250,000.

The young physician must think very, very hard before changing practices. It will cost two years or more of your financial life. Someone once told me that one way to get rich is to keep your first home, your first spouse and your first job.

BUYING A BOAT

Don't.

How do you make a million dollars in boating? Answer: start with ten million.

Boat stands for *Break Out Another Thousand*.

The same advice applies to an airplane or similar toy. It is difficult or impossible to accumulate wealth with the purchase of depreciating assets. The only boat you should consider buying is a 12 ft. john boat for the lake on your recreational property.

BLACK SWAN EVENTS

I suggest you read *The Black Swan: The Impact of the Highly Improbable* [1] and *Wealth, War & Wisdom* [2]. Both address how to prepare for those once or twice a century, unexpected catastrophic events that occur. Their main point: such events do occur, do not be lulled into complacency. What if there had been 100 planes on September 11th and they had also hit Hoover Dam, the rail yards at Chicago, the oil refineries outside of Houston and the lock and dams at Granite City and Alton, Illinois, blocking barge traffic on the Mississippi, Missouri and Illinois rivers? Our economy would have ground to a halt. Keep a percentage of your assets in the safest of investments, such as gold, both in your possession (even buried in your back yard), and in a safe deposit box outside your country of residence (make sure you have adequate documentation when you go to retrieve the money), Treasury Bills, and land.

Also keep a small percentage in an otherwise high-risk investment, but that would pay off big-time should the Black Swan visit, such as put options. The other important point: geographically and financially diversify your assets, and do it yesterday.

VACATIONS

The most expensive part of a vacation is not the travel, lodging, meals and entertainment but the income lost from not working. So, within reason, go where you want and have a good time.

EMBEZZLEMENT

You are a hard-working, honest physician, so you presume others are honest. Sorry, but there is *significant* embezzlement in at least one-half of physician's offices. I am not talking about paper clips and rubber bands, but 5 and 6 figure sums. And what will really shock you, and personally disappoint you, is that it is not the marginal, disgruntled worker, but one of your most senior, trusted employees, because they have the opportunity. They are the ones you entrusted with your signature stamp, to conduct your business, and who have access to the cash and checking accounts.

Several suggestions: First, 49% of the fault is the physician's for providing the opportunity. Second, all offices should have a *forensic* audit, and with this audit, the consultant should recommend specific controls so that your employees are not tempted.

Lastly, if you run personal expenses through your business or do other things you should not, and an employee who has knowledge of this is caught embezzling, they will blackmail you not to prosecute them.

They didn't teach you this in med school, did they? Welcome to the real world.

MARQUIS DE TALLEYRAND

Talleyrand is considered to be one of the "slickest" politicians ever. He was able to remain in power, and keep his head (literally), through the regime ancien, the revolution, the empire, the restoration and the second empire. He said "never write a letter, never destroy a letter".

My point: Never put anything in writing that can later be used against you, and save anything written by others. It seems that every week there is an article in the paper where someone is convicted of something by what had been written in emails. Computers have long memories.

INVESTING IN FOR-PROFIT FACILITIES

As your direct income from seeing patients gets squeezed, and your expenses continue to rise, returns from investing in a for-profit facility in your area of practice, such as a free-standing surgery center, endoscopy suite, etc., will become an increasing percentage of your take-home pay.

There are several issues to consider:

1. The profits can be mind-boggling, with the returns, or distributions, of 100% per year, or even more. Aside from your education, this may be the most profitable investment of your life. It could easily add another 50% to your income. But something's greatest strength can also be its' greatest weakness. The real potential of such astounding gains can blind even the most sane, rational person, especially a younger, more naïve physician. Beware of greed.

2. Remember the concept of alignment of interests. The best situation is when the developer/manager makes money when you make money, and loses money if you lose money. Beware if they can make money while you could lose.

3. It is almost always easier to get into something than to get out, the exit strategy must be well defined from the outset.

4. You must also consider what could happen if things go wrong:

   a. What if the center opens, and your biggest producer is involved in a serious auto accident (take it from my personal experience – auto wrecks happen)? Could you write a check every month to meet overhead?

   b. What if the government changes the rules (always your greatest concern)?

   c. What if the center is a complete loss? Could you pay off your share of the debt?

Investing in this type of for-profit facility can be amazingly profitable, but never lose sight of your potential liability.

GAMBLING

It is called gambling because you can, and usually do, lose money. You work too hard for your money to just throw it away. Do not underestimate the addictive power of gambling, it can destroy your life.

An occasional person does strike it rich, although it is invariably lost sooner rather than later. It is much easier to get ahead by working hard and saving your money.

True gambling is games that involve independent events over which the participant has no control. A perfect example is roulette. There are 38 spots on the standard wheel, 1–36 plus zero and double zero (rare wheels still have only one zero, you lose your money only two-thirds as fast). Although there are 38 spots, the payoff on a specific number is only 35 to 1, giving the house a better than 6% advantage. The house is in business because over the long term the house always wins.

The state lottery gives pathetic odds, usually paying out about half of the take. If you do hit the jackpot, you will be third in line to collect after the IRS and your state Department of Revenue. Think of it; you could be the first doctor to win your state's lottery. All of your patients would see you on the TV and in the newspapers and even on billboards along the highway.

There are games where skill, strategy and knowledge can result in winning over the long term. These include poker, blackjack, bridge and craps (if you are able to control the degrees of freedom of the dice as they spin through the air, it is possible to gain the desired number often enough to beat the odds [3]. Skill at such games is actually desirable when some companies recruit executives because it indicates an ability to identify, handicap, control and manage risk.

SPEAKING FOR PHARMACEUTICAL COMPANIES AND REVIEWING MALPRACTICE CASES

I discuss these together because I did the same thing with the money received, I donated it to charity. To me (others disagree) this negates any semblance of a conflict of interests. In a malpractice case, charge what you wish for your time, but I believe donating the money directly to charity provides you with more credibility.

Whenever doing legal work, I *strongly* suggest you insist on a retainer (i.e., an up-front payment). This is mandatory when working with a new attorney (many attorneys insist on this when working with a new client). I know of two situations (not me) where people were stiffed on their fees.

When speaking for pharmaceutical companies, keep your talk generic. I lose respect for people when they sound more like "hired guns" than physicians.

CUT YOUR OWN GRASS

I feel you, or a family member, should mow your own lawn. I see people out jogging while they pay someone else to cut their grass. The exercise is just as good or better, and you have saved $40 or $50. A little manual labor from time to time that is smelly, hot, loud (be sure to wear adequate ear protection, sun block, etc.) and boring is good for everyone. It helps a high income professional such as a physician maintain perspective on what the vast majority of the other people in the world must do to make a living.

SUMMARY OF CHAPTER THIRTY-NINE

- A physician must defend their employees.
- Push decision making as far down the line as possible.
- Your time is valuable. Do not waste it doing anything someone else can do.
- An executive must stay focused on the primary objective.
- Changing practices will cost you 2–5 years of your financial life.
- Do not buy a boat or airplane or similar toy.
- Prepare for Black Swan events yesterday.
- The most expensive part of a vacation is the income lost from not working.

- Embezzlement occurs in at least one-half of physician's offices, usually by your most trusted employee.
- Never write a letter (or email), never destroy a letter: Watch what you put in writing.
- For-profit facilities will become increasingly important as a source of income.
- You work too hard for your money, don't gamble.
- Donate the money from speaking honoraria for pharmaceutical companies and reviewing malpractice cases to charity.
- Mow your own lawn.

REFERENCES

1. Taleb N N. The Black Swan: The Impact of the Highly Improbable. New York: Random House, 2007.
2. Biggs B. Wealth, War & Wisdom. New York: John Wiley & Sons, 2008.
3. Sharpshooter. Get the Edge at Craps: How to Control the Dice! Los Angeles: Bonus Books, 2005.

Chapter Forty
The Importance of Charity

Noblesse oblige is "the obligation of honorable, generous and responsible behavior associated with high rank or birth" (Webster's). This elegantly and succinctly states what I feel are a physician's responsibility to their community and to society.

I feel physicians in academia and private practice need to expend more effort in their support of charities, fraternal organizations, and public service in general. Physicians are a little more generous with their money than their time, but overall I would categorize their effort as somewhere between very poor to just plain inadequate. Many businessmen, who carry similar workloads yet devote significantly more time to community service, and other generous physicians I know, share my opinion.

By any standard, physicians make a significant amount of money, in general, about five times the national average salary. Your children enjoy the Boy Scouts, Girl Scouts and the YMCA. If there were a disaster, the Red Cross would help you just as they would anyone else. You enjoy the opera, the symphony, the arts, and the parks in your community. Someone has to make these things work, to spend their time and money to make their community and their country a better place to live. Physicians make their living from the community, and I feel should give back more time, energy, and money.

Other people cannot be asked to contribute their time and effort if you are not willing to do the same. You say you are

R.M. Doroghazi, *The Physician's Guide to Investing,*
DOI 10.1007/978-1-60761-134-9_40,
© Humana Press, a part of Springer Science+Business Media, LLC 2005, 2009

busy. Well, who the heck isn't? Make time to help out and contribute your money. If you do not contribute, how can you justify your children joining the scouts, or you going to the park or the museum or the symphony? If your home burns down, you should refuse any help from the Red Cross or any other relief organization.

How much should you donate? My general rule is that you are at least starting to reach your potential when you do without things you desire. Aim to donate at least 3 to 5% of your income, hopefully more. If you do, I congratulate you and I am proud of you.

I suggest you read *Titan: The Life of John D. Rockefeller, Sr.* by Ron Chernow [1], and *Carnegie* by Peter Krass [2], from which most of the following information was obtained. Rockefeller and Carnegie are two of my heroes. Although they certainly had their faults (as we all do), I believe they were great men who helped build this country, and provided the jobs for immigrants such as my grandparents. They also defined philanthropy in the United States. Rockefeller, and his son John Jr., endowed the University of Chicago (my medical school alma mater), Spelman College (Rockefeller's wife's maiden name was Spelman. Rockefeller supported education for black women almost a century before it became chic and fashionable), Rockefeller University, The Rockefeller Institute for Medical Research, The Rockefeller Sanitary Commission (hookworm project), Rockefeller Park (and multiple other charities in Cleveland), Jackson Hole National Park, Acadia National Park, Grand Teton National Park, Colonial Williamsburg, Shenandoah National Park, and Great Smokey Mountain's National Park. The Flexner Report, which defined medical education in the United States, was implemented with $130 million of Rockefeller money. Rockefeller said "Make as much as you can, save as much as you can, give away as much as you can".

When I was growing up in Granite City, Illinois, before going to school in the morning, we turned on the radio to KMOX (1120 AM on your radio dial, 50,000 clear-channel watts from St. Louis, MO). Richard Evans' "Thought for the Day" was just before the "March of the Morning". In one message, Evans emphasized that one gift of a million dollars can do infinitely more good than a million gifts of one dollar. Carnegie made the same point when he said "wealth, passing through the hands of a few, can be a much more potent force for the elevation of our race than if distributed in small sums to people themselves".

The point: you must have a strategy, charity must be focused. The great philanthropists, from Rockefeller and Carnegie, to Feeney and Gates and Buffett, spend considerable time and effort to ensure their gifts will have maximum potential impact. Be very patient, you will have to and should turn down most of the requests for your money. Research the charity or cause as intensively as you would any investment, and when you finally discover something that could change the course of humanity, or maybe just make a few peoples' lives a little more bearable, enjoyable, or fulfilling, give it your best.

Carnegie thought it was a sin to die wealthy. He thought the only acceptable way to dispense wealth was to give it away before dying. Waiting until after you are gone not only diminishes the deed, but as Carnegie both accurately and cryptically noted "they would not have left it had they been able to take it with them".

Carnegie's essay *Wealth*, first published in the *North American Review* in 1889, and his other work and deeds, had a great influence on Chuck Feeney, co-founder of the Duty Free Shops. Beginning in the 1980 s, Feeney *anonymously* gave away billions, leaving himself with only several million dollars [3]. People such as this are worthy of our admiration.

Bill Gross, head of bond giant Pimco, holds the same opinion. In an interview on CNBC on May 15, 2008, Gross, who was in the process of auctioning off arguably the greatest stamp collection in the world, with the proceeds going to charity, said "What's the point of dying with your money ... There is no benefit of trying to move up the list of the Forbes 400 to 325 as compared to 375". Gross said the real benefit of the collection is that he and his wife have the enjoyment of seeing the good things the money will bring.

I also stress the satisfaction you will realize from personally seeing the results of your work. Several years ago we gave a sum to endow the Doroghazi Clinical Teaching Award at my Alma Mater, the University of Chicago, Pritzker School of Medicine. Last year my sons and daughter-in-law attended the banquet when I presented the award. It was a proud day for my family. What difference does it make if you have enough to spend in two lifetimes or 10 lifetimes? All you need is enough to spend in one lifetime.

There are also several practical issues. When Buffett made his gift to the Gates Foundation, he noted that someone still alive will undoubtedly make better decisions than someone six feet under. Distributing your money only after you die may also expose your will to challenges. Relatives who think they deserve more may not share your joy of leaving a bushel of money to the Salvation Army or the Boy Scouts.

Unfortunately, but not surprisingly, scams occur even in the realm of philanthropy. In the 1990 s, the Foundation for New Era Philanthropy defrauded donors of $135 M. Check out the recipients of your charitable donations as thoroughly as you would any investment. Websites for this purpose include BBB Wise Giving Alliance www.Give.org, Charity Navigator www.Charity Navigator.org, Philanthropic Research Inc. www.GuideStar.org, and the Internal Revenue Service www.IRS.org.

In addition to the goodwill generated by your unselfishness and good deeds, being active in the community will also pay off both personally and professionally. I have met as many nice people and made as many friends through the Boy Scouts, Rotary, United Way, University of Chicago Medical Alumni Association, and other activities, as I have anywhere else.

Note that when these people or their families get ill, because they already know and respect you, they will want you as their physician. Such people are desirable patients. They are often influential, have good insurance and pay their bills, show up for their appointments on time, take their meds as you suggest, are appreciative of your excellent care, and their recommendation is golden with other potential patients. There is also very little more gratifying as a physician than to take care of people who are also your friends. Being active in the community *will* have a very positive effect on your practice.

There may also be tax advantages for the money spent for charitable activities (but you must discuss this with your accountant). Almost all charities have Galas, dinners, parties, etc. The fee to attend is usually at least partially tax deductible (but beware purchasing items at charitable auctions, already mentioned in Chapter Thirty-Four). You are doing good things, having fun, meeting nice people you may not have met otherwise, and Uncle Sam at least partially helps pick up the tab (that will not happen very often).

I also feel that charitable giving should be from your own personal pocketbook, and not through your practice. I am not referring to a charity in your area of practice. For example, it would be good charity, and good business, for a group of cardiologists to donate to events sponsored by the American Heart Association. Rather, I am referring to any charity or cause not within the direct sphere of your practice. In *Unconventional Success* [4], Swensen relates the story of how the chieftan of a very large financial institution directed corporate charitable donations towards his pet charities. That is exactly what will happen in your practice. The most influential person in the group will be able to direct the money (i.e., *your money*) to their pet charities. Keep charitable donations, political contributions, and perks, such as sports tickets and club memberships, out of the practice and in the pockets of the individual members.

Physicians need to give more back to the community. You are one of the privileged few given the opportunity to make a difference, possibly a big difference, and it will make you feel good inside. Set an example for other physicians. Please be generous.

SUMMARY OF CHAPTER FORTY

- Charity is an obligation of honorable people.
- You are approaching your charitable potential when you do without things you desire.
- Charity must be focused.

- Give your money away before you die so you see the benefits of your generosity.
- All you need is enough to spend in one lifetime.
- Unfortunately, scams occur even in philanthropy. Be careful.
- Being active in the community will pay off personally and professionally.
- Keep charitable donations out of the practice.

REFERENCES

1. Chernow R. The Life of John D Rockefeller, Sr. New York: Random House, 1998.
2. Krass P. Carnegie. Hoboken, NJ: John Wiley & Sons, 2002.
3. O'Clery C. The Billionaire Who Wasn't: How Chuck Feeney Secretly Made and Gave Away a Fortune. New York: Public Affairs, 2007.
4. Swensen D. Unconventional Success: A Fundamental Approach to Personal Investment. New York: Free Press, 2005.

Index

About the Author

Dr. Robert M. Doroghazi was born and raised in Granite City, Illinois. He paid his own way through college and graduated in three and one-half years from the University of Illinois, Champaign-Urbana with High Honors and was elected to Phi Beta Kappa. He paid his own way through medical school, and graduated from the University of Chicago, Pritzker School of Medicine with Honors and was elected to Alpha Omega Alpha Medical Honorary Fraternity. Dr. Doroghazi completed his Internship and Residency in Internal Medicine at the Massachusetts General Hospital in Boston, and his Cardiology training at Barnes Hospital in St. Louis, MO. In 1983, he and Dr. Eve E. Slater co-authored *Aortic Dissection*, published by McGraw-Hill. Dr. Doroghazi retired at age 54 after 23 years of practice with Missouri Cardiovascular Specialists in Columbia, MO.

Dr. Doroghazi is an Eagle Scout and has received the Silver Beaver Award. He is Past President of the Great Rivers Council, Boy Scouts of America, Columbia Northwest Rotary, Job Point (Advent Enterprises), and has served on the Board of the Columbia United Way. He currently serves on the Boards of the Great Rivers Council, the Boone Hospital Center Foundation, the Columbia Civic Orchestra, the Museum of Art and Archaeology at the University of Missouri, Columbia, and is Vice President and President-elect of the University of Chicago, Medical and Biological Sciences Alumni Association. He plays in the first clarinet section in the Columbia Community Band.

Dr. Doroghazi has endowed the Doroghazi Outstanding Clinical Teaching Award at the University of Chicago, Pritzker School of Medicine.

. Dr. Doroghazi has two sons, John and Michael, and lives in Columbia. He publishes "The Physician Investor Newsletter" and has developed the website: thephysicianinvestor.com